Examining Tuskegee

The

JOHN HOPE FRANKLIN SERIES

in African American History and Culture

WALDO E. MARTIN JR.

& PATRICIA SULLIVAN,

editors

SUSAN M. REVERBY

Examining Tuskegee

THE *Infamous*

Syphilis Study

AND ITS *Legacy*

The University of North Carolina Press CHAPEL HILL

Parts of this book have been reprinted with permission in revised form from "History of an Apology: From Tuskegee to the White House," *Research Nurse* 3 (July/August 1997): 1–9; "Rethinking the Tuskegee Syphilis Study: Nurse Rivers, Silence, and the Meaning of Treatment," *Nursing History Review* 7 (Fall 1999): 3–28; "More Than Fact and Fiction: Cultural Memory and the Tuskegee Syphilis Study," *Hastings Center Report* 31 (September–October 2001): 2–8; and "'Special Treatment': BiDil, Tuskegee, and the Logic of Race," *Journal of Law, Medicine & Ethics* 36 (Fall 2008): 478–84.

The University of North Carolina Press has been a member of the Green Press Initiative since 2003.

Designed by Courtney Leigh Baker and set in Minion Pro with Letterpress Text Display by Tseng Information Systems, Inc.

The paper in this book meets the guidelines for permanence and durability of the Committee on Production Guidelines for Book Longevity of the Council on Library Resources.

Library of Congress Cataloging-in-Publication Data
Reverby, Susan.
Examining Tuskegee : the infamous syphilis study and its legacy / Susan M. Reverby.
p. ; cm. — (John Hope Franklin series in African American history and culture)
Includes bibliographical references and index.
ISBN 978-0-8078-3310-0 (cloth : alk. paper)
1. Tuskegee Syphilis Study. 2. Human experimentation in medicine—Alabama—Macon County—History. 3. Syphilis—Research—Alabama—Macon County—History. I. Title. II. Series: John Hope Franklin series in African American history and culture.
[DNLM: 1. Tuskegee Institute. 2. United States. Public Health Service. 3. Syphilis—History. 4. African Americans—History. 5. History, 20th century. 6. Human experimentation—History. 7. Informed consent—History. 8. United States government agencies—History. 9. Universities—History. WC 160 R452e 2009]
R853.H8R48 2009
174.2'80976149—dc22
2009016648

13 12 11 10 09   5 4 3 2 1

For   LIZ SIMS &

CYNTHIA WILSON,

who keep making history,

and in memory of

CHARLIE WESLEY POLLARD &

HERMAN SHAW

Contents

A section of illustrations appears after page 108.

Acknowledgments

Big books take big time, and this was no exception. I never imagined when it started as a short article about the key nursing figure that it would take over my life for so long. For those who joined this journey and supported me, I have only gratitude for your patience and willingness to understand why it mattered.

I am well aware of the political economy that makes scholarship possible. My full-time position in Women's Studies at Wellesley College is my bedrock and allowed for sabbaticals. I have held three "folding" chairs—the Whitehead Associate Professorship in Critical Thought, the Luella LaMar Professorship in Women's Studies, and the Marion Butler McLean Professorship in the History of Ideas—during the time it took to research and write this book. The Social Science Students Summer Research Program provided three student assistants. I am deeply grateful that a number of fellowships made my research and writing possible. The American Association of University Women, the National Endowment for the Humanities, the Radcliffe Institute and the W. E. B. Du Bois Institute at Harvard University, and the National Library of Medicine (Grant number 5 G13 LM009227-02) bought me the time to think and write for more than a few hours at a time. I started the research when at the Du Bois, began to write when I was at Radcliffe, and finished the first draft again at the Du Bois. I hope that Drew Gilpin Faust, Judy Vishniac, Skip Gates, and the other grantors think they invested wisely. The Du Bois fellows and staff members who became friends as I finished— Gretchen Long, Catherine Manegold, Patricia Sullivan, Patricia Hills, Hudita Mustafa, and Donald Yacovone—all listened and critiqued this work while sharing food and ideas.

Many other scholars and writers have published on the "Study"—I am just the latest in this effort. I could not have done this if it had not been for

Jim Jones's groundwork and historical imagination, which glistens in his book *Bad Blood*. I am deeply grateful for his endless support and willingness to listen when I was in moments of writing despair and for just being fun to pal around with. Allan M. Brandt took my previous edited book on the Study into his series, answered questions, and encouraged my inquiry. Barbara Rosenkrantz's review of Jones's book initially taught me how to think about the question of treatment and the need to see change over time in the story as more significant. In particular, Ronald Bayer, Thomas Benedek, Christopher Crenner, Gregory Dorr, Jonathan Erlen, Amy Fairchild, David Feldshuh, Vanessa Northington Gamble, Fred D. Gray, Evelynn M. Hammonds, Darlene Clark Hine, Susan Lederer, Paul Lombardo, Sandra Crouse Quinn, David Rothman, Benjamin Roy, Richard Shweder, Susan Smith, Stephen Thomas, Harriet Washington, Robert M. White, and Tywanna Whorley have all added to the historical debate. I am appreciative of how our differences influenced my thinking and forced me to be clear about my ideas.

Since the 1990s, I have tested my ideas out around the country at lectures, conferences, and public forums in places too numerous to mention. I learned from the challenges these presented, the debates I got into, and the energy I gained from the interest. The Race, Medicine, and Science Workshop provided years of support and thought, especially on the link between biological ideas and race. To Evelynn M. Hammonds, Alondra Nelson, Anne Fausto-Sterling, Lundy Braun, Duana Fulwilley, Everett Mendelson, Bill Quivers, Jon Beckwith, Jenny Reardon, Alexandra Shields, and Jennifer Hamilton — thank you for all the stimulating discussion.

Friends and colleagues made this a much less lonely journey. In Women's Studies at Wellesley, Elena Creef, Sealing Cheng, Charlene Galarneau, Irene Mata, Nancy Marshall, and Lara Freidenfelds all listened tirelessly and forgave me the times I was in Alabama in my head rather than at Wellesley. Jo Ann Citron provided endless legal ideas, hours of argument, and very good food. Lise Vogel always asked key questions. Rosanna Hertz, my close friend and Wellesley colleague, taught me to appreciate sociology, accepted my historical imagination, brought me into her family, and kept me focused on the two important social science words — "so what?" Sociologist Susan E. Bell and I each finished our own massive book projects at the same time while trying to balance the demands of our teaching at small liberal arts colleges and our lives. Susan and Rosanna are the best kind of professionals and friends: thoughtful, caring, and tough.

Help came in many forms. No one does this kind of work without the archivists who save the materials and then make sure you can find them.

To Robert Richards at the Southeast Regional National Archives, my gratitude for all he does to preserve the men's medical records. Archivists at the National Archives in Washington, D.C., Tuskegee University, Fisk University, the National Library of Medicine, the University of Pittsburgh, Johns Hopkins University Medical School, and the University of Michigan were of great assistance as well. Harold Edgar allowed me to see a smaller subset of the medical records he obtained during the lawsuit. John Parascandola, former Public Health Service historian, provided answers and primary documents on numerous occasions. Joel Howell read over the medical data and talked to me about what they meant, and Harry Marks supplied his never-ending expertise whenever queried. Stanley I. Music provided good scotch and lively discussions on research. Karen Buhler-Wilkerson answered any and all nursing history questions.

This would not have been possible without the interlibrary loan and research librarians at Wellesley College, who found articles, obscure facts, and citations for me, year in and year out. Wellesley's technical geniuses were just great to work with, often on short notice. Thanks to HanSu Kim, Alana Kumbier, Betty Febo, Irene Laursen, and Claire Loranz, in particular. My access to Harvard University's vast libraries filled whatever lacunae were left.

Numerous research assistants helped me to find things, filed the endless documents collected, and listened hard. I am particularly grateful to Jackie Mahendra, Katie Seltzer, Elian Rosenfeld, Joan Huang, Laura Choi, and Carmella Britt. Rachel Stern spent a year working as my assistant when I was at the Du Bois Institute and then a grueling week in the National Archives coding the medical records. Donna Stroup, a professional biostatistician in Georgia, took the data and made the statistics work. I may not be the last historian to thank eBay, but I may be among the first to keep typing "syphilis" into the search option. It brought me copies of some of the earliest textbooks on syphilis, as well as actual vials of arsphenamine and bismuth, posters, and ephemera often otherwise impossible to find.

Editors and readers all made this a much more finished project. Kennie Lyman, who meticulously read and critiqued an earlier draft, pulled out her hair at my passive sentences and then did a masterful job of transforming the endnotes into a new format. She made me realize time and again what facts needed to be emphasized, and she railed against fuzzy thinking. This book is all the better for her effort, and I take responsibility for the advice I did not follow. The editors and staff at the University of North Carolina Press waited for this project to come to a close. My editor, Sian Hunter, has been a marvel at encouragement and patience. Beth Lassiter made my sentences and ideas clearer and the book shorter, and Dorothea Anderson provided superb copy-editing. Paula Wald and others saw it through the production process. Karla K. C. Holloway and an unidentified reader became my interlocutors. In having to respond to them, I think I made this a much sharper book. Merlin Chowkwanyun waded through the penultimate draft, providing his usual pointed and thoughtful queries while giving me great hope for the new generation of historians.

This would not have been possible without the friendships and connections I formed with individuals both at the Centers for Disease Control and in Macon County. David Sencer and Don Millar, now retired from the Public Health Service and the Centers for Disease Control, gave generously of their time and connections, never questioning whether I could be entrusted with their sides of the story. Bryan Lindsey and Bill Jenkins were guides to materials they knew about through their roles as heads of the Centers for Disease Control's Tuskegee Syphilis Study's Participants Health Program. In Macon County, I developed another family at the National Bioethics Center, the Tuskegee Human and Civil Rights Multicultural Center, and the Shiloh Community Restoration Foundation. To Liz Sims, whose stamina and organizational prowess made Shiloh happen, and to Cynthia Wilson, knowledgeable in all things Tuskegee at the National Bioethics Center—I cannot express enough my gratitude for your help and my overwhelming admiration for what you both do. The friendships of these two women have been sustaining. The Study's history and legacy could not happen without them. Fred D. Gray and his family have also made a monumental effort to keep the Study central to Macon County's history in the museum they have organized.

This book was in part encouraged by medicine in some form as my family's "business." My late father, Reuben Mokotoff, was a cardiologist who died before the book was finished. I missed being able to talk it all over with him, but he taught me about medical passion and diagnostic acuity. My mother, Gertrude Fox Mokotoff, a former bacteriologist, college teacher, and politician, is indomitable. I thank her too for her stories of doing syphilis serologies in the 1930s. My sister, Eve Mokotoff, HIV/AIDS surveillance manager for the state of Michigan, answered epidemiology questions, while I relied upon doctor brothers David Mokotoff and Eric Quivers for more cardiology advice. My youngest brother, Charles, was a guide to all things Macintosh and musical and the intricacies of the National Institutes of Health. Dr. William W. Quivers Sr. told me wonderful stories of being in Tuskegee during World War II when he was a supply officer for the Tuskegee Airmen and when he married his wife in the Macon County courthouse.

My children, Mariah Sixkiller and Micah Sieber, really did grow up with this project. They had to explain what I did to their friends and in-laws and are now adults with lives, partners, and careers I can really appreciate and honor. I especially thank Mariah for giving up her bedroom to the books and thousands of files. She cooked fabulous meals with her husband, Casey, for me and provided her connections in Washington that brought me information. Micah spent more than half his life with my obsession with all things "Tuskegee," and I will cherish forever his historical imagination and trenchant humor. To my family and friends who "slept with syphilis" in Mariah's old bedroom/guest room/office, my gratitude for your understanding of why this was necessary.

Bill Quivers gave up trips (even to Paris) so I could finish chapters, waited patiently for this to end, and provided an ear always for words, thoughts, and confusions. He came with me to Tuskegee on several occasions (despite insisting he was an urban man), slogged through an earlier draft, and promised me I would not embarrass the family. I celebrate science nerds falling in love in middle age and the surprise benefits that come from serving on a faculty committee.

Above all, there are the men of the Study. I was privileged to meet a few of them before they died, to be welcomed into their homes, and to be present at the White House for the federal apology. I continue to stay connected with family members and feel honored to know them. I, and all of us who are protected in medical research because of their sacrifices however unknowing, owe them more than I can say.

Examining Tuskegee

Introduction

Race, Medical Uncertainty, and American Culture

"He who knows syphilis, knows medicine," famed early twentieth-century Johns Hopkins physician Sir William Osler is often quoted as saying.[1] The contemporary adage would be different: "Those who know 'Tuskegee' know racism in medicine and injustice." Yet these simple maxims belie their connected longer versions and not-so-simple truths. A twentieth-century medical research study of African American men with the sexually transmitted disease of syphilis, in which the hundreds involved did not know that treatment was supposedly withheld, has led to many stories where conceptions of race, uncertainties in medicine, mistrust of doctors, and the power of the state intertwine.[2] This book is about what made the study possible, why it continued, and the histories and stories told after it ended. It unravels the political and cultural purposes served when a complicated experience has many narratives, but the tale is told simply as a straightforward allegory for all time about racism, medicine, and mistrust.

At first glance, the crucial facts seem clear: white government doctors from the U.S. Public Health Service (PHS) found approximately 400 African American men presumed to all have late-stage, and therefore not infectious, syphilis in and around Tuskegee in Macon County, Alabama. After some initial treatment was given and then stopped, the PHS provided aspirin and iron tonic, implying through deception that these were to cure the men's "bad blood." PHS doctors also told nearly 200 controls—men without the disease—that they were being cared for with the same simple medications. The only permission asked for was the right to autopsy their bodies after the men had died in exchange for payment for a decent burial.[3] Doctors and a nurse connected to the county health department, the venerable black educational institution Tuskegee Institute (now Tuskegee University), and the Tuskegee Veterans' Administration Hospital provided assistance and did the x-rays, tests, and autopsies.[4] Syphilis is a complex disease, and many of the men survived their disease while others were felled by it. Those still infectious could have passed it on to their wives or sexual partners, and through them to their children.

The study went on not for one year but for forty, between 1932 and 1972— through the Depression, World War II, the Cold War, into the civil rights era—as administrators, doctors, and nurses made it possible. It began at a time when there was "modern treatment" for syphilis in the form of heavy metals and continued into what is usually considered the curative penicillin era of the post–World War II years.

Since 1972, the study's cultural malleability has gained it a central position in the American pantheon of experimental monstrosities and racial injustices. Sometimes in the stories the horror deepens as facts disappear, rumors take over, and questions abound. There is absolutely *no* evidence, for example, that the men were injected by the PHS with the difficult-to-culture bacteria that causes syphilis, although this belief continues to be held regardless of the facts or the endless corrections that appear. There absolutely *is* evidence that the PHS tried, yet *not always* successfully, to keep the men from extensive treatment.[5] Those who focus primarily on the medicine sometimes attempt to separate out the morals of the study from the actual syphilis and the complicated questions over which treatments would have helped and when.[6] As the power to prolong life or cause early death is combined with the American obsession with governmental control and racial politics, it is no surprise that the stories of what happened during the study have taken on ever-changing and mythic proportions.

The Great Pox

If the study had been on any other disease, it might not carry such heavy cultural baggage. Syphilis—the great pox, lues venerea, or bad blood—was dreaded for nearly half a millennium until the age of modern antibiotics. Debates linger over where syphilis, caused by the spiral-shaped *treponema pallidum* bacterium, first appeared. It is alternately seen as the disease of the "other" brought to the New World by Columbus's debauched men or, it is as strongly argued, taken to Europe in their bodies as a form of biological revenge. It first came ashore in Naples and then swept through country after country in the endless wars of the early sixteenth century, causing "the syphilization of Europe" and acquiring its reputation as the disease left behind by marauding armies.[7]

Over the next five centuries, the disease's "natural history" began to be mapped, although not without medical debate, and its transmission modes came to be acknowledged. The disease's virulent effects on human bodies changed over the centuries as disease and host accommodated to one another, but by the twentieth century knowledge of its phases was beginning to be understood, even as debates raged over this complex disease. In its earliest and most contagious stage, syphilis is primarily passed through sexual contact. The bacterium can also enter a fetus or an infant at birth through its infected mother or transfer between an infant and a wet nurse.[8] In adults, a few weeks after the spirochetes enter the body a chancre or primary lesion that is often not painful or even noticed appears, usually at the point of exposure. Infected fetuses can be stillborn, die as infants, or develop blindness, deafness, abnormal nose and teeth formations, and neurological complications as children.

Several weeks to months later, either before or after the chancre disappears, the disease enters its second stage. An eruption of lesions in the form of a rash occurs more generally across the body, accompanied by weakness, headaches, and severe pains. This too abates and with it the disease's ability to be passed along to others. In the third stage, there is a latency period where no visual signs of the disease exist and the health of the individual does not seem in jeopardy. This may last anywhere from several years to decades to the rest of the life of the infected person.

Once this period ends, however, in late latency the spirochetes can attack almost any organ or structure of the body. Syphilis was an ugly and loathsome disease made more so by the stigma of its primary transmission through sexual contact and its ability to emerge years later elsewhere in the body, causing a sufferer's eyes to be blinded, a heart to stop, or a mind to be obliterated. Received medical wisdom when the study began posited that racial and sexual differences affected the disease's path, with African Americans "expected" to have more cardiovascular complications while various neurological defects were supposedly experienced by whites.[9]

Treatments began as soon as the disease emerged. Mercury as a cure for skin diseases was imported to Europe from Arab physicians by the early 1500s and was used extensively, along with a host of other herbal, medicinal, and biologic agents—from guiac tree bark to sarsaparilla tonics. Its usage led to the adage, "A night with Venus, a lifetime with Mercury." By the early twentieth century, the spirochete had been identified, serological tests to determine its presence seemed to make certain diagnosis possible, and German research led to the focus on arsenic compounds as the "magic bullet" for the disease. By the 1920s, months of treatment with various combinations of heavy metals—mercury, arsenicals, and bismuth—shaped what was seen as the "modern" treatment, especially for the early stages of the disease in adults. A focus on fever therapies, particularly the introduction of malaria, was thought to aid in treatment of neurosyphilis.[10]

By the time the study began in 1932, concern over treatment, debates over racial and gender differences, and the problematic accuracy of the blood tests filled medical journals and texts. It was becoming clear that not everyone died from the disease or even became seriously sickened by it. From a public health perspective, as Surgeon General Thomas Parran argued in 1938, "with one or two doses of an arsphenamine, we can render the patient promptly non-infectious, [but] not cured."[11] The medical debates continued for the next decade until it was found that the new "miracle" drug, penicillin, could usually eradicate the disease in its earliest stages and perhaps even in latency *if* organ damage had not yet occurred. Even after penicillin, the study continued for another three decades until media attention and public outcries brought it to a close.

Collective Memories

When the study ended, the stories began. The knots that tie racism to experimentation, a fearful disease to the black male body, sexuality to the state, and gender and class to claims of racial collaboration give the stories their cultural staying power and their deep place in collective memories. New events renew and reinvigorate its telling. The varied and culturally embedded stories invoke anger, pain, guilt, shame, sorrow, or apology when remembered or learned about for the first time.

The stories carry so much power because they are about betrayals of trust and death. Some tell of intentional duplicity that rests primarily on racial identities: one more example of whites taking advantage of seemingly helpless poor African Americans and black professionals refusing to tell the truth to the country folk. In some versions, the problems are professional and institutional: doctors using their trusting subjects and federal, state, and local health authorities abusing their power. Many see the study as a failure from a different time when physician hubris, moral understandings of informed consent, and experimental norms were less sophisticated. There are also stories of betrayals that work the other way: of historians and members of the public who do not understand how medicine treated syphilis in the years of the study or of those who cannot comprehend the context of racism and violence that shaped what happened.

The study has become a site of collective memory and a contentious ground for a civic—rather than a civil—war battlefield. The nearly forty years the study has been in the public realm of history, imagination, and rumor must now be added to its forty-year existence.[12] As its story gets repeated, its truths pass between different communities, as fictions become facts and rumors become truths.

The past, present, and even the future do not form linear stories. For many African American patients, as bioethicist and lawyer Patricia King has argued, "experiences with medicine and biomedical research are not separate."[13] The history of maltreatment, even among those whose knowledge of the actual study is weak or nonexistent, carries forward into contemporary explanations for the health disparities that separate the life chances of blacks and whites. As medical researchers now confront the study's supposed legacy in the fears of potential subjects and patients, they must understand its shifting temporal nature.[14] This requires, as lawyer/critic Karla F. C. Holloway argues, balancing historical knowledge of a memory of "direct vulnerability that is culturally constructed and culturally passed on" with the needed autonomy for individuals in each given medical encounter.[15] The stories of the study are not always about history in some abstract objective sense. They are, as with many other historical controversies, about how we treat one another, about how we make progress.

Ultimately, what happened in the study is about how varying kinds of assumptions about race can fill in the uncertainty that is central to medicine. It is impossible to separate the shifting ideas and beliefs about race from the complexity of the changing medical questions about syphilis and the ethics of doing research. It is the demands of research that call forth the need for more and more information. It is hesitant trust that shapes many encounters between blacks and whites and allows differing truths to be told.

This book is not a summary of the older versions of the study's history, although clearly those who know it will find some familiarity here. The other histories are still available, and they are full of analytic insights and excellent detail.[16] This is a rereading and reanalysis to understand what happened and why this study has such power. It is about why the study happened, how it might have been stopped, and why the stories go on and on.

Doing History

In many ways, the study has become both invisible and hypervisible. Its details and beginnings tie it to the long history of the use of black bodies in medicine and the hidden nontherapeutic nightmare medical tortures carried out in concentration camps by Nazi doctors.[17] Yet what makes the story so powerful is in fact its visibility on American soil. The researchers published their results and cataloged the disease's toll over the years in more than a dozen articles in respectable journals. The study was made more visibly public in 1972 when a disease investigator finally gave the story to an Associated Press (AP) reporter. The outcry that followed led to a federal investigation, Senate hearings, a lawsuit, and new federal regulations about informed consent, which still shape medical research. In the last decades, the study has also generated or been part of rumors, historical monographs, documentaries, plays, poems, photographs, music, a TV movie, photomontages, a surgeon general's nomination hearings, a presidential apology, and the creation of the National Bioethics Center at Tuskegee University and plans for several museums in Tuskegee itself.

To tell all these stories requires the usual skills that are part of the telling of history. Historians always struggle to find out what actually "happened" in the past and write books because sources open up, methods of analysis change, and new questions develop. Always working with incomplete information, there are also differing interpretations of the same "facts."[18] For this book, the availability of the men's medical records changes some of what can be known. The time that passed between when the study ended and I began this research in the early 1990s meant that some individuals had passed away and that others could only tell the same stories over and over inflected by the fictions that abound no matter what I asked. Their memories become central to one of the concerns of this book: Why is the study remembered in particular ways?[19] It is an effort to understand why, over time, with the "subjective and embellished telling of the past, the past is constructed—history is made."[20] I underline the contingencies of lives lived, and therefore of history, and why the messiness of both past and present is often ignored and never fully capable of articulation. It is a reminder of what critic Saidiya Hartman calls "the impossibility of reconstituting the past free from the disfigurements of present concerns."[21]

I have tried to make clear the distinctions here among "race" (a constructed social identity), "racism" (a set of beliefs and behaviors and individual and institutional structures used to disempower and keep African

Americans from equality), and "racialism" (the use of racial categories without emphasis on hierarchy). Throughout the history of the study and its aftermath, differing racial assumptions operated that used social power, biological beliefs about difference, and perceptions of sexuality as the lens to justify or explain what had happened. I delineate when differing kinds of assumptions are used and how they are shaped by the context of state power, shifting medical ideas, and scientific zeal.[22] My questions thus reflect the current focus on disparities and the problems with the "use of race as a proxy for genetic relatedness," as well as the growing literature on race, gender, and health care.[23] In other words, there is a socioeconomic and political context to the history making and storytelling, which changes over time.

Telling the Stories: Testimony, Testifying, and Traveling

My approach requires the telling of what I am calling the "testimony," the "testifying," and the "traveling." By testimony, I do not mean just depositions given in the lawsuit or the statements at a government hearing. I have been collecting and reading the letters, reports, articles, and words of those who were involved in the study to write a brief for a historical understanding of what happened.

In writing about a historical trauma such as this study, I am also looking for the "testifying." I mean this in the African American vernacular religious and communal sense of the word. Usually thought of as testifyin', it is what linguist Geneva Smitherman defines as "a ritualized form of communication in which the speaker gives verbal witness to the efficacy, truth, and power of some experience in which [the group has] shared" that speaks to a more complicated reality. When someone "testifies," they are speaking out loud about a set of truths and beliefs that are usually part of a self-revelatory experience. Testifying is about "celebration, affirmation of beliefs, and a way to criticize society or the church that is open to all."[24] I am not arguing here that the testimony comes only from the white doctors and the testifying only from the African Americans. Rather, I am looking at what the testimony tells us about what happened and how the testifying captures what might be differing communal explanations for the truths.

The first section of the book is "Testimony." The opening chapter introduces Tuskegee Institute (now Tuskegee University) and the PHS and explores how the concern with syphilis renewed a relationship developed more than a decade before the study. For those unfamiliar with the basic details, the second and third chapters go through what appears to have happened. I argue that the study was much more uncertain than the usual focus on the power of the PHS allows. I provide evidence of the study's messy science, how it became a study of "maltreatment" and "undertreatment" rather than "no treatment," and the implications this had for the men who were the subjects and controls. The fourth chapter explores the many unsuccessful individual efforts to make the study stop and why it finally did end. The fifth chapter explains how the story was told in the years immediately after the study ended — in the media, in a federal investigating committee, at a Senate hearing, and in a lawsuit — as the study made its first move into cultural knowledge after 1972.

The second section is "Testifying." It opens with a chapter on the men who became the study's subjects and controls, culling analysis from their words and those of their families and the quantitative and qualitative information their medical records provide. The next three chapters explain the study from the viewpoints of some of the white PHS physicians, the black doctor who supported the study in Tuskegee, and the black nurse who has been the subject of much speculation and concern.

The final section is "Traveling." It concerns the decades after 1972 and how the study moves about in American lore. There was a cultural process to the study becoming an icon, and its details matter. I begin with the study's life in bioethics, history, and rumor. I then move to the fictional forms the stories have taken and to the political spectacles and efforts at apology. I explore the "counter-narratives" that have developed to provide an alternate take on what happened. I close with an exploration of the problems of using "Tuskegee" to cure racism and where we are now.

This is a long and sometimes confusing history with many names and dates. I have provided a chronology and a names list to guide the reader. The appendix also contains statistical data from the analysis of the men's medical records. More is available on a website.[25]

I struggled with what to call the study throughout the writing. Its cultural shorthand is now the Tuskegee Study or Tuskegee Experiment. In reality, it was never really an experiment in the sense of a drug, biologic, or device being tested.[26] It was supposed to be a prospective (going forward in time) study of what the doctors called the "natural history" of late latent syphilis, even though the PHS created much of this "natural history" through their actions. Its name varies in the published articles. The word "Tuskegee" appears in a number of the published articles by the PHS doctors as a location, just as the long-running major heart study still ongoing today is often called the Framingham Study. With the effort to organize a federal apology in 1996–97, the call came to rename it the "U.S. Public Health Service Study at Tuskegee" because this would be more accurate. But in truth the word "Tuskegee" is what circulates and is known.

I dealt with this problem in three ways. Before the study is fully organized, I apply the term "study," as I have here in the introduction for the sake of clarity. After it is operational, I call it "the Study," to make its formal presence known. When it is appropriate to explain its metaphoric existence, I use "Tuskegee," in quotes. The study as an idea, the Study as facts and lived experiences, and "Tuskegee" as a cultural icon are what this book is about.

I also need to acknowledge that because I have worked on this for more than a decade and a half, I too have become part of the story, as I have written articles, given lectures, and answered myriad questions from students, reporters, bloggers, colleagues, callers to talk radio, the general public, and once even the White House counsel's office. I have explained my own role when appropriate to exemplify how a historian can emphasize certain facts and create analysis that become not just history but memory.

I do think there are truths here—facts that fit the evidence better than do others. I will stay as faithful to these as I am able.[27] Historians, of course, provide their own form of testimony and testifying in what stories we choose to tell. Over the years, my feelings have ranged from horror and anger to sadness and acceptance. Doing the research brought me into contact with a few of the men who became the Study's subjects and their families, as well as some of the doctors who made it possible. I sought to understand their viewpoints.[28] I continue to work with multiple museum and oral history projects at Tuskegee University and in Macon County that tell the stories in other ways.

I believe that assessing varying perceptions is central to a historian's task. I know from experience that I will make many people angry through what I have written if it does not accord with their understandings, memories, or interpretations, just as I please others. It is the nature of the Study's power and importance that parts of this book may be controversial, and I accept that. There will always be more to say.[29]

Retribution and redemption are another matter. It is not something a historian can provide in a text, although in the end "rendering an historical verdict . . . requires drawing a moral bottom line."[30] In the United States, we do not usually have Truth Commissions to address past crimes perpetrated by those with state-sanctioned power.[31] At best, at the national level, we set up federal investigations, or special prosecutors, or call a congressional hearing. At the local level, attorneys file lawsuits. Media coverage, a television documentary, or a movie might focus national attention. In this case, before all the men died, there was even a presidential apology in the White House.

There is still mostly just rumor, fact-dropping, and political usage of the Study, whether in a fiery sermon or a quick bioethics lecture. There are physicians who believe that medicine has been maligned in the tellings and in the taking out of historical context. There are family members of the men who still feel no real closure and who use the Study's power to provide a narrative around which to organize ills of subsequent generations. There is widespread anger that the criminal courts never meted out punishment to those still alive who established and perpetuated it.[32] That kind of judicial assessment is impossible to provide now, if it ever was possible.

Knowing what happened and why it matters in medicine and American life might get us a little closer to a goal of justice. It is a task worth taking up.

PART I

Testimony

Historical Contingencies

Tuskegee Institute, the Public Health Service, & Syphilis

"Why us?" a family member of one of the men in the Study asked me at a meeting at the Shiloh Missionary Baptist Church in Notasulga, Alabama, just outside Tuskegee in 2007. The Study could perhaps have happened elsewhere. But, in many ways, the long-standing and complicated ties between Tuskegee Institute and the federal government over health care and disease in the black community provided the historical contingencies that made the Study possible, while only a disease as linked to sex and the black body and as widespread as syphilis could have brought them together for so long both in history and in imagination. The relationship between the PHS and Tuskegee Institute began de novo with the Study, but it had roots deep in the American ways that both had grown up and in the ties of disease to blackness.

The Contingency of Place

Tuskegee Institute was built in a small southern town in a county carved out of the huge southern lands of Native American peoples.[1] When Alabama was admitted to the union as a frontier state in 1819, death by bear attack or in childbirth or through the cruelties of slavery in the fields, mills, and mines defined daily realities.[2] In the 1840s, when the Indian wars ended with treaties that were broken over and over, Native American peoples were driven out and their land was given to whites, but not before they left their legacy behind in the bloodlines of both blacks and whites and in the names of towns like Tuskegee and Tallasee.[3]

By 1860, those identified as black Americans (both free and slave) outnumbered whites in Macon County by more than two to one. Small log or shotgun cabins outnumbered plantation homes in the red clay back ways, as barely 12 percent of Macon County's white population identified themselves as slave owners.[4] As in other parts of what became known as the Black Belt, cotton covered the fields made fertile by slave labor and trees filled the forests on the hills.[5] Other enslaved African Americans worked in sawmills. Intense farming depleted much of the soil of the county, and small landowning white farmers had a hard time meeting even the minimal taxes to keep hold of their property.[6] Except among the large plantation owners, a southern way of hardscrabble making-do dominated the working lives of most of Macon County's black and white population.

Union soldiers during the Civil War did not make it into Tuskegee. But a battle a few miles out of the town at what would be the railhead at Chehaw was part of Sherman's goal of making the resupply of Atlanta difficult. Purportedly, the college friendship between a northern officer and a planter, Edward Varner, kept the Union army from burning the town of Tuskegee down.[7] As with much of the history of both the town and the institute, the vagaries of location, the link to the North, and the political skills and connections of the populace made things happen.

Reconstruction dashed many of the hopes of Macon County African Americans. Much too soon it became clear that, for many, slavery would be exchanged for a system resembling serfdom. The Alabama chief of the Freedmen's Bureau advised the state's newly freed men and women that they should "hope for nothing, but go to work and behave yourselves."[8] Work in this case meant contract labor that left most former slaves deep inside of a crop-lien system and outside of a cash economy.[9] Migration in search of better land and more political power was on the minds of many Macon County African Americans: "A local Democratic paper . . . reported in 1876 that one party of forty blacks had just left the county, having been preceded by another group only days before, and that an emigration agent was working secretly in Tuskegee." Between 1860 and 1870, the black population of the county dropped by over 5,000, but the fears on the part of white landowners that they would lose their entire black workforce proved baseless. Macon County's black population remained at about 13,000 in the 1870s and 1880s.[10]

The African American men who did stay in the county made use of the new franchise by electing one representative to the state legislature as soon as possible. White conservatives vied with black and white Republicans for control over the county, often searching for ways to curry the favor of black voters. As elsewhere in the South, threats, terrorizing, and violence began to follow black voters who used their electoral power. By the end of the 1870s, white conservative control over the electoral process through both fraud and intimidation solidified.[11]

Tuskegee Institute itself was often subject to the vagaries of friendships and fortune, efforts at continued enforced racial compromise, and more hidden growing economic and political power.[12] Many southern African Americans turned their hopes to education in the face of post-emancipation difficulties.[13] Despite divisions over this, many white southerners also came to believe that at least some elementary education would be necessary to retain their black workforce and that teachers would have to be trained.

An ex-Confederate colonel and lawyer in Macon County and an ex-slave made a political deal that traded the promise of state aid for black education for voter support among black men to elect a white man to the Alabama legislature.[14] It worked—the Alabama legislature made $2,000 available for "the Normal School for colored teachers in Tuskegee" in 1881. The funds, however, could not even cover the cost of the site of what Tuskegee Institute's famed leader Booker T. Washington referred to as "'the Farm'... 100 acres of spent farmland on which stood 'a cabin, formally used as a dining room, an old kitchen, a stable and an old hen-house' where the 'big house' had burned down during the war."[15] Washington chose an apocryphal image when he recalled that the first animal given to the school by a local white patron was "an old blind horse."[16]

On this plantation land, Tuskegee Institute began in Booker T. Washington's imagination and in what he believed were the reflected hopes of both whites and blacks. Over the next three decades, Washington created what would become a vitally important educational institution in the rural South. As he told the story in his ghostwritten and carefully crafted 1901 autobiography, *Up from Slavery*, it was his ability to define and realize the needs of the black rural masses while translating them publicly to the local white population and to the noblesse oblige beliefs of northern and midwestern philanthropists that made Tuskegee Institute possible.[17] By the time he died in 1915, there were, stunningly, "two thousand acres and one hundred buildings, with a faculty of nearly two hundred and an endowment close to $2 million."[18]

On that original land rose buildings built brick by brick by the students and an education that emphasized respectability, cleanliness, and manual labor.[19] Washington's well-known iron-fisted control focused on the most minute details of the institute and its citizens' daily lives, down to his supervision of tooth brushing and his weekly exhortations at chapel about behaviors. Policing of his students' black bodies was critical to his effort to obtain what one critic calls the "recuperation of dirt" and the maintenance of "self control," which led to "politicizing the domestic to gain social control."[20]

Tuskegee Institute maintained a complicated relationship with the nearby rural "folk" as well, reaching out to teach, uplift, and serve through what was called the Movable School program, and yet condemning what was seen as the "dirt" and sexuality of black rural life.[21] Containment of the "corporeal" black body and the "contagion of 'sexuality' as disease," both inside and outside Tuskegee Institute, was absolutely central to Washington's efforts.[22] He tried to create what came to be called "a New Negro," in a break from the perceived "stereotypes" of licentiousness and "minstrelsy."[23]

On the surface, Washington cooperated with the tightening hold of Jim Crow segregation, which denied black Americans political and voting rights, underfunded a separate educational system, sustained economic peonage, and kept power through frequent eruptions of state-sanctioned violence.[24] The need to carefully gauge the appropriate balance of the needs of blacks and whites and meet the financing of the institute continually haunted Washington's efforts. Teachers and students at Tuskegee acceded to "elaborate rituals of segregation" when whites came to visit. They kept the institute away from those blacks who directly challenged the system. They presented white philanthropists with an institution for African American education they could fund without compromising the sensibilities of the majority of southern whites.[25] In doing so, Washington was able to build up a black educational institution with black faculty and an increasing local black middle class of teachers, professionals, and small landowners.[26]

Even as Tuskegee Institute made education and economic progress possible for some, however, it never overcame the real dangers that shaped the violence of daily life. Despite expectations and promises, African Americans in and around the town of Tuskegee had to be very careful not to cross carefully delineated lines of white beliefs about racial appropriateness. A "hard look," as one Tuskegee resident noted, from a white man, could spell danger.[27]

And, in the end, even Washington could not hide from the myths of black male sexuality and the cultural meaning of the black body that was embedded in parts of American culture. His serious illnesses (kidney disease, arteriosclerosis, and high blood pressure) led to his collapse and hospitalization on November 10, 1915, in New York City. The St. Luke's Hospital physician he saw told reporters: "There is a noticeable hardening of the arteries and he is extremely nervous. Racial characteristics are, I think, in part responsible for Dr. Washington's breakdown." Such terminology infuriated Washington's supporters. As one of his doctors wrote: "[Racial characteristics] . . . means a 'syphilitic history' when referring to Colored people." Washington was never tested for syphilis, and he died of kidney failure brought on by high blood pressure. It was not until ninety years later that a medical review finally confirmed that he was not syphilitic.[28]

Washington's power gave him the means to institutionalize his focus on the body and discipline in Tuskegee and beyond. In 1902, Washington brought surgeon John A. Kenney Sr. to Tuskegee to run a small hospital and the nurses' training program, which had begun a decade earlier. Health facilities at Tuskegee remained very sparse until 1912, when Boston philanthropist Elizabeth Mason gave the funds to build the John A. Andrew Memorial Hospital, named after her grandfather and Massachusetts's governor during the Civil War.[29] It provided both acute and preventive care, serving as Macon County's health department until 1928 and even after 1928 providing physical space. Although it was a private hospital for the institute's students, faculty, and staff, it was increasingly called upon to be a community hospital for needy black people throughout the Black Belt.

Under Kenney's leadership and with his connections to the National Medical Association (formed in 1895 because racism kept black physicians from membership in the American Medical Association), an annual clinic was organized that brought patients and physicians together. At the first clinic in 1912, the visiting doctors treated 440 patients, performed 36 operations, and announced happily that everyone "recovered." By 1918, the John A. Andrew Clinic became the John A. Andrew Clinical Society, dedicated to "the advancement of physicians and surgeons in the science and art of medicine and surgery and the study and treatment of morbid conditions affecting thousands of needy sufferers in this section of the South."[30] The annual meetings provided one of the few post–medical school training opportunities for black physicians, surgeons, and dentists—under big-name white doctors, who were invited to lecture and demonstrate the latest techniques. It gave patients from black communities throughout Alabama, barred from care elsewhere, a chance to receive treatment. However, unwittingly, as for poor people, white and of color, from throughout the country, they became "teaching material" as well for those learning the newest methods.[31]

Washington understood that freedom required health and that self-improvement had to be linked to the provision of services.[32] He was not alone. As understandings that germs caused disease layered upon older sanitarian notions, the *Atlanta Constitution*'s astute phrase "germs know no color or race line" served as a warning to the white community that physical segregation, regardless of Washington's public statements, had its limits and that social separation could not keep microbes from connecting everyone.[33] Tuskegee Institute's focus on the black body spread beyond the campus.

Improving the Black Body

Better race relations through attention to health care was an even more central concern of Washington's successor. Robert Russa Moton, a big, imposing man with a voice to match, stood and acted with the military bearing that reflected his years as the commandant of the cadet corps at Hampton Institute in Virginia before his move to Tuskegee.[34] During World War I, President Woodrow Wilson sent Moton to France to ensure black soldiers' loyalty in the face of segregated service, to check "rumors" over "unmentionable crimes," and to explore whether "social diseases" were more rampant in the black military camps. Moton's reports emphasized the cleanliness and morality of the black soldiers.[35]

Just before he died, Washington pushed for what would become National Negro Health Week, where cleanup, clinics, and health messages were organized in communities across the country. Moton had begun work on its precursor while he was still at Hampton, but it needed support from the federal government to spread. Surgeon General Hugh Cumming agreed to allow the PHS to help with the planning of the "week" and issued a bulletin explaining why it was necessary. Moton argued, "It is the state's business to see to the public's health."[36]

Moton's connections to the federal government and the PHS came into sharper focus during the 1921–24 battle to site a blacks-only veterans' hospital on Tuskegee Institute land. The institute, the National Medical Association, and the NAACP, in a well-orchestrated, often contentious campaign, made a concerted political push to have the hospital staffed and run at the highest level by African Americans. As historian Vanessa Northington Gamble has written, some black newspapers editorialized that, without assurance of black professional leadership, there was fear that "white Southerners wanted control of the hospital as part of a racist plot to kill and sterilize African-American men and that the hospital would become an 'experiment station' for mediocre white physicians."[37]

Despite fierce opposition by many in the white community, which led to death threats to Moton and Kenney and their families, an ambivalent PHS and Veterans' Administration (VA), and a Ku Klux Klan march near the campus, which was met by armed Tuskegee cadets, black professional control of the hospital was won by 1924. Moton's willingness to compromise to get federal support was roundly criticized, even if it proved necessary to attaining black leadership at the VA Hospital.[38] It became one more plank in solidifying the relationship between Tuskegee Institute and the federal government over health care issues for African Americans. In the end, however, this was a hospital for veterans. It could do little for the local community (other than provide jobs), even lacking a clinic for their care. But by 1932, when the study began, Tuskegee already had a decades-old relationship to the PHS and a record as a key institution that pressured the government to participate in improving the health of rural African Americans.

The PHS Partnership

Tuskegee's leaders found the PHS a powerful, though sometimes hesitant, partner. The PHS, chartered in 1798 as the Marine Hospital Service, started as a loosely connected series of hospitals for sick merchant seamen. By the end of the nineteenth century, it had expanded into a commissioned corps of medical officers with a national mandate and the surgeon general at its head.[39] By the early 1900s, the PHS was involved in medical research, quarantine, and the control of infectious diseases from flu to syphilis. "Cleaning up" was always central to the service's expanded role; the provision of privies and clean water was often at the core of its public health work. Its role in enforcing quarantines and stopping the spread of disease gave the PHS power to police borders. The Public Health Service, its formal name after 1912, became crucial to the linking of the "dangerous" immigrant to biological stigmas and the labeling of the diseased as the "other."[40]

The PHS commissioned officers corps was built on a military model. The exams to become an officer were considered even more difficult than state medical boards and gave those who passed a sense of elitism.[41] Once in the corps, officers moved from station to station and were taught by more "experienced administrators wherever practicable." As Ralph Chester Williams, a former commissioned officer, who wrote the first full-fledged history of the PHS, observed, "There was an unwritten policy . . . that officers should be 'caught early and treated rough.'" "Such efforts, it was assumed, provided the officers with both 'discipline' and an 'esprit de corps.'"[42] Loyalties were directed toward the PHS itself rather than to local projects or issues.

Private physicians and their powerful professional organizations frequently thwarted the PHS's efforts, as they did those of other public health agencies. Governmental agencies' attempts at the delivery of care were often denounced as the beginnings of "state" medicine. In the face of such opposition, public health authorities were forced to tread narrow paths in choosing how to improve health care and its delivery. To do its work, the PHS could not function without the financial assistance of foundations willing to fund health initiatives and the political assistance of local and state health authorities. PHS officers often helped to start state and local health departments and were "loaned" out to begin or continue public health work, where their "diplomatic" skills were as essential as their scientific ones.[43]

The media romantically portrayed them as doing battle against invisible disease foes and lauded their efforts. As a media paean declared in 1941, the PHS was a "cross between a military organization and a monastic order," which provided its officers with "probably the most heroic job in the U.S. today."[44]

Given the nature of the diseases to which the PHS turned its efforts, fieldwork and laboratory work came together.[45] The PHS began to conduct biomedical research in 1887 with the opening of the Hygienic Laboratory in one room at the Marine Hospital on Staten Island. PHS officers believed that statistical proofs came from observations and collection of morbidity and mortality data, as well as from clinical field experiments. Research on prisoners and inmates of state mental asylums and observational studies in rural communities became more common, although tensions with local physicians and state and local health departments often required their vaunted diplomacy or the intervention of the surgeon general. In the South, suspicion about the "outsider" federal agents and their foundation allies could prove dangerous.[46] In 1922, for example, Birmingham's health officer, who was also a PHS official, was dragged from his home, placed against a tree, and whipped because of his "Kaiser-like and high handed actions."[47]

Danger was built into the research in both the laboratory and the field, as the PHS's martyrs "Killed in Action" list attested. Officers frequently contracted the diseases they studied in the laboratory or died in the field. Taliaferro Clark, the PHS physician who would suggest the organization of the study, for example, had contracted yellow fever while in the field earlier in his career.[48] In PHS laboratory and clinical research, doctors' intentional self-exposure in the cause of science was common.[49] This kind of direct research added to the PHS's "esprit de corps" and created a sense that martyrdom in the name of science had become expected and necessary.

These practices had become the norm in medicine by the 1930s. Such self-experimentation, intentionally or not, worked in part to stave off long-standing public worries about experimentation and to convince researchers that their efforts served a noble purpose. Medicine's public approval ratings soared in the 1930s as this form of bravery became the subject of celebratory books, radio broadcasts, films, and plays.[50]

Heroics also served, however, to hide unwitting martyrs from view and to justify their sacrifice. Not all subjects knew they were contributing to what researchers thought of as scientific progress. Permission—in the vague sense of that word—often came from those in charge of the vulnerable rather than from the subjects themselves.[51] And there was always some unease about all of this research. As historian Susan Lederer noted, "The staff of the Veterans Administration explained, 'We don't like to use the word 'experiments' in the Veterans Administration; 'investigations' or 'observations' . . . is the approved term for such a study in the VA hospitals."[52]

Scientific Muscle

In the opening decades of the twentieth century, clinical research became an increasingly crucial part of medicine's armamentarium, even if the infrastructure to make it work remained limited. Much of it depended upon the use of "reliable men" in the elite medical institutions who might "err" but "not deceive."[53] As historian Harry Marks has argued about research in these years, "Experimentation was meant as an exercise in morality as much as intelligence."[54] Science was truth; there were to be "no other gods."[55]

The opening years of the study took place while the PHS was winning its campaigns over infectious diseases.[56] And the PHS's work was not done in a vacuum. PHS officers either trained under leading medical researchers or sought their imprimatur for their work. Letters, visits, and advice moved back and forth across the country between major medical schools and clinics and the PHS.[57] The connections put PHS doctors into the center of the scientific effort and garnered accolades and a sense of professionalism. The medical schools and clinics, in turn, could look to the PHS for funding and organizational prowess.

The status conferred by these connections supported the PHS as it threaded its way through the minefield of public health projects. When a county doctor's objections could delay a treatment program or a state's politicians could deny the findings of a well-run study, having links to what appeared to be "science" was critical to PHS physicians and helped them through the moments when all their work seemed for naught.[58]

PHS efforts to prove its abilities with surveys, self-experimentation, and mortality statistics did not always work. Despite its efforts to find scientific proof for the causes of hookworm and pellagra, for example, the PHS had to contend with alternative explanations of disease causation that fit political needs and older medical beliefs. Deeply seated understandings about eugenics, racial differences, or even contagion meant that even with the increasing "testable scientific findings," the PHS could not always translate its conclusions into policy.[59]

Nor were the PHS's "best men" immune from the prevailing cultural and scientific assumptions that shaped beliefs about race and disease.[60] Indeed, they helped to create them. It was an era when what historian Evelynn M. Hammonds has called "the logic of difference" permeated both medicine and public health. The colors that could be supposedly read on the skin and the myriad comparative measures taken of various body parts and organs defined biological racial differences and set up typologies.[61] In the post–Civil War era, southern physicians in particular were certain that the African American population would eventually die out because of inherent biological inferiority and susceptibility to disease.[62] But racial categories and biological differences were as likely to be seen in Jews and Italians as they were in African Americans. Doing the medical inspections as waves of immigrants passed through various ports, PHS physicians determined who was healthy and who might bring in visible or hidden disease.

Many of the PHS leaders in the Venereal Disease Division went to medical school at a time when eugenic understandings of race were central to their education.[63] Eugenics theory was used to explain hereditary differences in intelligence and disease, especially by race, and called for both increased breeding of the more intelligent and state-sponsored sterilization of the "unfit."[64] Into the early 1930s, PHS doctors would have been steeped in the beliefs that gave "bad blood" a meaning beyond its vernacular use as a name for syphilis. Assuming that behavioral and disease traits could be passed on through families and races, eugenicists believed in a hierarchy of races and that "bad blood" reflected a racialized "blood taint—a propensity toward moral and medical degeneracy."[65] PHS physicians, picking up their medical journals in 1932, could also read about "observations on the bones of the skull in white and Negro fetuses and infants" or "epileptic reactions in the Negro race." If they wandered into the physical anthropology texts, there was more to be learned about what biometrician Raymond Pearl labeled "comparative racial pathology," such as on the "kerato-cricoid muscle" in blacks and whites or in Pearl's own famous study on "the weight of the Negro brain."[66] "Having 'bad blood,'" as historian Martin Pernick has written, "meant you were contaminated and contaminating, whether the specific agent was a germ or the germ plasm."[67] Nowhere was this clearer than in the case of syphilis.

A Wily and Fascinating Spirochete

By the early twentieth century, syphilology had become a medical specialty. Individuality in treatment required balancing metals treatments (mercury, then forms of arsenic and bismuth), fever therapies, drugs proffered by non-specialists, and the home remedies and patent medicines that promised to be "blood purifiers."[68] Silence about the disease was pervasive, and the very word "syphilis" was kept out of polite conversation. Instead, terms such as "bad disease" or "bad blood" circulated in American communities, along with the old euphemism "the pox" and the alternate medical term "lues venerea." Syphilis's stealth became its hallmark, both from the refusal to discuss it openly and from its ability to lie dormant in the body and then become dangerous.

Syphilis generated interlocking concerns over medicine and morality.[69] Debates over whether lectures on morality, chemical prophylaxis, or prophylactics would be most effective in combating syphilis's damages abounded. The disease provided endless research questions to consider: How much treatment and when? Why were some organs and not others affected? Could the body develop an immune reaction to the spirochete? Was reinfection possible or just relapse? What was the meaning of negative serology in a long-term case? Could the blood tests be relied upon? And, of course, what were the differences among races and genders?[70]

Given the PHS's beginnings in providing health care for mariners, syphilis had long been one of its central concerns. With the growing focus on venereal disease during the war, Congress authorized $2 million in 1918 for the PHS's new Venereal Disease Division. The funding rose quickly in the immediate postwar years and then, with no troops to protect, dropped precipitously throughout the 1920s. The lack of funds, however, did not lessen the PHS's concern.

The standard public health focus in the first half of the twentieth century was "not whether the person is syphilitic but whether he is in a contagious state." Worry that syphilis would be passed on to an "innocent" spouse or lover and then congenitally to a child had informed much of the early twentieth-century public health effort to stem the disease.[71] "Every syphilitic person must be considered as a *focus of infection*, as a potential danger to the community, in the same category with the 'typhoid carrier,'" wrote the authors of a major 1922 study of "syphilis of the innocent."[72]

Before penicillin became available, Surgeon General Thomas Parran and the PHS's Raymond Vonderlehr wrote in their 1941 text *Plain Words about*

Venereal Disease that syphilis was no longer considered contagious when the patient had had "at least 20 injections each of an arsphenamine and a heavy metal" and in "untreated patients . . . in whom it is certain that syphilis has been present for more than five years." The danger remained, they warned, that a woman could still transmit to a child more than a decade after infection, and she should be treated during pregnancies.[73]

Even as funding for venereal disease dropped away in the late 1920s, the PHS focused on the facts. The Venereal Disease Division's *Venereal Disease Information* journal reported the statistics that the PHS and local and state health departments had begun to gather on prevalence. Debates over how much treatment and which arsenicals and other metals to use, when, and at what dosages filled medical journals. More than anything else, syphilologists wanted to understand the disease's natural history and to determine how much treatment was really needed and for whom and when.

Facts and Knowledge

Thomas Parran, who became the Venereal Disease Division's head in 1926 and surgeon general in 1936, made the battle against syphilis his most famous accomplishment.[74] His emphasis on both clinical research and syphilis in the black population served to provide the ties that would bind the PHS and Tuskegee Institute together in practice and memory forever.

Recognizing the need for more research, facts, and uniformity in treatment, Parran became the PHS's representative on the Committee for Research on Syphilis organized by research scientists, the PHS, and the American Social Hygiene Association and funded by anonymous wealthy philanthropists. In 1929, in hope of providing models and reports on appropriate care for syphilis's many manifestations, the committee formed the Cooperative Clinical Group, composed of the heads of the country's five leading university-based syphilis clinics with Parran as the chair. The specialists' treatment recommendations relied on the difficult-to-handle arsphenamine and were almost useless to the general physician. This was problematic for the PHS officers, since their concern was implementation as much as scientific perfection. In turn, Joseph Earle Moore, head of Johns Hopkins's famed syphilis clinic, worried that if the PHS made recommendations for treatment without appropriate data, the wrong form of treatment would become the standard of care.[75]

Much of this was moot, given the expense and time needed for treatment. The best recommendations for early syphilis suggested a year of injections with costs that "averaged between $305 to $380 but could range as high as

$1000. Even public clinics often charged as much as $80 for a curative level of therapy." As health economists in the early 1930s found, "eighty percent of the population could not afford the cost of adequate care [for syphilis] . . . from private physicians."[76] Despite publication of the Cooperative Clinical Group's numerous reports, the PHS was, by the early 1930s, still deeply focused on what treatment was appropriate, for whom, and at what stages of the disease and how to make the facts known to the public and the general physician.[77]

Parran and the PHS needed to break the silence about the disease. They initiated a major campaign in the 1930s to make the public aware of syphilis and to seek blood tests and treatment.[78] Parran spoke openly about the disease everywhere he could, even when CBS radio refused to let him broadcast an address in 1934 because he intended to use the words "syphilis" and "gonorrhea" on the air.[79] His best-selling book, *Shadow on the Land*, his articles in popular magazines, and the numerous public information and film campaigns put out by the PHS made information on syphilis more readily available and encouraged open discussion.[80]

Getting the "facts" of syphilis out proved to be doable but difficult.[81] The PHS accumulated data on the disease's occurrence from examinations of army inductees, from blood tests done in various cities and counties and college campuses, from clinical data, and from death statistics. Collecting facts, standardizing data, and completing surveillance became essential. But the statistics were never as accurate as the PHS and its supporters would claim. The data was never complete and never without underlying assumptions that often led to diagnosis in some individuals but not in others; the reporting of data by race but not by class; and the collection of statistics from urban clinics but not from private doctors.[82]

Ideologies about race shaped both the collection of survey data and the way it was understood. During the surveys conducted during World War I, black soldiers were purported to have higher rates, although the basis for the diagnosis was not always clear, and blacks with syphilis were allowed into the armed forces but white syphilitics were kept out.[83] By 1930, one of the first major surveys would claim that "estimates as to the infection rate in this race vary widely. No large series of accurately studied cases has been reported."[84]

Syphilologists thought they might have a "gold standard" of knowledge in what became known as the Oslo Study. At the turn of the century (1891–1910), Caesar Boeck, chief of the syphilis clinic at the University Hospital in Oslo, Norway, hospitalized some "2000 patients with primary and secondary syphilis until lesions healed without treatment, believing that the patient's own defense mechanisms alone could better combat the disease than the anti-syphilitic treatment of his day." Fifteen years later, the new chief, Boeck's former deputy, tried to follow up on the same patients. He was able to find information on 21.7 percent of the patients: 309 men and women who were still alive and another 164 who had died. Nearly 40 percent were symptom free (about half still had blood that was seropositive), 14.1 percent had heart disease, and approximately 4 percent had neurological complications.[85]

This data would pass "from textbook to textbook and from one scientific paper to the other," so that the standard wisdom became, as American syphilologist John Stokes would claim, that, of those, black and white, who were untreated in the disease's early stages, "two-thirds will pass through life unharmed."[86] For many syphilologists, the Oslo Study showed that although patients had to be treated individually, the majority could be expected to not die from the disease. The physicians' old adage, "if a man has survived syphilis for twenty years he is to be congratulated not treated," was now provided with research confirmation.

Syphilis as a "Sanitary Sin"

But the Oslo Study still was a problem for American syphilologists. As the PHS's Raymond A. Vonderlehr put it clearly in 1938 in his racialist terms: "Our present information indicates definite biologic differences in the disease in Negroes and whites."[87] The obsessive concern with both the danger of "Negro blood" and the hidden dangers of syphilis combined to make the disease a presumed racial menace. Tales of black "sanitary sins" filled popular and medical journals.[88] Such "sins" were especially feared because they could easily spread across racial lines. A Mississippi doctor told fellow members of the American Medical Association in 1910 that danger, especially from syphilis and gonorrhea, was actually greater from "mulattoes, octoroons and quadroons." Miscegenation, this physician warned, would spread the "immorality" and diseases of the "pure Negro" and eventually "Africanize this country" with a "Frankenstein monster."[89] At a Southern Medical Association meeting in 1915, a Texas physician declared "the negro a menace to the health of the white race." Venereal disease was in particular the gravest danger, the physician concluded, for which "the negro must bear the largest share of responsibility." "It is appalling," he noted with great alarm, "the venereal infections among the nurses of our children, the cooks in our homes, the servants who drive our automobiles, wash our clothes and have daily ingress into our home, where personal contact greatly enhances the danger."[90]

Much of the claim of the widespread existence of syphilis and its link to the black community came from the PHS's efforts to do surveys by taking blood. After a one-day census in 1926, the PHS reported that the rates were "4 per 1000" for whites and "7.2 per 1000 in blacks." These numbers, the PHS concluded, failed to capture the real prevalence since so many people with the disease either did not know they had or it or were not under treatment.[91]

Community-wide surveys with Wassermann dragnets (in which everyone was given a blood test) were sought to get a better approximation of syphilis's pervasiveness. In 1930, O. C. Wenger, from the PHS's Venereal Disease Clinic in Hot Springs, Arkansas, and Paul S. Carley, a physician staffer with the Rockefeller Foundation, reported on the use of blood tests of "apparently healthy Negroes in Mississippi" in an attempt to devise a baseline to measure against, once control efforts were started.[92] Carried out in the heart of the black South in three Mississippi Delta counties, the surveys found a rate of nearly 20 percent. Carley and Wenger argued that the figures were "an underestimation of the problem." They noted, "In the Negro, the administration of from two to four doses of some arsenical, intravenously, often causes a positive Wassermann reaction to become negative." They gave no comparative evidence as to whether changes in the serological reaction differed in whites. By extrapolating the data to include all African Americans in rural Mississippi, they concluded that "syphilis is probably the major public health problem among rural Mississippi negroes today."[93]

Claims about social behavior infused the report. "The rural negroes of Mississippi are unmoral and prodigal," the authors asserted. "As a group these negroes are carefree, happy and peaceable; crimes of violence unassociated with a sexual background are rare; their prodigality is inordinate and their sex appetite is enormous."[94]

Within a few years, the PHS and Wenger were back in the Mississippi Delta. They were brought into cotton-growing Bolivar County by the Delta Pine and Land Company to survey nearly 2,000 of its black workers. Nearly one-fourth tested positive for syphilis, but neither the employer nor the state could pay for a full round of treatment. The prohibitive cost of a private physician meant that rural African Americans were never treated or that they received, if their employers paid, inadequate medication.

As always, the PHS had to balance medical need, southern race relations, and economic reality. The PHS hoped to get funds to treat those workers who were infectious; anything more seemed impossible. The PHS approached the Rosenwald Fund, a Chicago-based foundation that had a commitment to improving both rural black education and black health care. The Rosenwald Fund wanted an expanded demonstration project that could use statistics on prevalence to persuade legislatures and then state and local health departments to provide treatment and convince employers to pay for it.

After much negotiating, the Rosenwald Fund and the PHS designed the first major serological survey *and* treatment program for syphilis in the country. It was to be undertaken in six counties in six different southern states and was to be jointly sponsored by local and state health departments, the PHS, and the Rosenwald Fund. Thus, under the banner of research, treatment, public health administration, and disease control, the PHS arrived in Macon County for what was to become a decades-long stay. Infection was the focus; racial differences were the underlying assumption; obtaining knowledge about the disease was the central concern.

2

Planned, Plotted, and Official

The Study Begins

Macon County proved to be an ideal site for one of the Rosenwald Fund Demonstration Projects.[1] In 1930, the county was 82.4 percent
black, spread over 650 square miles, representing what Taliaferro Clark, the
PHS's lead physician/researcher for the project and head of its Venereal Disease Division, labeled the "broad extremes in the development of the Negro
race."[2] Tuskegee Institute was presumed to represent the "best." Much of the
rest of the county's black population, caught up in grinding rural poverty,
seemed to be the "worst."[3]

Little health and education infrastructure to support the demonstration
work existed—mainly a newly minted county health department and the
assistance of officials at Tuskegee Institute. There was no public hospital or
clinic, and there were only sixteen doctors (only one of whom was black)
outside the VA Hospital and the institute's John A. Andrew Memorial Hospital, which was primarily for its staff and students. As elsewhere in the South,
few had access to basic health information, even with the institute's efforts to
teach health and hygiene to rural African Americans beyond its walls.[4] Most
black children spent more time in the fields than in overcrowded grammar
school classes as school followed the crop cycles. Illiteracy rates were high.
Root doctors, midwives, and healers provided most medical care; regular
doctors were used only for emergencies or when funds were available.[5]

The various roadways of the county captured the difficulties of rural life
and its separation from officialdom. Dirt roads that turned to soggy red clay
mud during the winter rains outnumbered the paved ones. Beyond this was
what renowned Fisk University sociologist Charles S. Johnson, brought in

by the Rosenwald Fund to study the community, described as "another, narrower, and less obvious network of footpaths which—unplanned, unplotted, and without official recognition—intersect, connect and supplement but never compete with the public highways."[6] The lives of many of the black residents were also "unplotted," since their births, illnesses, and deaths often remained "without official recognition" from the state or the doctors.[7]

Macon County's residents lived their lives on those roads forming various kinds of physical and mental maps through crucial forms of connections. For those in and near Tuskegee, who were part of Tuskegee Institute or the VA Hospital, the nearby rail line and the automobile made the outside world accessible. For the poor on the farms, license tags for their aging cars proved so expensive that they were given up or shared, while mules, wagons, and feet still defined the possibility of travel.[8] Tuskegee Institute, only a few miles away from the farmlands, was rarely visited by these rural people and might as well have been in a foreign country.[9] Perceived color and class lines within the black communities also kept them apart. As one rural Macon County man reported in 1930, "That school ain't got no race pride much. They only like yellow and red folks. They ain't so much on the black ones."[10] The reverse was also true. To those who came to study and try to understand them, local residents, with falling-down homes, lack of sanitation, and overcrowding, seemed to come from another time and place.[11]

Alabama was a dangerous land for African Americans when the Study began. In March 1931, the nine young black men who became known as the Scottsboro Boys were arrested in Jackson County in northern Alabama on false charges of raping two white women. Over the next few years, they were subjected to trials that focused much of the world's attention on assumptions about black male sexuality as being part of an "essential" nature—assumptions that were used to prop up the Jim Crow system.[12]

Elsewhere in Alabama, sharecroppers and industrial workers were organizing. In July 1931, in Camp Hill in nearby Talladega County, a shoot-out between local sheriffs and sharecroppers who were protesting their own situation and that of the men in Scottsboro left a black church burned down, a sheriff wounded, a sharecropper killed, and a posse to put down the "uprising" traveling throughout the county. In December 1932, in Reeltown in Tallapoosa County on the Macon border, another shoot-out over land foreclosure put the Sharecroppers' Union organizer in jail for thirteen years.[13] News of these protests and the resulting violence trickled into Macon County in the columns of the local newspapers and traveled by word of mouth for those who could not read. These eruptions served as a constant reminder of how much law and violence underlay the power of Alabama's white supremacy.

Against this backdrop and led by the PHS's Taliaferro Clark and O. C. Wenger, a demonstration project on syphilis treatment came to Macon County. It was expected at first to help and encourage investigation. The testing and treatment was only for African Americans, but the hope was that the model for care could then be spread across the country. Race mattered in terms of difference, and then it did not matter in terms of using the results.

Conditions in Macon County

In the depths of the Depression, sickness and death seemed to stalk the rural black population of Macon County. Illness was expected in the overcrowded and drafty one- and two-room cabins, with no running water or even glass in the windows. In the poorer homes, light often came in the form of a flambeau made of a kerosene-filled soda bottle and a rag. Tuberculosis, pneumonia, and influenza (but not syphilis) became the biggest killers in the Depression years. Malnutrition and intestinal diseases took young children who made it past the danger of miscarriages and stillbirths.[14] "They survive on grits, rice, grease, syrup and cornbread," a doctor reported.[15] As one man put it bluntly, "We don't git no money. This is the country."[16]

Macon County's men and women who became the patients in the Rosenwald Fund Demonstration Project spoke willingly about their illnesses and expectations for health care to Johnson and his research team. In turn, the sociologists tried to write their words down in the patois and vernacular they heard.[17] These narratives reflected folk beliefs and the problems of access. Most ills were described in terms of the pains or symptoms—chills, fevers, sores—in the vagueness of "heart" or "woman" troubles, or in what residents thought the doctors told them.[18] Henry Daniel explained, "Course I knew I had bad blood already cause my brother had scoffla [scrofula] when I was born." George Edwards told his interviewer that his wife had "high blood pressure[;] some calls it the 'two bumps' [tuberculosis]."

As with patients everywhere, treatment was expected as part of a medical encounter. When the doctor told Louis Cowan his blood was "good," Cowan was not pleased. Even with his "good blood," he stated, "I went back up dere lots of times to see the doctor cause I tho't dere was really something wrong with my blood. I ain't no count, my head swims, heart beats fast and I gits real nervous." Even when they received drugs, many patients misunderstood the connections between their symptoms and the treatments. As Amos Foy reported, "I had a terrible misery in my throat. I was sorry for the time to come to drink water it hurt me so bad. I have taken 20 shots and it certainly has helped me."[19]

The interviews led Johnson to conclude that there was a resignation and fatalism: "The heavy fall of death prompts to reliance upon both herbs and something akin to magic, in the attempt to bring about cures."[20] With little or no money, Macon County's residents borrowed from one another's medicines or used charms, teas, and potions to stave off ills or to ease the pains. When her daughter had whooping cough, Anna Belle Keys explained, she gave "sheep nanny tea and kerosene with sugar and I got a bottle of oil." Emma Morris had two children die of "yellow thrust" (yellow thrush), and she made them "thread salve" from yellow berries, to no avail. George Edwards's wife "put dis string around the baby's neck to keep off sickness. The three buttons and the penny helps her to tease [teethe]. The piece of black leather keeps off de whopping cough." Jimmie Smith's wife relied on "pomegranate hull tea and broom straw root tea" for the "weakness of the back," and Abraham Deloach's wife bought "Hoffman medicine for all run down women."[21]

With almost no public funds or insurance, visits to or from doctors were infrequent or nonexistent since local charges were "$2.50 to $3.00 plus mileage one way, which for a ten mile trip might amount to $12.00."[22] Doctors were called only in emergencies. Frank Jerriedoor reported, "The doctors . . . wont come to see you less you got the cash or will pawn something." Hilliard Boyd agreed with this: "You phones them and they say, 'Is you got the money?' If you ain't you need not supect them." John Harris explained that it was time for his wife to go for treatment at the clinic, but without shoes it would be difficult to walk the two miles.[23]

Yet others found doctors willing to wait for payment or with other motives. Hayes Jones's wife explained: "I sure has a big doctor's bill but Dr. Lightfoot is reasonable. He'll just wait and wait until the money comes." Matilda Mackie said with pride that a private doctor told her that "if you ever feel any pain again just ring me up cause you show pays your bills." Charlie Johnson's wife said her husband had been treated for his malaria by Dr. Cowan, explaining: "I don't know exactly whether he [Dr. Cowan] was in any way connected with my father Elbert Cowan, but I 'spected it comes from slavery time. You knows how they were all mixed up like that." Even the midwives had trouble getting paid. Midwife Rosa Lancaster reported: "My regular price is $10.00 but I don't always charge that for it. I would bees ten years getting it. They all aint paid up yet."[24]

Even with the Rosenwald Demonstration doctors, there were differences among the patients in understandings and expectations. Lucinda Gilmore recalled: "When I took treatments I don't know what I was being treated for. They just told me I had bad blood." Bennie Williams had "good blood . . . but I don't believe it," he said. "I think I need the treatment too." Oliver Harris's wife asked a very reasonable question: "Every time your blood report comes back good, does it mean you really got good blood, or can you have bad blood and get a good report?" Abraham Deloach reported: "Seems to me dey oughta trat you fur something else cide blood. Dey promised to treat us for our 'plaints but every time we goes over there they don't do nothing for us." Robert Neal's son got sick from the shots, and his father agreed he didn't have to go back.[25]

In describing the financial duress and fatalism of the families, Johnson failed to discuss the fears of medical care that may also have kept away even those who could pay. Will McQueen was sure that his first wife had been "killed" in a local hospital because, he explained, the nurses told him they cut the wrong "viscicule" near her tumor. The doctors frightened Cora Gosha, and she admitted that "I just wouldn't go."[26] Pelly Alexander reported that "Dr. Davis was a nice doctor," but another of the physicians "lay your arm down like he guttin a hog. . . . I told him he hurt me. . . . He tole me 'I'm the doctor.'"[27]

Richard Pitts raised the most pointed question when he was interviewed outside of the hamlet of Hardaway. "I bee sick sometime. Biggest times I am hungry. No it aint' take me long to answer them questions. The biggest thing I want to know is, what you going to do with all this when you get through?"[28]

Demonstrating Treatment

The Rosenwald Fund and the PHS doctors thought they had an answer. The goal of the Demonstration Project was to prove to health departments and state and federal legislatures that syphilis was prevalent but that it was possible to control its spread.[29] Even though local physicians in Macon County who had both black and white patients reported that "there was considerable syphilis in the community at large," the focus was only on black men, women, and children.[30] Johnson's interviews demonstrated that there were blacks and whites living together in the community and that some were suspicious of the focus on blacks. "Why you all ain't going to everybody if [you] wants to find the sick ones," one man asked. "White folks is sick just like us."[31]

With local and federal support, the PHS moved in for the year and a half between February 1930 and the first of September 1931, talked to employers, plantation owners, ministers, and doctors, and began their case finding through testing in as large a population as they could bring in. To the land-owners and employers, the PHS promised treatment for syphilis that would mean fewer stillbirths, less time lost among the black workforce, and im-proved worker "efficiency."[32] Education extended to the local physicians as the PHS explained that the common policy of giving only a few treatments would not stop the disease's spread.[33]

The effort became a concerted drive to bring public health into the back-country. Black men, women, and children — the PHS counted 3,684, one-sixth of the county's black population — turned out in school yards, churches, and stores and under trees at crossroads in hamlets with names like Nebraska, St. Paul, Chesson, Downs, and Liverpool.[34] "As a group," one doctor in the project thought, "they were susceptible to kindness, and there may have been an inducement of implied official authority, although there was no volitional effort to create this impression."[35] The doctors took blood and urine samples, performed minimal physical exams, and made efforts to obtain case histo-ries. The hope was to provide at least "20 injections [of the heavy metals] and 192 mercury rubs" to keep down transmission of the disease.[36]

The physicians gave the shots and sent the patients home with a written instruction sheet that told them how to get the mercury into their skin using a rubber belt. These rubs, central to what syphilologist John H. Stokes called "self-medication," were considered "highly effective but messy."[37] "Rub the salve into the skin on your stomach when you get out of bed in the morning," they were told. "Then put on the belt. See that the belt fits snugly. Wear belt all day and take it off before you go to bed at night."[38] It seemed to work. "The belt came to be regarded by many as a sort of magic," one physician reported, "and the number of faithful adherents was thereby augmented."[39] As Will McQueen told his interviewer, "Course I salvates myself and keeps fine."[40]

The project's triage-like focus was on those whose infections were pri-mary or secondary, active, and more likely to spread.[41] The PHS gave those with latent disease the rubs and smaller amounts of the injections more to bring in the entire family than to effect a cure. The rules were clear. As those doing the treating were told: "Remember the older patients should be treated with Neo [neoarsphenamine] or Hg [mercury], as a general thing unless they have only had their infections a comparatively short time or in the face of some definite lesion. Put these cases on KI [potassium-iodide] or protio-iodide and gradually eliminate them from the clinics, so you have more time for the younger groups."[42] George Graham's wife confirmed this experience to her interviewers. "My husband got bad blood. He didn't take no shots[;] he's too old for that." Henry Daniel Seal reported: "The doctor says I am too old to take dem shots, so he gave me liquish medicine. It does me lots of good." Others could not get off work to go to the clinics. Carter Ashberry's wife explained that her husband was told to take the treatments: "He didn't take them because Mr. Dozier [the landlord] said he wasn't going to feed us if he didn't work every day and we can't starve." Charlie Lee Washington "quit taking those shots cause they made me sick."[43]

The PHS doctors were shocked to find that 39.8 percent of those who came forward in Macon County tested positive for syphilis, although their sampling came from a small geographic area of the county and may have reflected a localized outbreak. This proved to be the highest prevalence rate in the six southern counties studied during the Demonstration Project. The researchers thought the high number was perhaps due to the 62 percent they believed had untreated congenital syphilis, although the medical basis for this claim was never explained.[44] The PHS's Taliaferro Clark was not surprised to find that "early syphilis formed a very small percentage of the cases found," as 1,400 men, women, and children were admitted into treatment.[45] No one seems to have questioned the findings, even though it was well known that the blood tests used could turn up high rates of false positives.[46]

Reassuring Robert Russa Moton, Tuskegee Institute's principal, about the county's high rate, the PHS doctors argued that Macon County's syphilitic numbers were "not due to inherent racial susceptibility" and could be explained by widespread poverty.[47] Views shifted between the assumption that blacks would be more syphilitic and the understanding that lack of education, crowded conditions, and little medical care encouraged the disease's spread.

As the Demonstration Project continued, obtaining money for supplies and getting people to return for their injections proved to be difficult. The plan for treatment unraveled and failed to meet the schedule.[48] Rains, planting seasons, marketing demands for crops, and difficulties in getting to the sites all interfered. The clinics set up in the county could not provide the continuity of care nor the structure to supply appropriate treatment.

In Macon County, fewer doses of neoarsphenamine were given than in any of the other southern counties (only 5 doses per person on average) but more of the mercury (106.1 rubs), which the patients were expected to apply. Clark claimed, however, that patients did better "with little arsenical treatment than with a large amount," in terms of reversing the positive blood tests, although whether they still harbored the spirochetes was uncertain.[49] "Increasing knowledge leads to the belief that the greatest infection of syphilis occurs in the early stages," he noted in his final report. "It would appear that the medication administered in these demonstrations, where most of the cases were noninfectious, should have been fairly adequate."[50] In other words, Clark thought the smaller amounts of treatment would help those in the later stages of the disease, and these were the patients they were uncovering in the county. Given that they were not following the patients for any length of time, it is surprising that he seemed so sanguine about this outcome. Even the instruction sheet to the patients had warned: "You must continue treatment for twelve months if you hope to get your blood pure."[51]

The Demonstration Project doctors tried to provide other care to the families. In addition to detecting and beginning to treat the 1,400 cases of syphilis, "3,500 typhoid inoculations were given, and 600 children [were] immunized against diphtheria, and 200 [were] vaccinated against smallpox." Seeds for gardens and yeast to combat pellagra were also made available, with the Red Cross's help.[52] Even though the syphilis treatment program fell short of its goals, the entire Rosenwald Fund Demonstration Project was deemed a success by its organizers: prevalence could be determined and treatment begun.

But Dr. H. L. Harris, a black physician sent into Macon County by the Rosenwald Fund, was not convinced. He knew the project could not begin to provide the services of a real rural health program, and the more crucial illnesses that came from lack of food and failures of sanitation concerned him. He had his doubts even about what they were doing for syphilis. He saw that "the heat melted the mercury" before the patients could use it.[53] He questioned the PHS's O. C. Wenger's techniques, worried about patients' reactions to the heavy metals, and believed that at least two deaths were "attributable to effects of treatment."[54] Wenger responded to this criticism by claiming that Harris did not understand how to work in difficult conditions.

Despite Harris's concerns, which the Rosenwald Fund considered seriously, the project became a model for what might have been a national campaign.[55] It would be used to make claims for treatment regardless of race.[56] If there had been more money, it is possible it might have continued and expanded. Yet, as Harris had seen, it could never be a substitute for a public health program or for the kinds of individualized care the patients needed. The project doctors never even got a chance to care for the syphilis properly.

In 1931, as the Depression deepened and the Rosenwald Fund's stock portfolio dipped precipitously, even this small demonstration ended.

In many ways, the Rosenwald Fund Demonstration Project proved that race could *not* be used to explain either the prevalence of the disease or the willingness to come to treatment. Treatment of African Americans became the model for all Americans. "Mass control of syphilis among rural Negroes in the South," Clark concluded, "is both possible and practical, and offers a new and promising approach to the ultimate control of this disease in all classes of the population."[57]

Levels of income, education, and medical care in the various black communities that were treated explained the different disease rates. Desire for treatment crossed class lines as thousands came forward for the help. The racism that shaped socioeconomics in the counties clearly mattered in terms of how widespread the disease became. When needed, race would be ignored in order to generalize about the need for treatment. But in the end, the assumed biological difference based on race and the need to fully understand the disease proved even more intriguing. The availability of what was seen as a pool of disease proved to be too beguiling to be ignored.

Beginning the Study and the Provision of Treatment

When the Rosenwald Fund Demonstration Project closed, the PHS's concern with syphilis and Macon County did not end. As with other syphilologists, the PHS doctors saw the disease as a noble enemy that could be attacked and beaten.[58] To accomplish this, the disease had to be publicly named and openly discussed and its "natural history" had to be understood.[59] This meant more research as well as treatment programs. There were studies in urban clinics but not enough focus or follow-up on latent disease.[60] Only the Oslo Study stood as a measure. But its focus was on whites, and it was done retrospectively.[61] Most researchers were trained to believe in the racialist assumption that syphilis was, as leading Johns Hopkins syphilologist Joseph Earle Moore claimed, "almost a different disease" in African Americans and that prospective studies were better science.[62]

With the Rosenwald Fund Demonstration Project behind him, the PHS's Taliaferro Clark still was intrigued with what he had seen in Macon County and concerned about what could be done. He knew there was debate over treatment of those with late latent syphilis if they had not received treatment earlier in the course of the illness. He was a field-tested man looking for answers to practical questions. As the PHS noted in its annual report in 1933, in a section probably approved, if not written, by Clark:

The treatment of syphilis under ideal conditions is of utmost value in the control of this insidious disease, but, unfortunately, owing to various social and economic influences, the ideal method of therapy is seldom possible of attainment, and the vast majority of infected people receive treatment that is generally regarded as inadequate, or no treatment at all. *It is highly desirable, therefore, to ascertain, if possible, the relative benefits accrued from adequate and inadequate treatment* [italics added].[63]

Nearing the end of his career and in his sixties, Clark must have imagined he had one more chance to make a difference with the disease that had consumed his professional life. With little private, state, or federal money, he knew he could not reestablish a major treating program or provide the kind of health care Harris thought so necessary.[64]

Instead, he developed a plan to take advantage of a pool of what physicians often referred to as "clinical material." His idea took more than a year to work out in detail. It eventually became a two-arm study. In one arm, he would follow a group that had late latent disease but had received little or no treatment. The other arm would be a control group that did not have syphilis but that came from the same socioeconomic strata. He did not suggest a study where small amounts of treatment went to one arm and placebos to the others who were also ill. He never argued for giving anyone syphilis.[65] He thought there was enough syphilis in the bodies of the county's black men and women and enough people left untreated for a sample to be picked. He never considered looking for whites from a similar class with whom to compare the findings.

As Clark's ideas took shape, there was no written protocol and no consideration of what the participants might gain.[66] It would not have been expected at that time. Instead, letters went back and forth between Clark and the "best men" treating and studying syphilis in the fall of 1932, to determine what was possible and to make the science as acceptable as it could be.[67] His colleagues added signs and symptoms to be studied, refined the details of the measurements, and agreed to the importance of the research. Physicians inside and outside the PHS supported his developing proposal of taking advantage of "an unparalleled opportunity of studying the effect of untreated syphilis on the human economy."[68]

Clark's original plan was to find out what happened to individuals with late latent syphilis who did not get any treatment over the course of six months or a year. The research plan that developed in letters and conversations included multiple blood tests to detect the presence of spirochetes, procedures to listen to and x-ray the participants' hearts, and diagnostic spinal taps.[69] As with all venereal disease, histories of when the disease began had to be taken, although both Wenger at the PHS and Moore at Johns Hopkins believed that self-reported information could not be relied upon.[70] Wenger reminded Clark that "we are dealing with a group of people who are illiterate, have no conception of time, and whose personal history is always indefinite."[71]

With all the diplomacy the PHS was used to employing, Clark laid out his plans to the Alabama health officials whose support he would need to work in the county. Murray Smith, Macon County's new public health director, was particularly enthusiastic. State officials agreed to the research and extracted a promise: There had to be some treatment, but it could not be supplied by the state since the study was seen as stepping into medical care that private physicians provided.[72] Not only the state officials had to be satisfied. Clark knew that in order to get planters to allow their sharecroppers to be tested, "it was necessary to carry on this study under the guise of a demonstration and provide treatment for those cases uncovered found to be in need of treatment."[73] By this, he presumably meant those in earlier stages of the disease and still infectious. Clark also knew he needed the cooperation of doctors who treated black patients and a hospital for procedures.

Clark went to Eugene H. Dibble, medical director at Tuskegee Institute's John A. Andrew Memorial Hospital. He requested that Dibble "have one of your men carry out the relatively small amount of treatment at designated points in the county required by Doctor Baker of the State Board of Health as a prerequisite to his approval of the project."[74] Dibble could not give permission by himself within the institute's hierarchy, and he wrote a formal letter to Tuskegee Institute principal Robert Russa Moton, outlining Clark's ideas and explaining that the findings "would be of world wide significance." Dibble acknowledged how expensive the treatments were, suggesting, although not saying, that it might be possible less would be needed. He stressed how little the study would cost and how much it would benefit their nurses and interns. The PHS, he explained, would furnish "the necessary dressings, cotton, X-ray films and the Neo-Salvarsan for any treatment given."[75]

There would have been no reason for Moton to doubt Dibble. Moton's own World War I experience had taught him about syphilis in the black community, and he must have known of the syphilis rumors concerning his predecessor, Booker T. Washington. He was acutely aware of what was presumed to be the extent of the disease and its ties to assumptions about black immorality.

Surgeon General Hugh Cumming, holding this position just before Thomas Parran and who had worked with Moton before, followed up with a carefully composed plea for cooperation. Cumming reminded Moton of the extent of untreated disease and noted that the institute's hospital "offers an unparalleled opportunity for carrying on this piece of scientific research which probably cannot be duplicated anywhere else in the world." Cumming explained, "It is expected the results . . . may have a marked bearing on the treatment, or conversely the non-necessity for treatment, of cases of latent syphilis."[76]

Both Moton and Dibble were assured that this was a research study to examine the necessity of treatment. Coming from the PHS and the surgeon general, it seemed to offer the institute yet another chance to be center stage on significant work that could focus on the lives of African Americans and might help them triage medical efforts in a time of fiscal crisis. Within three weeks, Moton wrote back to Cumming and agreed to what he called a "worth while cause."[77] For Moton, this would bring attention to a serious "race" problem, federal assistance, and a modicum of health care. It followed the institute's decades-old commitment of doing something for the rural black masses and assuming a leadership role.

Clark still confronted key questions of what to do about treatment and of who should be in the study. There were no funds to re-create a Rosenwald Fund–like project to provide drugs over a length of time. He knew case finding and keeping people involved in the research would not be easy—he was not expecting to go back to those from the Rosenwald Fund Demonstration Project because many of them had been treated. He realized that women and men would come forward as they had before and that it would take time to find individuals who fit the criterion for inclusion then being worked out.

Clark and his advisers made a critical decision. Unlike in the Demonstration Project, they would be tracking only men, even though they were bringing in men and women as the study began and treatment was provided. Choosing men had several advantages. Getting a history of the first chancre would be easier since it usually appeared on the penis. It was more difficult to identify in women because the initial syphilitic sores might be inside the vagina. Eliminating women from the study meant less chance of congenital syphilis being passed to the next generation. Johns Hopkins's Joseph Earle Moore, who was consulted often, wanted more tests because he was not certain that the men could be relied upon to remember when they were first infected. As he told Clark, the existence of sores could not be determinate since "a mere history of a penile sore only would not be accurate in as much as the average negro has had as many penile sores as rabbits have offspring."[78] It was hoped that the additional tests would be helpful.

The assumption made was that the men included in the study would not be infectious. Moore counseled that they should take only those who were at least ten years from initial infection to be sure, but Clark decided instead to go with five years because such cases would be easier to find. Moore wanted men with a clear history of latency—other men found at earlier stages would be provided "subsequent anti-syphilitic treatment" if needed.[79] Families would be brought in, and infectious family members were to be treated, although no effort was made to find other female sexual partners or to imagine the possibility of male partners.[80] There was not going to be the kind of case finding that was typical in urban settings where sexual partners were supposed to be named and then tracked down by health care workers in order to be treated. The men's names would be kept for the records and followed up on. The title of the study at this point mirrored that of the Rosenwald Fund Demonstration Project: "The U.S. Public Health Service Syphilis Control Demonstration."[81]

Now the personnel had to be put in place. In October 1932, the PHS's Raymond A. Vonderlehr, an up-and-coming physician who had worked on the Rosenwald Fund Demonstration Project, was ordered to the county to begin the tasks. Vonderlehr proved dedicated to the work and became the head of the Venereal Disease Division the next year when Clark retired. It was clear from the Rosenwald experience and from Alabama law, which limited white nurses from caring for black patients, that an African American public health nurse would be needed to find individuals and serve as a liaison to the community. Dibble suggested Eunice Verdell Rivers, a Tuskegee Institute graduate from Jakin, Georgia, with public health experience who was then working unhappily as a night supervisor at the John A. Andrew Memorial Hospital. The PHS gave her the title of "scientific assistant."[82]

Vonderlehr and Rivers began to canvass the county for men *not* in early syphilis and willing to be tested.[83] Many refused. As Vonderlehr explained to Clark, "We must find a male prospect, ascertain his age and whether or not he has been previously tested, and then get his consent for a Wassermann [test]. It is necessary to find and interview several times the actual number finally permitting a test and it is a pretty good day's work to get 30 to 40 specimens."[84] None of the consents were in writing, nor did Vonderlehr make it clear what they were explaining.[85]

Case finding and history taking started from field stations set up under trees in places such as Cotton Valley, Eli, and Swanson and in the school next door to the Shiloh Missionary Baptist Church in Notasulga.[86] Even though the workers were primarily interested in the men, they still treated both men and women. The PHS was following through on what they had promised the local health officials: they were giving out injections of neoarsphenamine, mercury rubs, and the more old-fashioned drug protiodide (oral mercury pills).

Difficulties on the Ground

The Study proved even more difficult to manage than had been the case with the Rosenwald Fund Demonstration Project as it spread out through the county and brought in men and women from outside the county borders. "We were accused . . . of examining prospective recruits for the army," Vonderlehr complained to his superiors about suspicions in one community when the workers tried to separate out the men from the women.[87] Rivers owned a small car and was required to make trips back and forth to bring men into the institute's hospital to be x-rayed, slowing down the progress. Using syringes at first, rather than the more expensive Keidel tubes, to draw blood was laborious because syringes required sterilization and broke more easily.[88] Record keeping proved difficult, since it was not always clear what stage of the disease the men were in, whether the blood tests were accurate, or whether the heart sounds detected with the stethoscope were from an old rheumatic fever murmur or were the signs of syphilitic aortitis (inflammation of the aorta).[89]

Since everyone who was ill expected treatment, Clark was very worried about expenses. "It was never our intention to undertake the expense of treating the whole county," he reminded Vonderlehr.[90] By January 1933, Vonderlehr reported that they had given out 317 doses of "neo" to men and 359 doses to women, in part because the rate of women with positive blood tests was nearly twice the male rate. Nearly "50 pounds of mercury oleate" for the rubs had been used as well. By the next month, another 368 men and 351 women had received "neo," and pills had been given to "124 males and 76 females."[91]

Vonderlehr reported on the results after the first few months. Once the cases were identified, blood was drawn for testing twice and small amounts of treatment were doled out. "The figures include both men and women," Vonderlehr explained to Clark. "Of 50 patients retested after the first . . . course of treatment, consisting of eight doses of neoarsphenamine and more or less heavy metal, only 3 (6%) showed a serological reversal. We are now going to attempt to bring in the husbands of the women in this group by circularizing [sending out notices] them."[92] As Vonderlehr noted several years later, "We treated practically all of the patients with early manifestations and many of the patients with latent syphilis."[93]

The PHS was surprised to find much less syphilis than they had expected. Only between 18 and 19 percent of the screening blood tests were positive—about half what the Rosenwald Fund Demonstration Project had reported, Dibble confidentially told Moton in March 1933. Five months later, the surgeon general told the Alabama state health officer that the percentage was "approximately 28%," still much lower than the Rosenwald figures.[94] The high rates found earlier might indeed have reflected either false positives or a narrow outbreak in an isolated part of the county.

The high prevalence rate that had brought them back to Macon County began to look questionable. O. C. Wenger, who came in from the PHS Venereal Disease Clinic in Hot Springs, Arkansas, for a few months to help Vonderlehr, thought more cases could be found by using some of the men from the Rosenwald Demonstration. He asked the state health department's chief physician to help track down "any number of old male negroes who showed a positive serology, who had no previous treatment and who received no treatment during the Demonstration Project.[95] But, in fact, very few of the men from the Demonstration Project became part of the actual Study.[96]

Vonderlehr decided not to attempt to find the untreated cases that had been discovered during the Demonstration Project because he was concerned with how many would come to *expect* treatment even more than did the new people they were recruiting. If they went back to the men and women examined but left untreated, he reasoned, they would not cooperate unless everyone in the community was treated. Clark acknowledged the problem, noting that a large number had to be examined to find men who fit the Study's criterion.

The racial differences they assumed existed kept being commented upon. Even with fewer numbers than they expected, Clark told Moore at Johns Hopkins that they were "uncovering more pathology than I thought would be the case, particularly the cardiovascular system, which seems to be the Negro's vulnerable point in syphilitic attack."[97] But, without autopsies, it was difficult to know for sure if the cardiovascular complications they "heard" or "saw" came from syphilis, high cholesterol, rheumatic fever, hypertension, or a combination.

Worry about the expense of the project in the middle of the Depression suffused their letters.[98] Clark continued to pressure Vonderlehr to finish up the work and to use as few supplies as possible. Vonderlehr noted in January 1933: "In making the request for these drugs I believe that the added expense is justifiable for the great amount of good, which they will do per se to the negroes of the county, *irrespective of the effect their administration will have on the study of untreated syphilis* [italics added]."[99] Clark reneged on an order for iodide pills in April and warned of the "ominous situation now confronting us here in Washington."[100]

By February 1933, Vonderlehr appeared to be getting impatient too. There was an enormous amount of work to do to keep the treatments going and to find the men they needed for a robust statistical study. He complained about the women who kept showing up for treatment, and older women, in particular, were given nothing.[101] "Young men and women" were taking time for treatments, he reported. Murray Smith, the local health officer, proved inept at some of the blood work. Too much treating was getting expensive and interfering with them finding the men they needed.[102]

Technical Problems and Deception

After four months of case finding, the researchers began to discuss how and when to do the spinal taps to test for neurosyphilis. Although there was an assumption in the medical literature that whites developed the neurological symptoms and blacks the cardiovascular ones, there was a debate over whether these differences were due to "internal resistance to the disease . . . [or] difference in putative strains [of the bacteria]."[103] They wanted the neurological data as well.

Spinal taps were a dangerous and painful procedure that involved inserting a needle into the spinal column to remove fluid.[104] If done incorrectly or with too large a needle, severe headaches of several days' duration could result from leakage of fluid through the dura mater. Lying supine for twenty-four hours could lessen, but not prevent, pain from the procedure.[105] Vonderlehr thought the spinal taps were absolutely imperative. Because he was "not seeing much paresis [impaired movement caused by syphilis's neurological complications]," he thought about "writing to the local mental hospital to see if they have negro men from Macon."[106]

Wenger, probably still smarting from the criticisms about what he had done in the Rosenwald Fund Demonstration Project, continued to worry that the spinal taps would not be done correctly. He was concerned that any flaws in technique would be used against them by other scientists, especially if they were to find neurological changes, since, he reminded Vonderlehr, "the profession still insists that changes in the spinal fluid of negroes is comparatively rare because the clinical evidence of neurosyphilis in that race is not so pronounced."[107] Clark agreed because of the "hopelessness of recognizing mild paresis among these illiterate people of such circumscribed cultural horizon."[108] They needed the spinal taps, as historian Christopher Crenner has argued, to show what kind of neurological complication, if any, appeared in African Americans.[109] Neither man thought that the histories or their examinations of the men would provide the needed evidence. Only the technology of the spinal tap and examination of the spinal fluid would provide incontrovertible data.

The deception devised next was stunning and reflected the PHS's belief that it could not explain what it was doing to the men. In order to get the men to come in, Dr. Murray Smith, Macon County Health Department head, along with the PHS researchers, devised a letter. Reminding the men that they had already had a "thorough examination" with the "hope you have gotten a great deal of treatment for your bad blood," they promised, "You will now be given your last chance to get a second examination. This examination is a very special one and after it is finished you will be given a special treatment if it is believed you are in a condition to stand it." Because they "expect to be so busy," the letter continued, the men might have "to remain in the hospital over one night." It concluded, "REMEMBER THIS IS YOUR LAST CHANCE FOR SPECIAL FREE TREATMENT. BE SURE TO MEET THE NURSE." Appealing to the men's masculinity and strength, nothing in the letter made it clear that the procedure was purely diagnostic or anything less than a very good deal.[110]

The spinal punctures began in March, and some of the problems that concerned Vonderlehr and Wenger began to appear. It was hard to get the men to come in during the weekends because Saturday was seen as a day for "business and pleasure" and Sunday was a day for church.[111] Rivers remembered later how painful the taps had been and how difficult it was for the men to go home and stay with their feet elevated for twenty-four hours. "But, a lot of the patients failed to follow instructions and they had to be brought back to the hospital and kept in the hospital for the next twenty-four hours," she recalled.[112] Nonetheless, by the end of May, Vonderlehr reported that they had managed to obtain spinal taps from 296 men, although they were still worried about the men who had "defaulted" and refused to come in, were afraid, could not get out of work, or had moved away.

The Alabama heat seemed to be working against them as well. The National Institute of Health, to whom they sent the samples, reported that "39 of the 108 specimens of spinal fluids were contaminated and unfit for testing."[113] In the face of such spoilage, Vonderlehr redoubled his efforts to find enough men. Rivers was told to pack the samples in more dry ice. By June, with help from Smith, Dibble, and Wenger, the numbers were up another 15 cases. Wenger thought this total of "307 spinal punctures out of 375" was a "remarkable showing, and proves conclusively what a good piece of work Dr. Vonderlehr has accomplished."[114] No one mentioned that the deceptive letter might have helped because presumably it seemed so necessary.

With the serology, physical exams, fluoroscopes, x-rays, and spinal taps completed, the PHS researchers prepared to wind things up. In June they sent thank-you letters. Rivers returned to Georgia to visit her family, driving her new coupe with the rumble seat her salary permitted her to buy, hoping another job might appear. Dibble continued his work at the institute's hospital. Wenger was back in Hot Springs. Vonderlehr prepared to work up the data on what they knew so far and awaited a new assignment.[115] The year was up and the Study seemed to be over.

Continuing

Vonderlehr, however, was not content to move on. The data was too intriguing and the serious question—did latent syphilitics really need treatment?—was too crucial. His focus was on syphilis as a disease and less on the differences specific to African Americans. As early as April 8, 1933, he had written to Clark to begin to outline his ideas for a much more long-term study: "It seems a pity to me to lose such an unusual opportunity."

Vonderlehr's preliminary ideas were stunning in their ambition but fit accurately with what would probably be necessary for a full understanding of the disease. His new plan required a five- to ten-year study and included autopsies to discover the syphilis-induced damage on untreated men, with "interesting points for study" figured out along the way.[116] The objective was to find approximately 400 men and to keep them coming back. He proposed giving them small amounts of what would be called "treatment"—but mainly this was to be aspirins and tonics and some small amounts of oral mercury compounds if they asked. Vonderlehr suggested to Clark that the subjects who had received primarily mercury, and even small amounts of neoarsphenamine, during the previous months could be considered "untreated in the modern sense of therapy."[117]

Consultation began again with syphilologists and with Moton and Dibble at Tuskegee Institute.[118] Vonderlehr wrote to Wenger in a confidential letter that he thought he could organize the Study with Dibble's assistance, with the rehiring of Nurse Rivers on a part-time basis, and with a few hundred dollars for "incidental needs."[119] As the advice poured in, autopsies became crucial. With autopsies as a medical gold standard, the damage that syphilis could do to tissues and organs would be read on the bodies, even when it was difficult to find it clinically and from the blood tests.

Vonderlehr discussed his ideas with Wenger. As was usual for him, Wenger focused on the practicalities. His assessment of the research in a letter to Vonderlehr has haunted stories of the Study since the letter came to light: "As I see it, we have no further interest in these patients *until they die*," he informed his colleague.[120] Read at face value, his callousness is breathtaking. Yet, throughout the letter, he keeps referring to the men as "patients."[121]

Wenger's practicality and bluntness continued. Local physicians could be brought on board from Macon and the surrounding counties and asked to send anyone from the Study applying for treatment to Dibble. If they were close to death, their doctors would be asked to notify Dibble, Rivers, or the local health department. However, Wenger warned, "if the colored population becomes aware that accepting free hospital care means a post-mortem, every darkey will leave Macon County." A month later, he pointed out the difficulties again: "The only way we are going to get post-mortems is to have the demise take place in Dibble's hospital and when these colored folks are told that Doctor Dibble is now a Government doctor too they will have more confidence."[122]

Vonderlehr set to organizing support for his new plan. He received agreement from the state health department to send in death certificates from the men on the lists. Nowhere in any of the correspondence was there discussion of what a no-treatment research study would mean. There was no thought given to the ethics of leaving the men untreated, or at best with some tonics, aspirins, and an occasional oral mercury compound.

In some ways it would have seemed normative. Venereal disease clinics had begun elsewhere in Alabama in 1932, but by 1933 there were no funds for treatment of the indigent.[123] By 1934, the state made some money available to treat infectious indigent patients but only in health departments. Local physicians, almost all of them white, would not be expected to provide such care for any length of time. In practical terms, the PHS accepted the realities of the racism in the southern medical system in a time of financial duress and tried to make do.[124]

The PHS had no intention, or the funds, to detail physicians to Macon County for years, or even months, on end. As the Study continued, the PHS doctors would come for blood draws and full examinations on a sporadic basis. The autopsies would be done at the institute's hospital or at the VA Hospital. Rivers was the linchpin. She would stay in touch with the men over time and get the families to sign autopsy agreements, the only formal written consent within the Study.[125]

Under these circumstances, the PHS doctors assumed that the men would most likely never receive treatment and that in the end this might not be so bad. Vonderlehr, Clark, and Wenger must have thought that making the best of a difficult situation by salvaging a scientific study of great import was rational. No one would have considered asking the men who would become the participants what they thought of this new idea. There was no intention of telling them that treatment for syphilis had, for all intents and purposes, stopped. Under these circumstances and with no one yet raising questions about the morality of doing this at all, the PHS continued.

Research, Not Treatment

There were, however, soon scientific concerns. In the summer of 1933, Vonderlehr shared his research ideas with other physicians and sent questions about his plans to the American Heart Association. The association's H. M. Marvin thought Vonderlehr's examination would not differentiate disease caused by hypertension and arteriosclerosis from syphilis. A follow-up by an American Heart Association committee confirmed Marvin's assessment. This response by these leading cardiologists, as historian James H. Jones argues, "was devastating."[126] It was as if Vonderlehr was performing a kind of political cardiology in which every untoward heart sound or shadow on the x-rays of the black men's bodies examined in Tuskegee morphed into syphilitic complications.

Vonderlehr continued to believe he was following the right procedures and that he and his physicians could tell the difference.[127] He assumed the autopsies would solve the problem of determining syphilis because the disease's impact would be visible after death, as signs of syphilitic aortitis differentiated from other cardiovascular diseases.

Following the criticisms, he added another idea: controls. "I am planning to return to Macon County some time this fall," he wrote to Macon County Health Department's Murray Smith, "in order to examine about 200 non-syphilitic Negroes who can be used for controls." Without the controls, Vonderlehr noted, it would be "impossible to say how much syphilis is responsible for the cardiovascular disease."[128] They would have nearly 400 men with the disease and approximately 200 without.

He thought this would raise the Study's scientific bar and make syphilis's impact visible. Clearly his effort was intended to set up the best possible research with very limited funds. Damage to the men's hearts could be measured more easily through less expensive and less invasive procedures of fluoroscoping, x-rays, and auscultation until autopsies were possible.[129] He promised Dibble, now officially named a special consultant to the PHS for $1.00 per year, that there would be no spinal taps on the controls.

By October 1933, the plans for the continuation of the Study were more or less in place. A sense of urgency to begin appeared when several men died and autopsies were not obtained.[130] Supplies for performing autopsies were sent to Dibble and pathologist/x-ray specialist Jesse Jerome Peters at the Tuskegee VA Hospital, and he was asked to do the x-rays and perform the postmortems. Peters was told to send the tissue samples from the autopsies to be checked by pathologists at the National Institutes of Health, as the spinal fluid had been before.

But, despite all his efforts, Vonderlehr would not be coming to personally supervise. The PHS's John Roderick Heller Jr., who was at the time assigned to a health department in Tennessee and who had been in the county earlier, was detailed to do the actual work of examining the men selected as the Study's controls.[131] From Washington, Vonderlehr stayed in close contact with Heller and oversaw the details, just as Clark had done with him. Again and again, his letters show his concern with making this the best science he could. He chided Heller in one letter for substituting x-ray paper for the regular x-ray film that had been used before. He acknowledged that this was cheaper, but he argued, "It seems absolutely necessary from a scientific standpoint to continue their [x-ray film] use in spite of the additional cost." Since Vonderlehr was also planning to have Moore at Johns Hopkins read the x-rays, he was obviously concerned that his work pass muster with the master syphilologist.[132]

Vonderlehr had the money to spend to get clear data but not to provide a range of treatment. A little mercury was used as an inducement. Wenger, now back at the clinic in Hot Springs, Arkansas, was asked to send pill boxes, "some form of salicylates [aspirin] . . . for the controls and some form of mercury necessary for administration to the syphilitic cases should they apply for treatment." One thousand ¼-grain calomel tablets (a mercurous chloride) were sent as well.[133] It seemed to be left to the Study's men to determine what they needed.

Heller reported by late November 1933 that finding controls was going well. Only one man they had placed in the control arm had turned out to be positive for syphilis, and they were redoing his serology to check, he told Vonderlehr. Three men whose wives were under treatment were assumed to be possibly syphilitic and thus were not accepted as controls. However, Heller noted, "I don't imagine that we will have more like that."

Supplies were limited. "We are naturally handicapped in not having the protiodide pills and others on hand but Dr. Dibble lets us borrow from his supply until ours arrives," Heller informed his boss.[134] Later in the month, he reported, "All the supplies have arrived and we are giving pills out lavishly."

No one at the PHS seemed to assume that local doctors or even Tuskegee Institute would cooperate with the Study as a matter of course. They handled their relationships carefully, promising those that they needed a piece of this important work and meeting some of their wants as well. They carefully formed honest relationships with the professionals but not with the subjects and controls. Jesse Jerome Peters, the pathologist, asked for Vonderlehr's help in getting to Johns Hopkins for a special training program. At the time, Hopkins had no black physicians on staff. Vonderlehr intervened with Joseph Earle Moore, who promised, "We shall be very glad to have the Negro roentologist come to the Johns Hopkins Department of Pathology for a week to observe the methods employed." In turn, Peters told Vonderlehr how grateful he was for the opportunity but was unable to explain that racism and the lack of connections would normally have excluded him from such professional development.[135]

Nurse Rivers continued to tend to the men. For her, they were patients, not subjects. "The patients are responding very nicely," she wrote to Vonderlehr. "[They are] so happy to have someone take care of them that they almost swamp me, call for aid for every one in the family sometime." In return, Vonderlehr tried to make Rivers into the "scientific assistant" her job title seemingly made her. His letters to her (always written through "Special Consultant Eugene H. Dibble" and rarely directly to her) politely thanked her for bimonthly reports but also taught her how to make them more useful by adding in data on the control cases.[136]

Vonderlehr clearly wanted the work to continue. He told Heller he would join him in Macon County for a week to start examining a second set of controls at the end of January 1934. "My reason for coming to Tuskegee has not been precipitated by any deficiency which has been found in the work which you carried on last fall," Vonderlehr assured him. "But I still feel that the closer our association in the examination of these controls is, the more perfect will be the findings from a *scientific standpoint* [italics added]."[137]

Messy Categories and Clean Data

Even with their focus on the men as untreated subjects or controls, the researchers' categories were never clear-cut. The trope of "subject" could not always hold, and its tension with the concept of "patient" was always in play. John R. Heller worried about a man who was labeled a control, even though he had had syphilis in the past. "At his request," he reported, "I did . . . write his personal physician in Hurtsboro, telling of our findings, despite the negative blood specimens and offering to be of any assistance that we could. I also suggested to the physician that I thought Dr. Dibble would be glad to inform him of X-ray finding as we had already taken the picture."[138] When a man, referred to as Patient X (not Subject X), since his name is blanked out in the record, wrote to ask for medicine for his wife's bad blood, Vonderlehr told him to take his wife to see Doctor Dibble at John A. Andrew Memorial Hospital for her treatment. Vonderlehr reminded the man, "It has been possible for the Public Health Service to give your wife this treatment because we are cooperating with the Tuskegee Institute and the Macon County Health Department."[139] It is, of course, impossible to know how often this happened and whether the man was a control, a subject, or merely someone in the community.

But, despite these humane exceptions, the medical supplies Vonderlehr sent Heller show that the PHS was actively deceiving the men into thinking that they were being treated. In January 1934, a shipment of 5,000 pink aspirin tablets, a tincture to color 5 liters of aromatic elixir red, and a gross of 4-ounce prescription bottles arrived in Tuskegee. To provide some real treatment to some of the subjects, Vonderlehr promised, "we have requested Doctor Wenger to send you twenty ampules of .6 and ten ampules of .5 neoarsphenamine." This amount would hardly have provided more than very minimal treatment for a few.[140]

Vonderlehr continued to worry that the categories be kept as clean as possible. Heller asked about a man whose name he could not find in the files or lists. "You may recall him," he told Vonderlehr, "as the *patient* [italics added] who stopped you in the door-way at the Hospital one morning in the Lobby, and talked to you for several minutes. He has had a spinal, etc." Vonderlehr told Heller the man had been excluded from the current study because he received "three doses of neoarsphenamine during 1921." This man, along with five or six others who presumably were not clearly untreated, Vonderlehr explained, was, after "further consideration . . . discard[ed]" from the Study.[141]

In his correspondence with Peters and Dibble, Vonderlehr explained clearly which individuals were negative or positive for syphilis and how to check the lists against the autopsies being performed. Rivers was sent the names of the subjects and controls as well and told how to follow up.

To make sure the local physicians cooperated by sending cases to the hospital when death was near, the names of the syphilitic men and the controls were sent to the "practicing doctors" in Macon and nearby counties.[142] Vonderlehr told Dibble that this would pique "scientific interest" even if they would have no "financial reward."[143]

As historian Susan Lederer has pointed out, Vonderlehr was focused on making sure that everyone who died was autopsied. He scanned the lists, often chiding the local physicians if he learned of a death occurring and not brought to autopsy. Writing to the Macon County public health chief, Murray Smith, in May 1934, for example, he asked about an "old Negro . . . age 51" whose death certificate was missing but whose death Smith had mentioned. Smith wrote back to say the man was actually alive and "was in this office begging for more good pills."[144] At other times, the autopsies went well and were providing the data they needed. After an autopsy, Nurse Rivers told Vonderlehr, "The heart was so interesting to Doctors Peters and Dibble that they advised me to send the specimen intact."[145]

Rivers continued to send Vonderlehr her numbers and narratives on a bimonthly basis. She noted the men's various ills, the caring she provided, and the regrets she had when she could not obtain permission for autopsies. In her narratives, the men were always "patients." As she wrote Vonderlehr that summer, "The other patients that I have seen or heard from seem to be doing nicely."[146]

Nonetheless, Vonderlehr's efforts were not working as well as he had hoped. By the summer of 1934, he seemed concerned that the follow-up was not proceeding as he had envisioned. Somehow Nurse Rivers, despite her efforts, was not giving them the information they wanted. The PHS physicians came and went, none there for more than a few months at a time. Vonderlehr explained the problems to his higher-ups in the PHS: "It would be well to discontinue the project if local cooperation should fail to materialize."[147]

In September 1934, the PHS detailed John R. Heller back to Tuskegee and asked him to visit all the local doctors again.[148] Rivers was to report monthly on new forms instead of every other month. Wenger also arrived in September and was sent more needles, "24.6 gm ampules of neo and 5000 cc solution of mercury benzoate."[149] The extra effort seemed to work. Local cooperation ramped up. Rivers's extra reporting meant there was more contact with the families but not necessarily more autopsies.[150]

Realizing that her cajoling was not enough to get the permissions for autopsies from the families, the PHS took another step. Surgeon General Hugh Cumming asked the Rosenwald Fund to consider helping support a burial fund that would provide $50 to each family that agreed to autopsy. When this money was not forthcoming, the Milbank Memorial Fund in New York was approached. It agreed to support this part of the Study, in May 1934.[151] Rivers could now promise the families that if they cooperated their undertakers would be paid and a reasonable funeral would be procured. For those in a poor community, where burial was a key point of dignity, it was an important offer and incentive.[152]

The men and their families thought they were now part of what was called "Miss Rivers' Lodge," not unlike other fraternal organizations in black communities that covered burial costs. Many of these had failed during the early Depression years, and this new source of burial insurance was a comfort. As Rivers was to note in a report two decades later, "Free medicine, burial assistance or insurance . . . , free hot meals on the days of examination, transportation to and from the hospital, and an opportunity to stop in town on the return trip to shop or visit with their friends all helped."[153]

Untreated Syphilis in the Male Negro

In May 1936, Vonderlehr and Clark, with Wenger and Heller as the coauthors, presented their first findings at a meeting of the American Medical Association.[154] It would prove to be the first of a dozen reports over the next forty years—and the first that would lead to confusion over what the Study was about. The article purported to compare untreated syphilitics and controls from Macon County, with data on black men with limited treatment pulled from the earlier Cooperative Clinical Group study from the 1920s. All were divided by age and years out from infection.

The published article did not make it clear that a big percentage of the men who were assumed to be untreated in Alabama had been given inadequate amounts of treatment as well. Further, the data assumed that men coming from the five university-based urban clinics and the men in Alabama were comparable groups on the basis of race and syphilis alone. Nothing in the comparisons considered that urban and rural differences might affect what they ate, how they lived, and what kinds of complications they might have. Vonderlehr defended his basis for deciding what had caused the cardiovascular problems, relying primarily in this first report on his physical examinations and the x-rays. The PHS researchers also stated clearly that the untreated subjects "submitted voluntarily to examination," without any explanation that they submitted to treatment only at first, not to research without treatment when the Study continued.[155]

Nevertheless, the findings were able to show that lack of treatment had serious effects. Their data demonstrated both cardiovascular and neurological damage, which was "two or three times as common in the untreated syphilis group as in a comparable group receiving even inadequate treatment." In a modern study, findings this dramatic would lead to the declaration of the need for treatment and the dismantling of the research. In 1936, only the doctors' consciences could have brought this to an end. There were no models on how to stop a study. There was no money to pay for treatment. The rules were as "unplanned and unplotted" as Macon County's back roads. And there was the knowledge that stopping the Study did not necessarily mean that there would be treatment.

These findings are also remarkable for what they do not say and for what should have been thought about. It was received wisdom that there would be little neurosyphilis in a black population, but the Study found that 7.8 percent of the men with syphilis had clinical evidence of neurosyphilis and 18.3 percent had reactive spinal fluid, suggesting that the spirochetes were still present in their spinal columns. This meant, as a researcher was to comment several decades later, that "26.1% showed clinical or laboratory evidence of *neurosyphilis* [italics added]."[156] This led to a lively discussion when the paper was presented at the American Medical Association meeting as the attending physicians reported their clinical experiences with black patients and neurological problems. Their lack of evidence and scientific basis for their claims ranged from malarias to a vaguely defined "racial influence" interfering with the disease's development. Only one physician from New Orleans noted that "central nervous system syphilis isn't rare in the colored; in fact, it is almost as prevalent in our clinics as in the white."[157]

The argument made was clearly directed at encouraging more treatment for syphilis—elsewhere. The researchers acknowledged that most indigent Americans of any race had had no access to adequate treatment for more than a decade. Their evidence was directed in part to physicians and health department officials who thought a few shots of neoarsphenamine or mercury rubs were sufficient. To researchers, the PHS physicians pointed out that only "an observation period of at least 20 or more years is necessary to give a true picture of the value of therapy." It was the hint that they might be expecting the Study to go on and on.[158]

By 1936, the pieces for support of the Study were in place. The funds to create it had been approved by the PHS, and the Milbank Memorial Fund had agreed to cover the costs of the burials. Controls and subjects alike were being given the same medicines: tonics and aspirins—with some mercury given to the subjects who "asked."[159] The findings were reported at medical meetings and then in publications. It now had a public name: "Untreated Syphilis in the Male Negro."[160] No one seemed to ask whether or not all the treatment at the beginning, even if it was limited, was making any difference in the men's disease. Nor was anyone asking whether the men understood what they were involved in. Or if, as the American Heart Association cardiologists had told Vonderlehr in 1933, other diseases than syphilis could really explain the findings of so much cardiovascular disease.

This was deep in the Depression years, when not treating those with latent syphilis was a common reality, given the complexities of the disease—and especially for those of all races who could not afford a regular doctor or a syphilis specialist or whose health department had scant funds. For the PHS, here was the possibility of getting to understand this form of a dreadful disease over a long period of time. Faced with black bodies and cardiovascular complications, there was little questioning of the cause of the illnesses and of the false readings on the serologies, or of whether the tissues and organs examined at the autopsies proved their diagnoses.[161]

The Study continued, even as the men who came out of the fields and small hamlets to meet the doctors and nurse in the chapels, churches, and schools were never asked if they wanted to participate in a nontreatment program.[162] Nurse Rivers kept calling on them over the months and then over the years. They were handed aspirins and iron tonics, which must have had a positive effect on ordinary ills.[163] And they thought they were being treated.

3

Almost Undone

The Study Continues

Even though the PHS secured the cooperation of the Macon County Health Department and Tuskegee Institute, the Study almost came undone over and over. Nothing in Macon County was simple. Even the southern climate worked against the PHS. Tissue samples arrived at its laboratories in poor condition. The men's bodies were sometimes embalmed or had deteriorated before they made it to autopsy.[1] The great migration of black men and women out of the rural South that began in the interwar years threatened to undermine what was supposed to be a controlled environment and made follow-up difficult. Despite the assumption that the men were mere subjects, they behaved like patients who, even in an era when compliance was expected and even with the racial power overlay, did not always do as they were told. Not everyone would remain without some kind of treatment.[2] Questions of treatment and ethics that could have stopped the Study and undermined its science only served to underline its importance to the PHS. The men were needed to prove that treatment for syphilis was necessary.

Treatment Arrives Back in Macon County

After the initial effort to find enough men between 1932 and 1934, Nurse Rivers kept in touch with the families, but the Study went into quiescence except for her continuing effort to obtain permission for the autopsies and the collection of data. The PHS was no longer a regular presence.[3] When Thomas Parran became the surgeon general in 1936, the push by the PHS to do more about syphilis and other venereal diseases became a critical focus. New federal funds were allocated.[4]

Even as the financial recovery in the nation slowed the next year, the Rosenwald Fund's continued concern with syphilis in the South's black communities picked up too. Working again with the PHS, the Rosenwald Fund helped pay for "bad blood wagons." These buses were set up for testing and treatment and sent to public places in small communities.[5] Supplied with a variety of drugs, the new project gave out a mixture of neoarsphenamine and bismuth injections and often dispensed just the iodide pills and mercury inunctions to the older patients.[6]

The Rosenwald Fund leaders continued to follow the conditions in Macon County. In 1937, they sent physician William B. Perry to run a mobile "bad blood" program. Writing to M. O. Bousfield, the Rosenwald Fund's head of Negro Health, Vonderlehr asked that Perry stop in Washington before heading to Alabama to be briefed on the Study's importance, explaining, "We plan to continue it indefinitely."[7] There is no evidence that they expected that the men of the Study would now be treated.

Armed with information about the Study and with the knowledge that stopping contagion was crucial, Perry entered Macon County. His focus was on early, not late, syphilis. He was able to treat 594 patients in the first eleven months—at least 30 were pregnant women.[8] The county health department, with the support of the PHS, then took over the program after the 1938 National Venereal Disease Control Act, which Parran had pushed through Congress, made funds available, even for Macon County. As the mobile clinic crisscrossed the county for the next several years with new doctors, two times as many women as men came forward for treatment.[9]

The program needed a nurse. There was too much for one doctor to do: drive the bus, find cases, follow up, send messages to the county's midwives to bring in pregnant women, and track down sexual partners.[10] With Nurse Rivers working only part-time on the Study, Surgeon General Thomas Parran personally arranged to have her work on the mobile clinic too.[11] This meant Rivers was now fully employed by the PHS, to do the mobile syphilis control and to continue to keep track of the men in the Study. As she worked for the new treatment program, she made up trays with often "a hundred syringes on each tray," heated the sterno for the alcohol stoves to sterilize the needles and syringes, and assisted the doctor.[12]

The new "bad blood wagon" was not intended to be for the men in the Study. Instead, they continued to be offered simple elixirs and the 10,000 aspirins (in pink and white) the PHS sent in, while Tuskegee Institute received a gallon of formaldehyde to preserve tissue sample and specimen jars. Also shipped to Tuskegee was 1,000 cc's of tincture digitalis, which would have been used for individuals who showed signs of heart disease, but it is unclear who actually received the medicine.[13]

Vonderlehr saw the increased value of the Study as open discussion of syphilis, and its treatment became more widespread.[14] He needed to know if all the treating was necessary. He must have known that it was not possible for the PHS, public health departments, or even the Rosenwald Fund to pay for all the treatment that might be needed across the country. Although his analysis of the Study's data had covered its first four years, this was not enough time to see if cardiovascular and neurological complications would emerge as the men aged. The PHS needed to know more.

Undoing and Doing the Science

Vonderlehr realized that he needed another skilled syphilologist if the PHS was to learn what was happening to the men. He sent the PHS's Austin V. Deibert to work with Moore at Johns Hopkins in 1937 to learn the latest skills. After nearly a year under Moore's exacting eye, Deibert might have been trained too well, because, all too soon after his arrival in Tuskegee in the fall of 1938, he began raising serious questions.

Since there was no protocol for the Study, Deibert read over the previous published article and looked at the medical records. Having examined the statistics and Vonderlehr's written claim that the Alabama men "never received treatment," Deibert was "quite amazed to discover that fully 40% of the group [163 men] had received some treatment [between 1932 and 1934], even though inadequate." In the face of this amount of treatment, Deibert argued to Vonderlehr that the comparison of the Study results with the Oslo Study data would not be acceptable: "I acutely fear that adverse criticism of the study would be justifiable." Clearly reflecting what he had learned from Moore, Deibert claimed that if the men had been given even inadequate treatment, this would "greatly lower, if not prevent, late syphilitic cardiovascular disease . . . [while] increas[ing] the incidence of neuro-recurrence and other forms of relapse. The effect of inadequate treatment on late syphilis is problematical."[15]

To solve this problem, Deibert proposed dividing the Study subjects into two groups, with the inadequately treated men in one group and "strictly new untreated men of comparable ages and infection dates" in the other.[16] As he was to chide Vonderlehr a few months later, "To be significant, the study must be stabilized by new men."[17] Concerned with making sure the Study passed muster, Vonderlehr checked with a PHS staff statistician and agreed that adding more untreated men was a good plan.[18] Deibert, after also checking with Moore at Hopkins, added at least another 18 untreated men.[19]

Vonderlehr seemed surprised that Deibert had not realized that there had been treatment at the Study's beginning, especially for the younger men.[20] He did not acknowledge that his own article never made this clear. He hedged on what else might be done by arguing that in the future they would have to "exclude all of those who were treated some years ago." Vonderlehr was also disconcerted to find out that two of the men in the control group had hearts that had developed aortic regurgitation, usually thought to be a consequence of syphilis. This was "interesting," Vonderlehr told Deibert. "I hope that too many of the controls do not show evidence of syphilitic infection before the project is completed."[21]

Six years into the Study, it became clear that the data could not support what they were claiming. Too many of the men might be "untreated in the modern sense," but it was not certain what the small amounts of treatment might mean. If more of the controls turned out to have syphilis and many of the untreated men with syphilis were found to have their illnesses affected by even inadequate treatment, the data would turn out to be difficult to manipulate statistically and might ultimately be meaningless in showing syphilis's deadly consequences.

Data was not the only problem. Deibert needed spinal taps from the new men to find any neurological complications. As he and Rivers moved into new communities in the county to recruit additional subjects, word of the spinal taps got out and refusals happened more often than they expected. Vonderlehr seemed unclear why this posed a problem. Chiding Deibert, he explained that it was "a surprise to learn that some of the patients objected to the 'back shots' inasmuch as these seemed to make a big impression on them after the study of six years ago."[22] Once Deibert promised that they were not "giving 'back shots,'" he explained, "they come out of the cane-brakes." He noted, without seeming to acknowledge that this might be a reasonable position to take: "They simply do not like spinal punctures." Deception helped. "A few of those who were tapped are enthusiastic over the results but to most, the suggestion of another [spinal tap] causes violent shaking of the head; others claim they were robbed of their procreative powers (regardless of the fact that I claim it stimulates them); some experienced memorable headaches. All in all and with no attempt at humor, it is a headache to me."[23]

Deibert was focused on the men as a data source. Yet he knew, as he put it, that to get things done he had to rely upon his sense that "I know something of the psychology of the negro . . . [and] I try my best to send them forth happily shouting the praises of the clinic to their friends at home," he promised Vonderlehr.

As he considered the difficulties, Deibert realized that even the inadequately treated men would have to stay if the Study was to have value. If such men were removed, he reasoned, "their fellow members on the 'list' will become suspicious." He assumed that having the inadequately treated men might prove useful to understanding syphilis. "To date," he observed, "I have found not a single case of 'disastrous syphilis' amongst them. . . . The paucity of clinical findings still alarms me, but I feel that the inadequately treated group accounts for this." Most of these men were between the ages of 25 and 35. He explained: "That none of them have developed aortitis fortifies my belief that even a very little treatment goes a long way in avoiding cardiovascular complications, tho admittedly it is a trifle too soon to make a definite statement to that fact."[24]

Deibert's findings raised serious questions. The PHS position argued for the need in the country for continuous extensive treatment in early syphilis cases. It hoped to use the results of the Study to show how dangerous the untreated disease was. What if Deibert was finding that the inadequately treated men who received some treatment in latency were not getting complications? Would this affect the PHS's whole effort to make the seriousness of syphilis known? Vonderlehr had an answer. He told Deibert that the lack of clinical findings was probably because "the patients who had the severe manifestations had died and a large percentage of the remainder may be beginning spontaneous recovery."[25] If anything, this was all the more reason to keep the Study going in order to see the complications much later on in the men's lives or to understand remissions.

Deibert's racial views and understanding of syphilis's cardiac complications may explain why he did not find the Study ethically disturbing and why he accepted the methodological problems. In 1939, before black doctors at the annual John A. Andrew Clinical Society meeting, he began with the assumption that black and white syphilitics had differing kinds of complications, which were often difficult to diagnosis. Never mentioning the Study, he argued against the overuse of the arsenic drugs, instead recommending early treatment and the use of bismuth, bed rest, and digitalis if cardiovascular complications arose.[26]

Although he did tell visiting doctors that treatment was necessary, it is possible he was following his own advice in the Study. If he thought that the men in the Study already had had enough inadequate treatment, to follow them for treatment of their cardiovascular problems could have made sense.

He had ever more reason to assume this might still happen since Rivers was in contact with the men and the John A. Andrew Memorial Hospital was there for backup. But, in the end, what happened to the men after he saw them was not seen as the PHS's responsibility.[27]

Deibert's worries should have given the PHS pause, at least on the scientific level. But there was no real model of how to do this kind of study. There were no ethical concerns expressed and no structure for oversight outside the PHS. The Study continued.

The Draft, the War, and Possible Treatment

Yet another set of events might have stopped the Study. As the country geared up for war after Pearl Harbor in December 1941, the draft for men 18 to 45 reached into Macon County. The draft meant physicals and blood tests and required treatment for syphilis.

After one man in the Study received a call-up notice, Murray Smith, the county health director, expressed deep worries that this would jeopardize the whole effort, since there were 256 men (although not all of them were still in Macon County) under the age of 45.[28] Vonderlehr was notified about the problem and counseled Smith to tell the head of the local draft board "that this study of untreated syphilis is of great importance from a scientific standpoint. It represents one of the last opportunities which the science of medicine will have to conduct an investigation of this kind."[29] Almost none of the men were drafted.[30]

Smith had another problem. Deibert found that 15 of the controls had developed "clinical or serologic evidence of a syphilitic infection." The known positives were supposed to be kept from treatment. Vonderlehr thought that controls who had contracted the disease "had lost their value to the study" and should be treated, unless Deibert thought otherwise.

Deibert did think otherwise and advised Smith that "I would prefer that these cases remain untreated." However, he noted, "patients in the control group who were infected after 1939 should be treated." When the men were no longer needed as subjects, they could become patients. Once again, Deibert was trying to salvage the validity of the Study—even though today, switching men from one arm to the other would be seen as hopelessly compromising the results.[31]

During the war years, as the PHS was commissioning venereal disease prevention films to be shown across the country and setting up rapid treatment centers (to decrease the time needed for treatment) for those deemed infectious, the Study's importance began to grow again in its eyes.[32] Surgeon General Thomas Parran explained this clearly when he wrote to the Milbank Memorial Fund to ask for the continuation of its funding for the burials. The men were needed for the PHS's other work. He was blunt: "This study, with its careful and complete physical examinations and subsequent observation up to and including autopsy at death, forms a necessary control against which to project not only the results obtained with the rapid schedules of therapy for syphilis but also the costs involved in finding and placing under treatment the infected individuals."[33]

All of this depended, of course, on continued follow-up. But the war also meant the lure of jobs in the industrial cities. Rivers kept trying, but some of the men were moving away, their families were losing touch, and the Study's ability to monitor everyone was diminishing. Vonderlehr's and Clark's assumptions that they could keep track of everyone for so many years were being undermined by the realities of African American life.

The war years meant, too, another kind of "experiment" in Tuskegee that would be a source of pride to this day. The first black men who successfully fought to become military pilots, under the aegis of the Army Air Corps and Tuskegee Institute, were training at Moton Field in the then-segregated army. Known as the Tuskegee Airmen, they had to combat the assumption that African Americans could not withstand high-altitude flight because of possible sickle cell traits or could not fight bravely.[34] The men of what was called the "Tuskegee Experiment" would go on to distinguish themselves with unprecedented success in bombings over Europe and against Jim Crow treatment at home.[35] The military men in this "Tuskegee Experiment" would be celebrated for their valor while the men in the Study continued to be watched.

What Did They Learn?

Having tried to protect their subjects from the war and from long-term treatments, the PHS again reported its findings. The second article on the Study, published in February 1946, reported on the men's mortality after twelve years. Written by a PHS physician and statistician, the article acknowledged that some of the syphilitics had been treated (which Vonderlehr had never reported in the first article) but argued that the amounts of medicine had been so small that they had made no difference, even though Deibert thought otherwise.

The article's claims about the data failed to acknowledge the difficulties of following the men or the accuracies of its diagnoses.[36] Constructing life tables out of the data, nevertheless, it argued that those who had received no treatment for their illness had had their life expectancies "reduced by about 20%."[37] Nowhere in the report, however, was it clear that the men thought they were being treated.[38] And still no one was raising questions about whether they should be told.

In the Study's third report, published several months later by Deibert and another PHS statistician, the dangers that syphilis posed were emphasized. The conclusions echoed the earlier reports: the untreated disease caused "a considerably greater amount of physical disability, not necessarily fatal, than [for] an uninfected person living under similar conditions." Although he understood the Study's limits, Deibert accepted that "an opportunity to study the natural course of the disease in individuals not subjected to specific therapy occurs so infrequently."[39] Deibert had been critical of the Study's assumptions and statistical manipulations, but this time he had accepted its premise.

It was to be another statistician two years later who questioned the Study's accuracy and legality. In 1948, Albert P. Iskrant, the chief of the Office of Statistics at the PHS, noted that "this study is not what I thought it would be," and it did not compare untreated with nontreated men. "Perhaps the most that can be salvaged is a study of inadequately treated," he concluded. Iskrant also disagreed that malaria was pervasive (which would have presumably affected neurological complications) and noted higher rates of neurological damage in "nonwhites" than in whites in the latest syphilis studies done elsewhere, undermining the racial assumptions of differences in complications. Further, he wondered whether the men had been treated, given the Alabama laws, the first time this kind of question was raised in written form. But his letter remained within the PHS, and the Study's premise remained protected. The medical and legal questions still went unanswered.[40]

Knowledge and Penicillin

Iskrant's concern reflected the major changes in research and syphilis care in the postwar period. The Study could have been ended because of other studies being reported, the discovery of penicillin, and the question of state-coercive experimentation—made apparent by the trial of the Nazi doctors at Nuremberg, Germany. Each of these held the possibility of questioning the reasons for the Study's continuance. Instead, each served to embed the importance of the Study deeper within the PHS.

The PHS never focused on the Study alone for research on syphilis, as the Venereal Disease Division sought answers to crucial lingering medical questions about the disease. Supported by the PHS, through the approval of both Vonderlehr and his successor John R. Heller, for example, Paul D. Rosahn began a systematic retrospective review of autopsies done from 1917 to 1940 at Yale Medical School, looking for the correlation among clinical symptoms, cause of death, and morphological evidence of syphilis.[41] Influenced, too, as his generation had been by Moore's assertions that "in spite of 400 years of study, we still do not know the actual importance of syphilis as a cause of death," Rosahn wanted to contribute to this knowledge by using the evidence on syphilis's complications, which autopsies provided.[42]

Rosahn's 1946 findings backed up what Moore and his colleagues had been arguing for years. Spontaneous cures were possible, and small amounts of treatment (20 injections) would affect the clinical outcomes of those in latency.[43] His study repeated what the Study's second paper had concluded: that syphilis seemed to have an effect on "host susceptibility to other diseases." Even with lack of treatment, he concluded, as the Oslo Study had before, "6 out of 10 untreated patients died with no evidence of syphilis at autopsy and another 2 probably were not harmed by it."[44]

He accepted that the Study at Tuskegee might provide better data than he had and that it would show, as he had not, "that syphilis probably lowers life expectancy significantly."[45] But, he also thought that it was possible that "environmental influences," a code term for social and economic conditions, might also have "an adverse influence on longevity."[46] Rosahn's findings could have led the PHS in two directions: treat everyone in the Study and call an end to it, or wait and see whether there was "spontaneous cure" or more damage. It chose the latter.

If further research did not bring the Study to a halt, a new miracle drug just might. Research on penicillin began in England and was stepped up during the war years. By 1943, the PHS's John F. Mahoney and his colleagues at the Venereal Disease Research Laboratory on Staten Island, New York, reported that penicillin appeared to be highly effective in killing the spirochetes of syphilis.[47] In the context of the war, this new antibiotic seemed a godsend. At first, supplies were limited. By war's end, as its manufacturing increased and supplies of the drug became more available, studies of penicillin's effect on syphilis took a central place in the debates on treatment.[48]

Leading researchers, however, were clearly worried about the overuse of what seemed like a miracle cure "before extensive scientific evaluations of its long-term results could be completed."[49] The initial excitement was tempered when reports of a "therapeutic paradox" appeared in the literature on cardiovascular syphilis. When treated aggressively, the active lesions in the aorta often came to be replaced with scar tissue, causing more cardiac damage. There was also the concern with allergic reaction to the drug itself.[50] Moore, at Johns Hopkins, remained suspicious of penicillin at first and continued to argue that knowledge from untreated syphilis was still needed as a control against treatments.[51] The data from his Hopkins clinic led him to argue that "the least satisfactory results of prolonged treatment are found in Negro men."[52]

Under the influence of these leading syphilologists, the PHS and other researchers in large medical center clinics began research into when and how penicillin should be given, in what mixtures, and at what stages in the disease. Most of the focus remained on early syphilis, since it reflected the major public health hazard due to infection and knowledge that treatment could keep later complications from occurring.[53] Expanding the rapid treatment centers, the PHS began providing penicillin to infectious syphilitics across the country, including in a major center in Birmingham, Alabama, two hours north of Tuskegee.

Most physicians agreed that penicillin mattered in early syphilis, but they were not as sure about latency. Thus a debate on the usefulness of penicillin in patients who had developed both cardiovascular and neurological complications went on through the 1950s.[54] In 1964, Dr. Rudolph H. Kampmeier, the famed Vanderbilt syphilologist known for issuing what would later be seen as a southern apologia for the Study in 1972, argued in a review article that "one enters an area of uncertainty and difficulty in evaluation of the effectiveness of treatment of the presumably late latent syphilitic."[55] Not everyone agreed with this position. Another public health official argued, "Substantial numbers of persons having untreated late latent syphilis constitute a public health problem, regardless of whether such persons have contagious disease."[56]

The uncertainty was there. Given the assumption that the men in the Study could probably not be helped because they were so many years out from their initial infections, the miracle of penicillin must have seemed irrelevant and the Study's historical importance more illuminated. The conclusion of so many other studies on syphilis that each patient should be evaluated *individually* was ignored. Thus, the changing science of syphilis research supported rather than ended the Study.

A Code for Barbarians

It was the commitment to "good" science raised at the trials of the Nazi doctors at Nuremberg that supported the Study's continuation and failed to create any sense of the parallels between coerced research in Germany and what was happening in Alabama. Between 1946 and 1947, twenty-three Nazi defendants, almost all of them doctors, came before American judges at Nuremberg to be dealt justice as punishment for their horrendous experiments on unwilling prisoners and concentration camp victims.[57] As the trial proceeded, it became clear that the physicians' ancient Hippocratic Oath "to do no harm" did not provide a code to cover research, especially when supported by the state.

The Nuremberg Trials became an examination of ethical conduct in research and of the limits of claims of "societal necessity."[58] The German defendants each argued that they were doing normal research, even citing American studies on prisoners in their defense and noting the difference between research and medical care.[59] Realizing that the American research community actually had *no* code itself but instead relied upon the "ethics" of the profession, American research physician and prosecution adviser Andrew Ivy wrote a committee report of one (later published in the *Journal of the American Medical Association*) to provide beginning principles, justify the American prison research, and testify against the Nazis.[60] The judges, in turn, using Ivy's report and the work of the prosecution's other doctor expert, promulgated a set of principles that now have come to be known as the Nuremberg Code.

The code, however, had little impact on research ethics in the immediate postwar years in the United States as Ivy's report supporting research, rather than the principles requiring informed consent and no harm to subjects, was more widely discussed.[61] American research and Nazi murder were never mentioned in the same breath; indeed, they were set up as opposites. In the context of the promise of penicillin and other antibiotics, as well as the increased federal funding and resulting expansion in medical research, what was done in the United States was considered good science. As ethicist Jay Katz so eloquently declared, the Nuremberg Code was seen as "a code for barbarians and not for civilized physician-investigators."[62] The PHS's John R. Heller made this perfectly clear more than thirty years later when he responded to historian James H. Jones, who asked whether or not the Nuremberg Code had given them pause in the Study. Heller took umbrage at the question and said to Jones, "But they were Nazis."[63]

More Than Ever

Meanwhile, Nurse Rivers still visited the men to provide what care she could and to encourage the families to allow autopsies. In the fall of 1948, the PHS sent its doctors to Tuskegee to do the third set of physical workups. This time

155 men were located. In their findings, which became the fourth article on the Study, 45 "inadequately treated individuals" were dropped from the data analysis. This article proved what had been shown before: that those who had untreated syphilis had significantly more mortality and morbidity, although there now appeared little difference among those who were 55 or older.[64]

In giving an unpublished report two years later to a group of PHS officers, O. C. Wenger summed up what had been learned. Although he agreed that syphilis was still causing illness and death, Wenger argued that "it is important to have the facts documented."[65] Unlike the published articles, however, Wenger acknowledged that 26 percent of the syphilitics and 35 percent of the controls had been lost to follow-up by 1948. Whatever the PHS's hopes had been for a captive population, Macon County was turning out not to be so contained.

Wenger's speech lay bare why the men in Alabama remained so critical. Knowing that not all cases of syphilis in the country could be found or treated, he reasoned, "It behooves the medical profession to 'Know for Sure' what happens if the disease is not treated." And the only way to know, he concluded, was "the correlation of postmortem findings with periodic clinical findings." Referring back to both the Rosahn autopsy studies at Yale and the work in Oslo, he concluded that this kind of correlation "can be done only in the Alabama group. What other way will we ever be able to learn the meaning of our clinical findings?"

Again it was Wenger who would write the chilling sentences that put into words the PHS's understanding of why the Study was important. "We know now, where we could only surmise before," he declared, "that we have contributed to their ailments and shortened their lives. I think the least we can say is that we have a high moral obligation to those that have died to make this the best study possible."[66]

Clinical Complexity

The PHS was not able to wall off the Study's men from penicillin, even if they thought their isolation and poverty would keep them from treatment. Macon County was not a concentration camp, and many of the men were by now either leaving the county or finding their ways to some treatment, even if it was not directly for their syphilis. Nor were all the local doctors who were told about the Study in 1932 still there.

By 1952, the fourth major survey began, and the PHS tried to find everyone. "In several instances, the patient was surprised during his morning plowing," the investigators reported, "and asked to step in the shade of the nearest tree for an on-the-spot history, physical examination, and blood-letting." A new male field investigator reported to the Study's leaders that 33 of 132 men examined (25 percent) had received penicillin.[67] In attempting to reassure the PHS officers that the Study still had validity, the field investigator concluded: "It is to be noted that economics has prevented the majority of our patients from receiving any consistent daily course of treatment; most of them receiving shots a week apart." Even Vonderlehr weighed in. Now a regional PHS medical director in Atlanta, he told the Study's director that "it is nice to know that the review of the surviving patients included in the study is going well. Hope that the availability of the antibiotics has not interfered too much with this project."[68]

Reports continued to be written about the Study's results during the 1950s. Peters, radiologist/pathologist at the Tuskegee VA Hospital, who worked on the Study for more than twenty years, became the senior author on a paper on pathological findings.[69] "It is a real contribution to our knowledge of the course of untreated syphilis," he wrote to the Study's director, adding rather immodestly, "I feel it is by far the best paper that has been published in this entire Tuskegee study."[70] At Johns Hopkins, however, Moore evidently thought the paper so bad that he shredded it at first—but then published a later version in the medical journal he edited.[71]

Peters was not acknowledging what others involved in the Study knew: that x-ray evidence had been lost, that "the clinical data was quite meager," and that there was a "surprising absence of syphilitic pathology" on micro-scopic tissue samples and gross anatomical findings.[72] A National Institutes of Health pathologist cautioned Peters that they had been defining "lung lesions as being possibly syphilitic without definite proof that they are. It seems to me we find ourselves in the present state of confusion in part be-cause of a past tendency to regard as syphilitic almost any lesions found in a patient with syphilis."[73] Peters also acknowledged that there was only a "50-50 chance" that cardiovascular complications would appear on autopsy.[74]

Many of the men, Peters knew, had died of other diseases. On the bodies he found disease caused by hypertension and myocardial degeneration, which were killing many of the men before their syphilis could do its dam-age. Peters worried enough about the extensiveness of arteriosclerosis that he thought Rivers ought to collect information on the men's "food habits."[75] Syphilis was clearly a major problem, but so were heart disease, pneumo-nia, and kidney disorders. As historian/physician Benjamin Roy has argued, "The a priori principle that explained the presence of disease also explained its absence. Because of biological differences blacks were more syphilitic than whites; because of biological differences, the absence of findings meant that blacks had syphilis that escaped detection until better means of diagnosis were available."[76]

Responsibility

The problems with the Study began to multiply. Two of the Study's new directors reported to the PHS in 1951: "Co-operation among the parties is painful and difficult to achieve, especially when fresh and suitable tissue specimens are sought. The more lay people involved, the more is the likelihood for unhealthy gossip and misunderstandings." Others were no longer sure Rivers was doing her job, as more of the men were lost to follow-up.[77] Efforts began to find men who had moved to other cities across the country. Letters went out to post offices, credit bureaus, and friends, as the men were tracked.

Sidney Olansky, John C. Cutler, and Stanley Schuman, the Study's new leaders in the 1950s, were concerned with carrying it on and getting the most out of it. In a curious way, they felt a responsibility: first to the PHS's Venereal Disease Division, then to science, and then to the men. Even though they knew the men thought they were in treatment, Olansky would write in a memo to Cutler in 1951: "We have an investment of almost 20 years of Division interest, funds and personnel; a responsibility to the survivors both for their care and really to prove that their willingness to serve, even at risk of shortening of life, as experimental subjects. And finally a responsibility to add what further we can to the natural history of syphilis."[78]

This sense of the Study's importance was confirmed when Trygve Gjestland, a Norwegian syphilologist who had reexamined the Oslo Study data, came to Atlanta in 1952 to meet with Olansky and Cutler. Gjestland, in this reexamination, emphasized both the Study's crucial nature and what a scientific mess it was because of unclear categories and uncertain criterion for much of the diagnoses. Further, he noted, "current clinical examinations should be more balanced than previously, when cardiovascular aspects were favored above neurological examination." In other words, the expectations of finding cardiovascular complications meant that the failure to do more spinal taps had left the area of neurological syphilis understudied.[79] With this advice, the Study's leaders decided that more spinal taps should be attempted so the comparisons could be made.[80]

As more papers were written and talks were given on the Study, the effort to understand syphilis's long-term effects became crucial. John C. Cutler wrote that the Study had taught them that "every individual in whom the diagnosis of untreated or inadequately treated syphilis is made requires, from the public health point of view, adequate therapy."[81] The Study's men represented the data needed to show the world what syphilis could do and what was important. Any sense of concern was mollified because Rivers was still visiting the families and helping with other ills.

Is This Ethical?

The PHS was not hiding the Study, and medical journals published the articles and reports. Unless a physician picking up the articles thought deeply, it would have been easy to see the men as "volunteers," and indeed in one report they were referred to as "people [who] responded willingly."[82] Reading between the lines would have been necessary since the reports did not make clear that the aspirins, tonics, and spinal punctures were being described to the men as "treatment." The language and titles of the articles—"untreated syphilis in the Male Negro"—easily distanced the medical reader. Another report called them "patients." The articles, as an analysis of them concluded, "depict the disease as dynamic agent whose impairment of the central nervous system takes place in the 'scene' of the patient." Terms like "'follow' and 'survey the patients'" made the PHS seem as if it were a bystander to a process that would lead to critically important knowledge. The men, referred to in this kind of syntax, literally disappeared.[83]

In 1955, as another round of the blood tests was done in the county, the Study received its first major criticism from outside the PHS orbit.[84] Georgia-born physician Count D. Gibson, an associate professor at the Medical College of Virginia in Richmond, heard the PHS's Sidney Olansky speak on the Study and make clear that treatment was being withheld. Gibson was so concerned about the ethics that he discussed them with Olansky, whom he knew from Emory University in Atlanta. Unsatisfied with Olansky's response, as a good scientist Gibson sent for and read all available reprints of the articles on the Study.

Then he wrote to Olansky: "I am gravely concerned about the ethics of the entire program," he told his former colleague. "The ethical problem in this study was never mentioned. . . . There was no implication that the syphilitic subjects of this study were aware that treatment was being deliberately withheld." After dismissing any criterion by which the Study might be justified, Gibson argued: "It seems to me that the continued observation of an ignorant individual suffering with a chronic disease for which therapeutic measures are available, cannot be justified on the basis of any accepted moral standard: pagan (Hippocratic Oath), religious (Maimonides, Golden Rule), or professional (A.M.A. Code of Ethics)." Making sure that Olansky understood his motives, Gibson concluded: "Please accept this letter in a spirit of friendliness and an intense desire to see medical research progress in its present remarkable rate without any blemish on its record of service to humanity."[85]

Olansky penned a handwritten response, the only insight into his views we have on its ethics before 1972.[86] He acknowledged Gibson's worries that the Study was "callous and unmindful of the welfare of the individual." But he explained: "I'm sure it is because all of the details of the study are not available to you." He confessed that when he had started with the Study in 1950 "all the things that bothered you bothered me at the time." Yet, he told Gibson, "after seeing these people, knowing them & studying them and the record I honestly feel that we have done them no real harm & probably have helped them in many ways." On the question of gender, Olansky reported, "no females were selected so that the question of congenital [syphilis] could be eliminated."

To buttress his views, Olansky repeated what would become the mantra: that the men had no chance to get treatment elsewhere when the Study started, that they "knew that they had syphilis & what the study was about, [and that] only those with latent syphilis were chosen. They got far better medical care as a result of their being in the study than any of their neighbors," and a nurse "takes care of all their needs."

Olansky did not avoid the issue of treatment. After explaining the choice of only those with the latent disease, he claimed, "All others were treated at great expense to the government." His answer expanded upon Deibert's worry from two decades earlier that many of the men had received some treatment. But the sentence leaves open the question of *how much* they were treated. Further, when he added that "any patient in need of medical care for [syphilis] or any other reason was treated," he is stretching the evidence and not dealing at all with the question of how many were treated, when, and for how long.

This is indeed a strange argument, since Olansky's article in the same year stated: "On the basis of the individuals examined during the 1951–52 survey, it is estimated that 70 per cent of the syphilitic group have remained untreated."[87] A year later, another of his articles made the claim that after 159 patients had been examined, "23 showed evidence of late syphilis . . . and that no one patient with late syphilis had received an adequate course of therapy."[88]

Olansky's reasoning may have been related to what he knew about penicillin. He told Gibson that at the stage it became available, the mortality between the men with the disease and the controls "had evened out and [there] was no real indication for therapy." To Gibson, Olansky acknowledged that "some of the patients did receive penicillin[,] but we are continuing to follow them," avoiding any sense that this compromised the Study or raised questions of why only some men were being treated.

Olansky seemed to be taking bits of the information—some of the men were treated, some got penicillin—and making them stand as a way to avoid the larger questions of the attempts to deny treatment. Having faced a set of moral qualms at the beginning, he had now told himself and Gibson that these were the truths. But he remembered what he had thought at the beginning: "I know exactly how you feel & what must be going thru your mind," he assured Gibson. And just as he had been brought into the Study's logic and come to accept it, he offered such a place for Gibson. Come join the "next roundup" he suggested or come to Washington so that "Dr. John C. Cutler . . . can fill you in on more detail than I can in a letter."

According to those who spoke to Gibson afterward, he was deeply disturbed by Olansky's response. But he was told at Medical College of Virginia "that if he wanted to get along, succeed and thrive in his medical career he'd better shut up about this and stop raising questions. He was going up against very senior and powerful men."[89] Gibson did no more at the time, but he did go on to become a major figure in the movement to build community health centers and a leading medical civil rights advocate. He never forgot his concerns about the Study and what he might have been able to do.[90]

Powerful men in a government bureaucracy, medical uncertainties, and racial beliefs kept the Study going. Olansky and others in the PHS convinced themselves that what they were learning was so important because it would help others. With no real sense of how to do this kind of Study, the researchers, fascinated by their "data," were undeterred by its scientific failings. The presence of Rivers, as a private public health nurse who could care for the families and meet needs, must have reassured their consciences. The debates over penicillin, and the understanding of late latent syphilis, convinced them that the men could not be helped at this point. No one was asking the men in the Study what they thought. No one inside the PHS or at Tuskegee Institute seems to have considered that they should.

4

What Makes It Stop?

In November 1957, in the twenty-fifth year of the Study, the PHS held a meeting to discuss what should be done next. The last major roundup of the men had taken place in 1952–53, although the blood draws were happening yearly. Aware of some of the continued difficulties and the number of men who were leaving the area, both retesting and finding new incentives were discussed.[1] It was agreed that "free hot meals" would be provided and that the iron tonics and aspirins the men thought were treatments would continue to be given.[2]

By the next year, each "patient" had received a special certificate signed by Surgeon General Leroy E. Burney for "completing 25 years of active participation in the Tuskegee medical research study" and a dollar for every year of "service."[3] Despite the language on their letters and certificates, the difference between medical research and treatment was not clear to the Study's men, as it often is even today in clinical trials.[4] Rivers wrote to a PHS official a few years later to explain: "All of the patients appear to be alright. They were thrilled with their examination, especially their cash awards."[5]

Rivers, too, must have thought it was really the right thing to do. The Department of Health, Education, and Welfare brought her to Washington and gave her their highest honor, the Oveta Culp Hobby Award, in 1958 because "her selfless devotion and skillful human relations . . . had sustained the interest and cooperation of the subjects of a venereal disease control program in Macon County, Alabama."[6] Rivers may have had no fear that the men would quit, but the assumptions and power that held the Study together were beginning to crack from both internal contradictions and outside pressures.

By the mid-1960s, discussions of ethics in medical research and the beginning promulgation of regulations moved from concern with the "barbarians" to those supposedly doing "good science."[7] The growing civil rights movement raised issues of racism and of what was happening in the Jim Crow South in ways that could not be avoided any longer. More publications and talks about the Study invited those outside the PHS's Venereal Disease Division to raise questions about the Study's morality and its science. The Study became more and more difficult to sustain. In this context of a shifting discussion of research ethics and growing societal distrust of governmental actions, individuals would again raise questions about the Study's morality that would make exposure outside the medical realm happen.

The Outside Peers In

Responsibility for the Study stayed with the PHS but moved into Atlanta and the oversight of what was then called the Communicable Disease Center (CDC). As the CDC grew into a medical giant running research worldwide, the Study increasingly became a remnant from a distant past. The PHS became interested in using the frozen tissue from the autopsies to test a stain for detecting syphilis spirochetes that it was developing, and the men's blood became the basis for newer serological tests.[8] In April 1965, a small group of PHS physicians and statisticians met at the CDC to consider where to go next.[9] There was increasing acknowledgment that some of the men were finding their way to penicillin but that the Study still remained useful.[10]

The notes from the meeting make it clear that they were aware that some controls had become reactive to the blood tests for syphilis, that subjects had wandered into treatment, and that follow-ups were becoming even more difficult. The physicians and statisticians accepted that the use of the older serology methods meant that they might have been wrong on the diagnoses and that the methods had been inconsistent. Eleanor Price, one of the statisticians, reminded the group: "Those with aneurysms died primarily during the first ten years and the trouble with the study is that there was no starting point. Makes it hard to analyze this." Anne R. Yobs, the chief of medical research at the Venereal Disease Research Laboratory who had long followed the Study, was direct: "If you can't evaluate it somehow, you better call it quits right now because it is not getting any clearer as time goes on."

The PHS's Sidney Olansky, however, had a different view: "This was meant to be a progressive study," he countered, "with the hope that as it went along we would pick up interesting things, with the important thing being what actually kills them." The men should be followed, he declared, "till dead do us part." There was acknowledgment that they were "fly[ing] by the seat of

[our] britches. May not find way immediately to use information but at least we ought to have it."

The 1965 meeting took place barely a month after the killing of civil rights workers, the beatings on "Bloody Sunday," and the marches in Selma, Alabama, only 100 miles from Tuskegee, and five years after the Supreme Court decision based on a Tuskegee case, *Gomillion v. Lightfoot*, declared that creating voting districts to disenfranchise black voters violated the Fifteenth Amendment to the Constitution.[11] The notes of the meeting, however, suggest that the doctors were not concerned about racial politics: "Racial issue was mentioned briefly. Will not affect the study. Any questions can be handled by saying these people were at the point that therapy would no longer help them. They are getting better medical care than they would under any other circumstances." These short notes became the centerpiece of the Study's defense for years to come. Indeed, Olansky had made this same argument to Count Gibson in 1955.

Irwin J. Schatz, a young cardiologist from Detroit, became the next person to attempt to influence the Study through a private letter.[12] It came in response to another article on the Study published in December 1964, this time in the more widely read *Archives of Internal Medicine*. It reported that "approximately 96% of those examined had received some therapy other than an incidental antibiotic injection, and perhaps as many as 33% have had curative therapy," backing up Olansky's claim to Gibson that the men had been treated. But the key finding reiterated the Study's main findings: untreated syphilis led to higher mortality and morbidity and particularly caused cardiovascular damage.[13]

Schatz, a cardiologist at Henry Ford Hospital in Detroit, reread the article several times to make sure he understood it. "I could not believe my eyes," he recalled, still calling up his anger more than thirty years later. He discussed the article with several colleagues and was met with shrugged shoulders and apathy. He wrote to Donald H. Rockwell, the PHS physician who had been the paper's senior author. Just a few years out of his cardiology fellowship training and well aware of the debates over the Holocaust and the Nazi doctors, Schatz made clear in three succinct sentences what he thought:

I am utterly astounded by the fact that physicians allow patients with potentially fatal disease to remain untreated when effective therapy is available. I assume you feel that the information which is extracted from observation of this untreated group is worth their sacrifice. If this is the case, then I suggest the United States Public Health Service and those physicians associated with it in this study need to re-evaluate their moral judgments in this regard.[14]

Schatz's letter was passed on to the paper's second author, Anne R. Yobs at the CDC in Atlanta. Schatz never received a reply, and Yobs made clear why in a memo to her superior: "This is the first letter of this type we have received. I do not plan to answer this letter."[15] Clearly, Olansky had never discussed Gibson's letter with others on the Study team and had kept any concerns to himself. Schatz never heard from the CDC but continued to be disturbed by the ethics of the Study.[16]

A New, If Unlikely, Crusader

The final push against the Study came from an unlikely place: a young venereal disease investigator in San Francisco working for the PHS. Peter Buxtun, a libertarian Republican, former army medic, gun collector, and NRA member with a bachelor's degree and some graduate work in German history, had taken a job with the PHS tracking down gonorrhea and syphilis patients and their sexual contacts in some of San Francisco's tougher neighborhoods. It was 1965 and he was 28 years old, an indefatigable investigator and a relentless storyteller. His supervisor wrote about him: "Because of his tenacity, his ability to 'crack' the stubborn patient, his readiness to 'take the patient out of the field' to obtain more information, his ingenuity and inventiveness, he is in fact our best interviewer, and for this reason he has been given the majority of the difficult cases."[17]

The skills that made Buxtun such a "crack" investigator were those of a man who planned to do things his own way. In his first monthly report, Buxtun claimed, "I hold that anyone capable of doing good epidemiology is capable of forming his owns [sic] opinions and choosing his own methods of all types of interviewing." His supervisor wrote in the margins, "Wrong."[18] His monthly narratives were supposed to be about what he was finding in the field. Instead, the early ones ranged from critiques of what he was being taught to disquisitions on syphilis's history. In his later reports, Buxtun was likely to quote from *Conservative Viewpoint* on Washington politics or from Dante's *Inferno*.

Buxtun argued that the PHS needed investigators who believed deeply in the morality of the work and who could operate free from a cog mentality. "Let us search for men whose self-respect and personal philosophy will make rules unnecessary," he urged. Buxtun's report from July 1965 included excerpts "from a letter written to me, by my uncle . . . while I was a student in college," which proved to be a hilarious story on how to tell if one's partner had syphilis. It drew his supervisor to comment: "A rather pointless bit of literary affectation, compounded from the styles of Ambrose Bierce, Thomas Mann and Lord Chesterfield. With some directions, his writing could be good though." His September report, rather than telling the story of his monthly experiences in San Francisco, proved to be a short explanation of German policy toward syphilitic prostitutes during World War I.[19]

Sometime between September and late November 1965, as Buxtun has told the story again and again, he wandered into the coffee room of his clinic to hear an older PHS officer finish telling a tale to a workmate.[20] The man was concluding, "And when the patient was insane we took him, this man, outside the immediate area of Tuskegee itself to a doctor and he didn't know about the Study and quickly diagnosed this man in his 60s as a) insane and b) secondary to long term syphilitic infection. The doctor of course immediately treated this man with penicillin and shortly thereafter had the county medical society and the CDC jump down his throat. 'See here doctor so and so,' I never knew his name, 'you have spoiled one of our subjects. You have *treated* someone who was not to be treated.'"

Buxtun was shocked by the story. Here he was, he recalled, "working five days a week in a tough part of town . . . where the cops didn't like to go" to track down men who had been named as contacts and dragging them in for treatment. I believed in it . . . and these men who would otherwise have been quite ill thanked us."

Buxtun pressed his PHS colleague for more of the story, and out poured the details of the Study as it had been handed down within the PHS and in the published reports. "I thought," Buxtun recounted, "we can't be doing this." The contrast between what he did every day and his knowledge of German history and of the Nuremberg Trials caught Buxtun up. He got on the phone to the CDC and asked the public relations person for any reprints. "Yah, sure," he says he was told. Thus he tracked down syphilitics during the day and read the published Study reports during the night. The contrast could not have been starker.

Buxtun reacted with horror as he formed his own image of the men in "dirt poor starvation prone Tuskegee" at the start of the Depression. His own sense of time in telling the story telescoped the decades-long study into a single Depression year. In his November 1965 report, Buxtun directed outraged prose at what he had learned. He contrasted quotes from the reports on the Study with parallels from the International Military Tribunal at Nuremberg. "Why should researchers patiently await and observe the demise of untreated American syphilitics when, in effect, they may be duplicating the 'research' of some forgotten Doctor at Dachau?" he asked. Addressing the "federal medical community," Buxtun sarcastically concluded, "Such a pity, that the public may never hear of the Macon County project. It will probably never receive its due credit as it surely would be misinterpreted by the Civil Rights people and the news media."[21]

Buxtun kept thinking about the underlying question: "What's wrong with getting the data." He argued, "It's the burning sword, if you will that the doctors keep falling upon." He knew it was a phrase that had been used to justify other horrific experiments in Manchuria by the Japanese as well as by the Nazis.[22] He also kept thinking about the racial tensions and the damage that knowledge about the Study would do to the CDC's "good programs."

Buxtun began by talking to people in his own office, all of whom told him to forget about it. Buxtun, who reported that he began to feel like Jeremiah crying out in the wilderness, could not. When his boss asked him about his concerns, Buxtun handed him the published reports. The next day his supervisor gave them back and, as Buxtun recalled, told him: "'These people are volunteers[,] it says so right here. Volunteers with social incentives, it says so right here. This is all nonsense.' And then he turned on his heels and walked away in disgust."[23]

But, unlike Gibson and Schatz, Buxtun persisted. Almost a year later, in November 1966, he wrote to William J. Brown, then the chief of the Venereal Disease Division at the CDC. Buxtun questioned Brown on the Study's ethics, ending with: "In other words are untreated syphilitics still being followed for autopsy?"[24] Brown drafted a reply to Buxtun, again arguing that there was divided "medical opinion" on treatment for latent syphilis in the 1930s and that the treatment was risky. The men were not infectious and were "volunteers and completely free to leave the study at any time." Further, Brown claimed that they had been treated with appropriate medications and been "entirely free to seek treatment at any time." He emphasized the fact that some of the men had found their way to treatment, and he used the word "freely" several times.

Brown made another claim that, while undermining the "science" of the Study, was used to explain why the PHS men thought no harm was being done: "This study has contributed greatly to the development of improved serologic tests and indeed numerous patients originally thought to be syphilitic on the basis of the old test procedures are now known to have not been infected." Brown reiterated a position that would come up over and over:

"We have felt a moral obligation to continue the study."[25] He neglected to mention that no one told the men who turned out to be disease-free that they did not have "bad blood."

In March 1967, Buxtun was called to the CDC for a conference. He was told, he recalled, to wait to be asked to join the meeting. Brought to a wood-paneled conference room, draped with the flags of both the United States and the PHS, Buxtun remembered being berated for at least five to ten minutes about the Study's importance, the great data, and the critical work of the PHS. He sat in silence while the tongue-lashing continued. Then he was asked, "Well, what do you have to say for yourself?"

Buxtun then read from the PHS reports, emphasizing the mess in the Study's science over time and how the men were "persuaded" to join with the free meals, promise of treatment, examinations, and burial insurance. Buxtun believed he had made them reconsider. But the only notes that mention his presence at the meeting were short and bureaucratic. Brown wrote at the bottom of Buxtun's November letter that there had been a conference: "This matter was discussed in much detail & Mr. Buxtun's specific questions were taken into consideration."[26]

About a year later, Buxtun quit his job to go to law school, still wondering what had happened. Almost three years after he had learned about the Study, in November 1968, less than half a year after Martin Luther King Jr. was killed and as riots blanketed the country, Buxtun again wrote to Brown. This time he emphasized the political problems the PHS and the CDC would have. Concerned about how it would play out politically, he reminded Brown, "The group is 100% negro. This in itself is political dynamite and subject to wild journalistic misinterpretation. It also follows the thinking of negro militants that negroes have long been used for 'medical experiments' and 'teaching cases' in the emergency wards of county hospitals."[27] Buxtun, no wild-eyed radical in the years of wild-eyed radicalism, was pointing out what should have been obvious by then: if there was more public knowledge, the Study's purpose and procedures would be read as racist and deceptive, and possibly illegal and immoral and even murderous.

The 1969 Review: What Next?
Brown did not immediately respond to Buxtun. Instead, he convened another meeting several months later, this time bringing in specialists from outside the PHS community. Brown must have realized that this was going to be a difficult meeting when he spoke with Dr. Eugene Stollerman, chair of the medicine department at the University of Tennessee Medical School.

Stollerman told Brown that "he was unfamiliar with the . . . study." Brown provided the details. Stollerman, Brown noted in a memo to his files, then told him that "this appears . . . to be a 'hot potato' from many standpoints — racial, public relations, etc. Wondered if we could be sued for withholding treatment. He thinks we should 'go all out to get this worked out as soon as possible.'"[28]

The meeting was considered important enough to be chaired by David J. Sencer, director of the CDC, a physician deeply knowledgeable about infectious disease and public health politics. As the list of invitees was compiled, however, no one seems to have considered that someone familiar with health issues in the black community, outside the CDC orbit, might be helpful.[29] The experts were mostly from within the PHS and the CDC or were researchers who were still quite interested in syphilis as a disease.

Sencer, after giving a history of the Study, declared that not treating at the beginning was not so much of an issue because of all the questions surrounding the use of the heavy metals and the stage of the men's disease.[30] He acknowledged, however, that the Study had now become "a political problem." Next, an attempt was made to separate the underlying science of the Study from its political context. Brown took over the meeting and summarized the Study's findings from the records and articles. "Syphilis," he declared, "was a primary cause of death in only seven [study subjects] as shown at autopsy," although he admitted that the autopsies were inaccurate because of the condition of the men's bodies. Clyde Kaiser, who represented the Milbank Memorial Fund, reported on the results of the Framingham Heart Study done on white men. He expressed his amazement that the men in Alabama seemed to be doing as well as those in the Heart Study, who had access to better medical care. J. Lawton Smith, a famed ophthalmologist who had worked on the Study two years earlier, thought only the tissue samples really mattered and expressed the need for "no treatment ('I doubt if you could cure them')," but later in the meeting he expressed the opinion that they should be given "shots of penicillin," should be told the Study was "being upgraded," and should be asked to provide their bodies at death. Sencer, however, thought this was "ghoulish," even though that very thing had been going on for years.

The doctors at the conference took the question of treatment seriously, as both a medical and a political issue. Olansky raised the concern that treatment at this stage would have "catastrophic [medical] consequences," "although," he claimed, "the original policy of the Study was that when medical treatment was indicated, they were pulled out of the Study and were given treatment." But Joseph Caldwell, who had done the most recent examinations, said that all they could do when someone had complications was to tell them "to get to a doctor to get better care." Smith recalled finding "two cases of glaucoma" when he had been there and of sending both men to treatment. The availability of the recently enacted Medicare was mentioned, suggesting the belief that the men would now have access to affordable treatment.

Again and again, Sencer asked the specialists if treatment at this stage was now indicated. Stollerman remained the most adamant: "I think they should be treated." He continued, "You should treat each individual case as such, not treat as a group." He believed that if they established criteria for treatment, decisions could be made on medical grounds for individuals.

There appeared, however, to be genuine medical disagreement over whether or not treatment would make any difference, except for those who might have active syphilis. Smith's work, and other work at the CDC, had shown that the syphilis spirochetes continued to exist in late syphilis, even after treatment with penicillin.[31] The consensus, in which Stollerman did not join, seemed to be that treatment in early and secondary syphilis mattered but that the men in the Study were now beyond its help. They worried about the Herxheimer reaction, which occurs when a drug kills off the spirochetes and releases toxins that can endanger the human host. At the stage of the disease that the subjects now had, it was thought more important to treat their other symptoms than to provide penicillin.

It was best, the doctors thought, to continue the Study to get out of it what could be salvaged. Once again, the sense that the Study was a "golden moment" never to be repeated trumped everything else. Explaining what they had been doing and offering treatment seemed a decision too complicated to enact because it was not clear where the CDC would get the authority to treat, and the doctors thought it might not even be worth it for the men. When they balanced the possible loss of more men from the Study against the probability that the final data might be medically useful, usefulness won out.

Sencer, clearly aware of how outsiders might view the Study, again raised the questions of how the decision not to treat would be "misunderstood." In the end, the members of the conference decided to send PHS advisers to speak with both the new county health officer and the local medical society in Macon County.[32] The medical society physicians were now all black except for one, but they were no longer feared as "troublemakers," as an Alabama health official put it. They would be asked whether they thought there should be treatment, "pro or con." Sencer thought that in this way there could be "better follow-up," and "the man who needs digitalis [for heart disease] could be taken where he could get it." At a time when doctors did not consult their patients and certainly not their research subjects, the only way the conference members thought of the problem was whether or not others might see the decision not to treat, as Buxtun did, as racist. They thought the referrals would now be best for the men.

Only after the meeting did Brown write back to Buxtun. The "highly competent professionals" had dealt with Buxtun's concern about treatment, Brown assured him. Brown argued that unless the men had "active disease," instituting treatment was "a matter of medical judgment since the benefits of such therapy must be offset against the risks." The implication here was that Buxtun was clearly not an expert and had no medical judgment. Brown also noted, however, that the CDC would be sending doctors out to meet with the local and state health departments, "to assure that all possible individual attention be given to people who participate in the study."[33]

Buxtun grudgingly accepted the CDC conference's conclusions about current medical treatment. But having left his job to attend law school, Buxtun took up a legal cudgel. Tracing out again what had happened over the decades and the damage that had been done to the "unaware men . . . allowed to die early and suffer disability in the interest of medical science," Buxtun asked Brown to reconsider the obvious: "What is the ethical thing to do? Compensate the survivors? Compensate the families of all the subjects? Or . . . await the quiet demise of the survivors and hope that will end the matter?"[34] Brown did not reply.

Buxtun persisted. He raised his concerns with two of his law professors at the Hastings Law School in San Francisco. One torts professor told him there was a problem with the statute of limitations. Another advised him "to write the whole thing up and send it to the ACLU." But Buxtun never did. "I could barely write a postcard home to mother. Sadly I didn't do that. Probably I should have," he recalled wistfully. His information went no further for another three years, although he kept telling people about it.[35]

The Criticism from Within

Another effort to make the story of the Study more public began at the CDC itself. Bill Jenkins, born in the Georgia Sea Islands and a 1967 graduate of Morehouse College, joined the PHS as a mathematical statistician and became the first Equal Employment Opportunity officer for the National Center for Health Statistics Training Institute. He went on to receive a master's degree in biostatistics, another master's in public health, and a Ph.D. in epidemiology, and then became one of the first African American professionals at the CDC.[36]

In the spring of 1969, as Buxtun was corresponding with Brown, a physician colleague told Jenkins about the Study. Jenkins remembered, "I didn't understand the implications at first," even though he had had civil rights experience.[37] Jenkins took his questions to Geraldine A. Gleeson, CDC health program analyst/statistician, who had become his mentor. But Gleeson had also worked on the Study, analyzing its statistics for publications.[38] Like the others who had questioned the Study before, Jenkins was told, "You just don't understand."

For Jenkins, as for Buxtun, the questions did not go away. He too kept reading the reports, trying to understand what they really meant, and he talked to friends. The "flicker" of light, he recalled, grew brighter as the implications of the Study became increasingly clear. Jenkins, with a group of other African American professionals, began a newsletter called *DRUM*, which was dedicated to ending discrimination within the Department of Health, Education, and Welfare, the umbrella department for the PHS and the CDC. The group wrote an editorial denouncing the Study's racism and ethics and sent it to the *New York Times* and the *Washington Post*, and then waited for something to happen.[39] Nothing did. At a time when such manifestoes were commonplace, and without the knowledge of how to call and conduct a press conference, Jenkins's and his colleagues' efforts went nowhere.

Jenkins later learned that the PHS had gone, as Brown had told Buxtun they would, to gain the approval of the local, virtually all black, medical society in Macon County. Jenkins was told that the society had apparently given its approval. It was 1969, and many African Americans considered black solidarity to be crucial. Jenkins's group did not want "conflict" with the Macon County medical society. As Jenkins was to say later, "One of my greatest failures occurred—we stopped our efforts." We should have "questioned, questioned, questioned."[40] When the leader of the *DRUM* group was killed, the group's effort on the Study ended.[41]

But these events did make the PHS and CDC officials aware that the climate had changed. In 1970, both the PHS's Arnold Schroeter and Anne R. Yobs argued that the Study should be stopped and that it had become, as Schroeter put it, "too highly charged."[42] But their higher-up, William Brown, disagreed, and the Study continued for another two years.[43] Once again cooperation was sought at the county, state, and Tuskegee Institute level for the Study, which had been languishing for several years.

The last organizing began. The PHS's Joseph Caldwell went back to Alabama in 1970 to do more follow-ups and to write up his results in what would become the Study's last report, published in 1973. Rivers, now increasingly infirm, helped train Elizabeth Kennebrew to take over her work, although she continued to circulate an up-to-date list of the men in the Study to undertakers, to arrange for examinations, and to help the PHS find about 20 other men who had left the area. Caldwell and Schroeter, who did the medical work, sent men in the Study to see other doctors when they recognized symptoms of heart disease or cancer that could be treated.[44]

While other workers from the CDC and the PHS continued to help Alabama provide treatment to its citizens with venereal diseases, the tracking of the Study's men continued.[45] A physician receiving a letter about a man in the Study, however, might not know what it was about. In February 1972, for example, Kennebrew wrote to a doctor in nearby Opelika to inquire about a subject's "diagnosis, therapeutic regimen (especially antibiotic), and prognosis." But she never said the Study was nontreatment. The man, she told his physician, was "a participant in a research study conducted by the Venereal Disease Branch."[46]

The researchers who oversaw the Study at the CDC and the PHS continued to be concerned about its shoddy science, but they could not determine how to abandon what they now saw as their "moral obligation" to the remaining men.[47] Caldwell's final report might have given them even more pause, when his data showed that most of the men still alive had gotten to some treatment. "Only one of the Tuskegee syphilitics has apparently received no treatment," he found.[48] Going back to the men and telling them it was all a sham seemed dangerous and unnecessary.

The Associated Press Gets the Story
In San Francisco, Peter Buxtun had not forgotten his qualms about the Study and its ability to undermine everything he thought his own work in syphilis control had been about. He kept talking about it. One night in 1972 he raised the subject over dinner with a group of friends, which included Edith Lederer, then a young AP reporter. This was not the first time Lederer had heard about the Study, but she had "glazed over," as Buxtun put it, when he had discussed it before. Buxtun told the story differently this time, or the company was more conducive to discussion. Lederer listened and asked if there were any documents. Buxtun was only too happy to supply them.

There was a story here, a big one, and Lederer knew it. Her boss thought she was too junior to write it and had her send the materials to a more seasoned reporter, Jean Heller, in the AP's Washington office. Heller held on to the documents for a few weeks, made a couple of phone calls to the CDC, and wrote the story. It went out on the AP wire on July 26, 1972, under the heading "Syphilis Victims in U.S. Study Went Untreated for 40 Years." Her lead sentence was shocking: "For 40 years the United States Public Health Service has conducted a study in which human beings with syphilis, who were induced to serve as guinea pigs, have gone without medical treatment for the disease and a few have died of its late effect, even though an effective therapy was eventually discovered."[49]

Heller picked up on the title given to the Study in a 1954 report.[50] The ungainly "untreated syphilis in the male Negro" evolved into three words: the Tuskegee Study. Once the story left the confines of medical journals and professional meetings, PHS and CDC ability to explain its actions or to contain its meaning was lost forever. "The Tuskegee Study" was about to enter American lore.

5

Testimony

The Public Story in the 1970s

From the day the first news story broke, the Study became notorious with "Tuskegee" its shorthand name. It came to light in the waning years of the civil rights movement when heated debates over the power and danger of medicine and the perfidiousness of government were commonplace. The story dropped onto a political landscape covered with concerns over sterilization abuse, birth control as black genocide, and approval of life-threatening drugs and attacks on insensitive medical institutions by feminists and civil rights activists.[1] Its very name "Tuskegee" reflected what was then seen as Booker T. Washington's accommodationist racial politics.

In the texts and subtexts of the early public story, the ways that race and experimentation intertwined formed the basis for only a narrow understanding of what had happened. Nuances that might explain complex actions got lost in the heated outcry. Historical facts that could have provided the basis for another narrative were left undiscovered. The sides backed into their respective corners and pitted racial justice against medical uncertainty and scientific inquiry. In the public rhetoric of the 1970s—the newspaper accounts, federal investigations, and lawsuit—one can see the stories that propelled the Study into history, bioethics creation narratives, and collective memory.

Reactions to the Story

The initial newspaper story set up the elements: the men, all black and primarily poor and uneducated, were "guinea pigs" who were left to die for forty years. The stage of the men's disease or any possibility that they received some treatment did not appear. Nowhere was there any sense that these men were other than poor hapless victims taken advantage of by a governmental medical machine.

The CDC made the initial response to the original article, and it was clearly improvising. J. Donald Millar, head of the Venereal Disease Division, acknowledged "a serious moral problem" when penicillin became available. Millar spoke a truth that seemed more like a prevarication: "Patients were not denied drugs," he said, "rather they were not offered drugs."[2]

The reactions were swift. There was a demonstration by employees at the Department of Health, Education, and Welfare (HEW) in Washington the next day.[3] Reporters began calling anyone who seemed to be involved. Outrage was the key element in almost all the responses to the news stories that multiplied across the country.

The CDC realized it was in trouble. By the second day, a CDC spokesman acknowledged that the Study "was almost like genocide. . . . A literal death sentence was cast on some of those people."[4] The term "genocide" appeared in many papers. Two months later, poet Zack Gilbert would use this term in a way that would become cultural belief: "So next time when I Talk to you of genocide, Shout my guts out about a White storm coming. Don't say I'm mad, brother."[5]

In casting around for an individual doctor to interview, the media was fed John R. Heller, the Study's director in the crucial years of 1933–34. Two days after the story broke, Heller, by then a special consultant to the National Cancer Institute and its former head, declared, "There was nothing in the experiment that was unethical or unscientific." He went on to assert that "it was not built into the project that treatment would be withheld," a claim that was belied, at the very least, by the title of the Study's reports. Indeed, Heller argued, "*all*" of the men had received "some form of treatment from private doctors and clinics," but he could not say how many or "whether the patients had actually gone to doctors to whom he said they had been referred [italics added]."[6]

Lashing out at the CDC's J. Donald Millar for saying that the men should have been given penicillin, Heller claimed, "Dr. Millar makes the assumption that it was the responsibility of the project to give treatment, which it was not." Heller also argued vaguely about the efficacy of penicillin for men with late syphilis, one of the first times the stage of the men's disease was mentioned. The reporter's questions made it patently clear, however, that Heller was morally blinded, or he was lying, or both.[7] Heller could not explain the responsibilities the PHS was supposed to have or the complicated medical picture. He did not acknowledge the deceptions.

Until there was a real person who had been in the Study, it remained an abstraction, however abhorrent. Names began to circulate in the community. Charlie Wesley Pollard, a farmer whose family had owned land for decades and a civil rights activist in Notasulga, just outside of Tuskegee, became one of the first subjects to be found. Tracked down by a reporter in a nearby stockyard, where he was trading cows, Pollard was told for the first time that the "treatment" program he had participated in had been set up to be a no-treatment study.[8]

When he returned home that night, the Study was in the newspapers and on the television news, and Pollard began to piece things together. He was a precinct captain for the Tuskegee Civic Association, a local civil rights organization, and he and his wife, Luiza, were no strangers to politics. Fairly quickly, Luiza Pollard got annoyed at all the "dozens" of reporters swarming around. "They'd run me crazy, asking questions, and taking pictures," she recalled. "So I just got fed up with it and decided I'd call Mr. Gray [a Tuskegee-based and well-known African American lawyer and civil rights advocate]. After that, Charlie went there . . . the first one to go to him."[9] Within days, as other subjects went to see Fred Gray, the possibility of a lawsuit emerged.[10]

One issue was whether the men even knew what disease they had. What had the PHS told them? Euphemisms for syphilis, of course, were part of the disease's history, even after Surgeon General Thomas Parran launched his 1936 campaign to break the taboo and name the disease in public.[11] CDC officials continued to claim they had used the appropriate slang. But did using the words "bad blood" really serve to tell the men what they had?

"Bad blood," a CDC spokesman announced, was a "synonym in the black community for syphilis."[12] Another PHS physician who worked on the Study admitted, however, the vagueness of this terminology in 1972: "'Bad blood' was a concern of some of the men . . . but they were sometimes asking about iron-deficiency anemia . . . sometimes about malaria . . . and sometimes about syphilis, and sometimes about the blood as 'thinned' by degenerative effects of the aging process."[13]

He did not say, or even know, that the term was not limited to the byways of Alabama or just black communities. Through the publicity surrounding the Study, "bad blood" became known as a local and specifically black vernacular. The use of the term reflected what sociologist Charles Johnson learned in the early 1930s: that the term *was* used for syphilis in Macon County, although "treatments for bad blood were expected to cure headaches, indigestion, pellagra, sterility, sores of various sorts, and general run-down conditions."[14] Charlie Pollard did not seem to think the term was clear: "I never heard no such thing [that he had syphilis]," he declared. "All I knew was that they just kept saying I had the bad blood—they never mention syphilis to me, not even once." Standing in the yard in front of his house, Pollard in his quiet way answered a reporter's question about "the possible infection of others," which was an affront to his dignity and a violation of southern politeness norms: "My wife hasn't had it—at least not that I know of—and I've been a clean-living man."[15] Another unnamed man in the Study was just as clear: "He said he had never heard of syphilis. He had heard of 'bad blood' but didn't know what it meant."[16]

Yet the term "bad blood" was not limited just to black communities nor was its link to syphilis ignored in the 1930s. In New York City, at the same time as the Study was beginning in Alabama, a Federal Arts Project poster put out by the Department of Corrections boldly made the connections: "Your Blood is Bad Means You Have Syphilis," and a 1930s flyer from the Arkansas State Board of Health with drawings only of whites on it read: "Syphilis is . . . Bad Blood . . . GET A BLOOD TEST."[17] But from the PHS statements, the men's interviews, and the Johnson community study, the lack of specificity in using the disease's actual name was added to the Study's lore. The terminology "bad blood" became the metaphoric vocabulary for the PHS's duplicity and a decade later the elegant title for the first major book on the Study.[18] The question of whether the words "bad blood" really were misunderstood, or were widely used, or were appropriate vernacular that we might now consider "cultural competency" was not explored.

As the story grew, focus shifted to the source of the men's infections. Some stories immediately jumped to the conclusion that the PHS had deliberately infected the men with syphilis.[19] Within a week, under the headline "Doctors Victimize Blacks: Blacks Used as 'Guinea Pigs' in U.S. Syphilis Experiment," National Black News Service reporter Jeanne Fox wrote: "600 black men from Tuskegee, Alabama—400 of whom had syphilis injections [were in the Study]."[20] It was clear from the story that she did not mean treatments. In a subsequent piece, Fox backpedaled and merely said that the men "had syphilis." But the story was already out. Nurse Rivers, in helping craft the local health department's response that July, said clearly: "At no time does the study show that . . . men had 'syphilitic spores' injected into their bodies as part of the study."[21] Her comments imply that the belief that the PHS was infecting the men must have been part of the Tuskegee community's buzz once the story broke.

The worry about deliberate infection was not paranoia. Coming after the death of Martin Luther King Jr., the killing of Black Panthers by the police, government spying on legitimate civilian protest groups, growing knowledge of "infecting" in other medical research studies, and the general unrest and distrust of the government, the idea that an arm of the state could have infected black men with a deadly disease was more than plausible. The idea that the PHS had intentionally infected the men became linked to the story. Any complicated understandings of why, if, and how many of the men had syphilis, and at what stage, quickly dropped out of the coverage, if they appeared at all.[22]

Physician Joshua W. Williams surfaced to tell his tale two days after the story broke. Identified by reporter Jean Heller as a local Tuskegee physician running clinics in the community, Williams had interned at John A. Andrew Memorial Hospital and had been the acting medical director when Dibble left for the VA Hospital in 1936. In his early 70s when he was interviewed, Williams recalled that the interns were asked to help with the blood draws during the Study but did not know the Study's "purposes or procedures." More ominously, Williams claimed that in the beginning of the Study, instead of giving the men the arsenicals, doctors might have been injecting placebos.[23] Although there was no other evidence to support it, Williams's story also became part of accepted lore.

In story after story, the PHS's "crime" grew more complicated. The number of deaths reporters claimed the PHS had caused ranged widely. The AP's Jean Heller was careful to give a low figure, implying that the number of 7 direct deaths might "go higher."[24] Noting that only 74 of the men were still alive in 1972, other newspaper accounts implied that the PHS was responsible for all of the other men's deaths. In the initial stories, the numbers ranged from the figure of 7 to 154 men with heart failure that may or may not have been "linked to the syphilis." A headline read "U.S. Health Experiment Kills 126 Black Men."[25] The newspaper story claimed (even though this was not a medical certainty) that had the men been given penicillin they would not have died. By September, AP follow-up stories that were based on the Study reports gave the numbers that would be used over and over: at least 28 and possibly as many as 107 deaths were deliberately caused by the failure to treat.[26]

As reporters delved more deeply, the question of penicillin's ability to cure the men began to appear more prominently. The CDC's story became complicated as the researchers tried to explain their science and downplay the racism charges. William Brown, by 1972 no longer at the CDC, explained to reporters that the Study was definitely known in medical circles, that penicillin would not have helped the men, and that the "risk of drugs . . . might out-weigh the benefits."[27] John R. Heller continued to deny that race was part of the story. Even in an interview with a black news magazine, Heller claimed: "There was absolutely no racial overtone, and this was not an attempt to exploit the Negroes. We told them what they had."[28] The Study's defenders hoped the rational voice of science would counter what they saw as a racialized overreaction. But Brown's and Heller's refusals to even acknowledge racial assumptions about syphilis, or that the availability of black bodies had anything to do with the Study, only made racial concerns an even more powerful element, to be seized upon by others.

The depth of the racialized story grew. In Macon County, the local health department parsed its reply to protect its venereal disease program. The health director stated: "We are not trying to justify or condemn the study. What we are trying to do is make it clear to the people of the county that the V.D. program we are undertaking now is in no way connected with the study, and that the subjects of the study still alive today are not dangerous. All the cases, even the ones not treated, are not communicable now."[29] One newspaper noted that there was a venereal disease program in Shreveport, Louisiana, that may be "a similar experiment," even though the story made it clear that there were no real parallels.[30] "Tuskegee" was on its way to becoming a condensed symbol of medical exploitation of African Americans that needed no explanation.[31]

The Tuskegee Syphilis Study Ad Hoc Advisory Panel

In the face of mounting concerns, the NAACP and the Black Congressional Caucus called for the Study to be halted and those who had perpetrated what the NAACP labeled "a racist crime" brought to justice.[32] In Congress, languishing bills mandating oversight of federal research received new life, and Alabama's two white senators, John Allen and James Sparkman, coauthored a bill to compensate the Study subjects, at $25,000 for each of the men or their heirs. Newspaper accounts denouncing the Study became part of the Congressional Record.[33] Swirling around with the anger over why the Study had targeted black men was the possibility that their wrongful deaths could be the subject of criminal prosecution as well as civil actions.

The Department of Health, Education, and Welfare had to act. Mervin DuVal, assistant secretary for health and scientific affairs, created an ad hoc panel with nine men and women (five blacks and four whites), all professionals from fields as diverse as psychiatry and religion.[34] DuVal, in a candid moment, later labeled the panel members "angry blacks and liberals who would thoroughly chastise HEW in a way so as to make it easier to expurgate this unpleasant bit of past history."[35] DuVal selected Broadus Butler, president of the historically black Dillard University in New Orleans and one of the World War II Tuskegee Airmen, as the panel's head. Dr. Vernal Cave, a panel member, New York–based venereal disease specialist, and former medical officer for the Tuskegee Airmen, promised a black news journal colloquially, "This ain't going to be no whitewash."[36]

As is common with citizen panels, DuVal both set up the questions they were to consider and provided the staff from within his department. DuVal gave them three charges: "Determine whether the study was justified in 1932 and whether it should have been continued when penicillin became generally available, recommend whether the study should be continued . . . and determine whether existing policies to protect the rights of patients" in HEW-sponsored research was "adequate and effective."[37] The panel struggled to make sure there was no "whitewash," but they were fenced in by the limitation of the charges, what they were able to find in terms of documents, and the format, which did not give them the power to deal with any form of compensation to the men.[38] They had less than a year to hold the hearings and prepare their report. Divisions soon tore the panel apart and caused disagreements on how to proceed.[39]

The panel's first priority came to be the recommendation that the Study be halted. Although the story had broken in late July, and the panel was set up a month later, the Study was still officially ongoing, and the men had not yet been provided with treatment. By October, panel members told HEW directly that treatment for the men of the Study should begin. But it would take until March 1973 and Senator Ted Kennedy's intervention for treatment to be offered.[40]

The panel was hamstrung because its staff did not know about, or even where to find, the initial correspondence among the PHS researchers.[41] The panel had the published reports, medical debates on treatment, later correspondence from the CDC files, and interviews. Ethicist and physician Jay Katz asked directly if there was information on the early years and was told, "There are no documents."[42] The HEW staffers did not know the whereabouts of the PHS's Venereal Disease Division records nor did the panel have a historian who would know to search the National Archives.[43]

The claim that the men had "volunteered," as the published articles had maintained, was therefore given more official weight. Likewise, because the panel focused on penicillin, its concern became the failure to provide the men with what was now presumed to be effective treatment. It did not consider the issues around providing (or failing to provide) what had been thought to be effective treatment in the 1930s and 1940s, and the horror over the Study was compressed into only the years after penicillin became available.[44] The medical controversy over penicillin use in the 1950s provided, from the vantage point of scientific research stripped of moral or ethical consideration, a way to consider why the Study went on. Further, the staff report to the panel continued to argue that there had been "scientific merit" in the Study. Without the early correspondence, the panel members did what they could with what they had.

Several panel members went to Tuskegee and made efforts to interview some of the men. Nurse Rivers met briefly with panel member Vernal Cave, but no record remains because panel chair Broadus Butler insisted that the tapes be destroyed—to "protect her."[45] Dr. Murray Smith, who had been the Macon County health officer tied to the Study in the 1930s and 1940s, was too ill to give testimony; Dr. Raymond Vonderlehr, who had started the Study, was too senile to appear, although he continued to want to set the record straight. Dr. Dibble, the Tuskegee Institute medical director, had died in 1968.[46]

When additional open hearings were held in Washington, those called before the panel spoke more about the scientific debates over treatment than about individual culpability at either the PHS or in Tuskegee or about who had approved the Study and why. Although this issue divided the panel, Jay Katz recalled, "no one wanted to implicate the black community."[47] Katz wryly noted, in looking back on his experience on the panel, "It is all too easy ... to fix your attention if you want to point some blame on the availability of treatment. And of course after 1946 as soon as it is admitted that we should have treated them then many people argued it was too late to treat them. It is much harder to fix blame on the conduct of human beings, particularly if they are physicians."[48]

Neither the men in the Study nor Fred D. Gray, who had become their attorney, ever spoke in public to the panel. When Study subject Charlie Wesley Pollard was asked to come to Washington, Gray sent a letter to the panel telling them Mr. Pollard would be bringing his counsel. "I received no reply to my letter," Gray later reported.[49] Rivers was invited but did not show up. Vernal Cave was so angry about the limitations on the witness list that he even boycotted one of the panel meetings. He told a reporter, "It is not clear to me whether these decisions were made by staff or by staff in consultation with the chairman of the committee. But we were not allowed to call everybody we wanted. We were limited."[50]

Using statistics from the last published articles, many of the CDC officials continued to insist that the men were better off not having been treated. PHS statistician Eleanor Price, working from her knowledge of the early Study days, told the panel's chairman that no one in the Study was still infectious and that their wives had been treated.[51] Well-known Duke University toxicologist Leonard J. Goldwater explained to the panel that treating with mercury would have been dangerous and speculated that many of the deaths attributed to syphilis historically may have been from mercury poisoning.[52] Looking at this "science" and the dangers of both the heavy metals and penicillin, famed Howard University physician and anthropologist W. Montague Cobb took a similar view. Perhaps protecting his dead colleague and good friend, Eugene H. Dibble, Cobb wrote in the *Journal of the National Medical Association* just after the panel had reported: "Evidence does not appear to have been brought forward any proof that anyone was subjected to avoidable risk of death or physical harm."[53]

This viewpoint, mostly articulated by the physicians within the CDC as a defense, however, was drowned out in the racialized atmosphere. Although no one spoke this out loud, it is clear that many in the CDC were stunned by the racial criticism of the Study. The warnings over the Study's ethics, which had been sounded at least since Gibson's concern in the 1950s, had been ignored. The racial assumptions that underlay the Study were not discussed. Those who either understood that there were differences concerning the various stages of syphilis or who knew that at least some of the men had been treated could not make their voices heard. It all sounded like rationalizations and medical coldness. Instead, hate mail began to appear in CDC mailboxes, and the CDC's director was hung in effigy at a Students for a Democratic Society demonstration.[54]

Some of the PHS physicians tried to explain what they had been thinking and doing. Stanley Schuman, an epidemiologist/physician who had worked on the Study in the early 1950s, was convinced there had been treatment for active cases. "As a physician, it was my understanding that I was free (and was expected) to diagnose and to treat any case of infectious or active clinical syphilis that I discovered." Explaining that he did use the term "bad blood," Schuman also told the panel that "after a complete and negative examination, a man with positive serology for syphilis was assured that he carried serological, not infectious traces of the disease." Nor was race the issue, he declared at the end of his testimony: "My clinical colleagues in Tuskegee in 1952 of black and white racial composition assisted me, consulted freely, recommended treatment whenever necessary, and were sympathetic to the long range objectives of the study."[55]

Not everyone who spoke before the panel agreed.[56] The sharpest divides came when both PHS researchers and two physicians who had worked in Tuskegee in the 1930s provided testimony. Their differences suggest the ways the racial and the scientific aspects of the Study were being constructed as polar opposites. Unfortunately, when this testimony was taken, only one member of the panel was on hand. All the other panel members only got transcripts. Their absence deprived them of any chance to question the differences that were being argued.

Tuskegee Institute physician Joshua W. Williams, who had told the AP about the "injections" several months earlier, gave more muted testimony. Gone was the story about injecting anything other than the antisyphilitic drug arsphenamine. Instead, Williams focused on the failure of the local health officials to follow Alabama law and to report the cases. As a lowly intern, he explained, he did not feel he could ask questions. Williams allied himself with the subjects, and his testimony suggested the pained sense of a professional who felt he should have known more and spoken up. Emphasizing the racial segregation at the time, Williams made it clear that he had felt powerless. Taking a "we had to do this" position, Williams linked race, medicine, and power.[57]

In his testimony, Dr. Arnold Schroeter, a physician who had been in charge of the Study in 1969, focused on these same issues by emphasizing, in contrast, the familiar narrative of scientific evidence in medicine. He believed that the PHS had not withheld treatment. His answer echoed that of others at the CDC: "Their goal [was] not to withhold treatment, but to observe what would happen; and at no time was treatment denied any of those patients if they sought it." Indeed, he concluded, "at the time that we reviewed the group in 1969–70, all but one had received some sort of chemotherapy." Further, Schroeter went on to say, he and cardiologist Joseph G. Caldwell did, if asked, tell a "patient" what medical problems he had. Schroeter testified that a man in the Study "was to be told in terms that [he] could understand; and if treatment was needed . . . we would seek treatment for him and see that he got it." It was, Schroeter continued, the doctors or "Nurse Laurie" (Laurie was Nurse Rivers's married name) who would tell the men what ailed them. He did not say whether or not anyone was certain how much the men understood the terms, although such checking on the "patient's" viewpoint would not have been common.[58]

Schroeter had himself argued to William Brown at the CDC, after the 1969 meeting, that the Study should be ended and the men treated. When Brown disagreed, Schroeter continued with his tasks as the Study's head. When he and Caldwell were in Tuskegee, he recalled that, for the last roundup in 1969–70, Caldwell in particular had worked hard to find the men, as did others within the CDC, not just to complete the research, he claimed, "but to find the ones who needed to be treated and treat them." No one asked him at the time why they still needed treating.[59]

It is possible that the CDC doctors who managed the Study in its last years had been treating, or at least recommending treatment for, the men's developing heart disease, and that the problems had been limited to earlier years. Maybe they were convinced that what could be done had and was being done. Certainly Caldwell's statistics from the last time the men were examined in 1968–70 showed that the men *with syphilis* were living longer, and with less illness, than the controls.[60]

Physician Reginald James, however, told a very different story. Seven years after the Study started, James was hired by the Alabama Health Department to survey and provide treatment for venereal disease cases in Macon County, following the program William Perry had begun with the Rosenwald funds in 1938. James worked with Rivers in their mobile treatment bus between 1939 and 1940. James made the powerful claim that if he saw a man from the Study, it was Rivers whose job it was to persuade the man *not* to take treatment with him. He never said why he did not protest this. But a HEW panel staff member asked him a crucial question: "Were they [the subjects of the Study] aware then that they had a disease that needed treatment?"

Here James suggested the difference between his treatment program and the Study. "Certainly all patients who came in the purview of my advice, they knew what syphilis was because I didn't hesitate to tell them. I even showed movies in the county where there was electricity. That wasn't in many places, but the word got around what syphilis was. There was no ignorance on the patient's part. They might have called it 'bad blood'; and I am sure that by word of mouth, they got information from the patients who attended my clinic." And by giving examples, James noted that his patients understood the relationship between syphilis and sexual activity.[61] In touting his statistics for prevalence and describing his treatment, James was making it clear that it was possible to name syphilis and treat it in Macon County.

Rivers, he argued, had done her job by keeping the men from treatment. No one asked James why Dibble and the others at Tuskegee Institute had not asked that the men in the Study be provided treatment through his program. Nor did they explore with the men themselves whether they had heard of James's program and whether they had any other information about their disease. Nor did anyone ask Rivers if she agreed with James's testimony.[62]

After James, the duel between the doctors began. John R. Heller, who had emerged as the key former PHS researcher and defender of the Study, gave his testimony next. Heller, having heard James's assessment of what had happened, disagreed. Hedging his answer and stating his position twice, he answered, "To the best of my knowledge, no patient was denied treatment. To the best of my knowledge." He, too, qualified his answer. "To the best of my knowledge," he said again in language that sounded as if it had been coached by a lawyer. Speaking of the men, he declared, "They were not particularly curious about their disease; but if they asked, I told them what the trouble was. If indeed it was syphilis and advised them to seek treatment, particularly those with early syphilis."

Heller clearly differentiated between early and late syphilis. As a public health man, he was claiming that those with early syphilis were treated appropriately, since it was assumed that they would be contagious; those with late or latent syphilis had to ask. He was also admitting what had become obvious: not all the men in the Study were beyond contagion. "If any of the others [with latent disease] . . . sought treatment," he told the committee, they were told to go to the VA Hospital, John A. Andrew Memorial Hospital, the county, or "more importantly, the private physicians." Again, no one asked whether the men understood what they had, the stages of the disease, or why they would need treatment if they thought it was already being provided. No one asked Heller these questions because only one panel member was there to hear him.

Heller was determined not to stand only in the medical world. He crossed the racial divide and tried to suggest that there had been approval of the Study from within the black community. Here, too, his argument was vociferously made and then modified. Perhaps realizing that he might have overstepped his claim, Heller backed down and said that the "community worked with us in the study," meaning this time only in getting "the people together in the various churches." Not only did Dr. Dibble and other civic leaders know and approve of the Study, he declared, but so did Tuskegee's famous scientist, George Washington Carver. "I personally worked with [him] in the laboratory attempting to get a perfect emulsion of mercury and peanut oil. We never succeeded, but this was merely an indication that there was in the black community knowledge of this study and knowledge of what we were doing."[63]

Even if Heller and Carver had discussed the Study, working together on a colloidal mixture is still not giving approval or knowing the Study's particulars. The panel's medical consultant asked Heller, "But if the people were not to receive it in the Tuskegee study, does it have any specific bearing?" Heller had to admit that he only used this incident to show that he and Carver had discussed the Study. By invoking Carver, Heller found a way to give the Study a famous black face of approval.[64]

In the absence of the other panelists, Dr. James and Dr. Williams became the interlocutors of the PHS physicians. It was left to them to raise the questions of race that the panel seemed so assiduously to be avoiding. To Heller, James raised the question of who constituted the black community and who had approved the Study. James made clear that the leaders in Tuskegee were "not the community." "Eighteen miles away [from Tuskegee]," James declared, "these people had never even heard of Booker T. Washington." Those in Tuskegee, James pointedly reminded the doctors, "weren't the community. They were not the community at all."[65]

Questioned about the participants, Heller finally had to admit the obvious: "They were told almost routinely that they had 'bad blood.' Now, some of them knew what 'bad blood' was but I would say the majority did not." Williams was even more adamant. When he had worked in the community no one was told what the men had, not even the interns.[66] The men knew, Williams declared, that bad blood or pox could harm you, but not many had other details.

James and Williams did not only attempt to speak for the black community in Macon County. They went directly to the medical questions to counter Schroeter's and Heller's testimony that none of the men had early syphilis. "They all had had late latent syphilis for at least three years," Heller had said. "How do you know that," James asked. "Were the reports always accurate? How do you know about the stages?" he continued to ask. "Can you actually and specifically and definitely state when and where syphilis begins and when did it go into this end of early latency?"

While James and Schroeter continued to spar over the timing of stages and treatment, Heller retreated to stories about his own clinical experiences. Recalling a case in which a patient had had a serious reaction to arsenicals, Heller clung to his argument that treatment was dangerous, especially for patients with late syphilis, and backing up his claim that only those with early syphilis needed treatment. But James would not let this go. Everyone was treating, he retorted. "They treated them but very cautiously. . . . That was done in Moore's clinic and Stokes' clinic."[67]

James and Williams had been there. They had known something, at least a little, about the Study when they were younger and had not stopped it. With all the experiences that their lifetimes had given them, they argued that the

PHS had treated the men in the Study differently. They were not moved by the argument that some in the black medical community had known what was happening, even if this were true about others—and about themselves. This was not enough to persuade them that racism was not at the heart of the Study.

Further, James and Williams were not convinced that scientific uncertainty and the need to understand syphilis were sufficient to justify what had happened. In their clinical judgments, the differences of opinion over the most effective treatment of syphilis could not justify the Study.[68] Nor was such a study necessary, given both the Oslo Study and Rosahn's autopsy studies. These exchanges could have given the panel members insight into the connections among racial assumptions, experiences, and science. But they seemed to have been ignored.

Instead, most of the members of the panel focused on the limited questions of whether the men were given any type of informed consent and treatment in the post-penicillin years. Well aware of the debates about research, the panel members were concerned that they not be seen as opposed to scientific progress. "The position of the Panel must not be construed to be a general repudiation of scientific research with human subjects," they wrote.[69] Many of the panel members clearly saw this as a chance to push for federal regulations, not just norms, to control research.[70] The panel examined the medical and ethical questions that were separate from issues of race. The racism of the Study and the ideas about race were taken more as a given than as something to investigate. As panel member Jay Katz recalled two decades after the report was written, "It is almost unbelievable that we said nothing about the racial implications of the study."

The final report of the Tuskegee Syphilis Study Ad Hoc Advisory Panel, issued on April 30, 1973, declared the Study "ethically unjustified" in 1932. It condemned the lack of informed consent and painted the Study as a breach of adequate scientific standards. Penicillin should have been provided by the early 1950s, the report declared. Better protections for human subjects, especially the vulnerable, were necessary. Without the early documents, the deception of the early years was not addressed adequately and the possibility that the Study had been needed was accepted.

The sign-offs on the report reflected the divisions that had riven the panel. Katz added his own addendum to the findings, charging that the violation of informed consent was much more serious than the panel's report made clear and arguing that the Study should have been closed down much sooner. He would continue to be an advocate for a national board to oversee experimentation.[71] Broadus Butler, the chair, refused to concur with the report. He transmitted it to HEW but stated in a private letter that the panel had become "advocates" and had "lost their objectivity."[72] Concerned with Butler's lack of support for the report, several panel members denounced him at a press conference. They need not have been worried. Even with its limitations and the innuendo of cover-up, the report was to have a major impact on mandated federal policy on informed consent.[73]

The balancing of patient autonomy with scientific progress was the axis upon which the report revolved. The public and academic communities were left to ponder questions of the relationship of race and the science of syphilis to racism and to research.[74] The Study gave new urgency to discussions that had been developing for decades about regulations within the federal health agencies, medical schools, and Congress. Pressures mounted on the government to consider how to oversee medical research, protect the vulnerable, and obtain informed consent.

The Kennedy Hearings and the National Commission

In front of more cameras and press, the Study's story landed in a congressional hearing on medical research and abuses in care already being run by Senator Ted Kennedy.[75] It added to testimony on sterilization abuse and experimental abortions, while providing a visceral portrait of medical research's long moral fault lines. As with many social reforms—from limits on work hours to drug control—these examples of innocent victims made governmental controls seem needed and palatable.

Kennedy's office made sure that officials from the CDC, the most critical members of the HEW panel, men from the Study, and whistle-blower Peter Buxtun appeared before the committee. Kennedy's insistent questioning of an HEW official made it clear that no one within the CDC or the PHS had moved quickly enough to see that the men got treatment, even though the story of the Study was being covered in the media. Despite the publicity and the HEW panel's October demand that the men be treated, the CDC had debated administrative questions about the legalities of paying for care but had not been able to come to a conclusion about this—for more than *eight* months.[76]

Hiding behind the assumption that the men were not infectious and now could make their own choices, CDC officials were caught up in the question of whether a public health agency that was responsible for prevention and research, not direct patient care, could now provide treatment legally to private individuals. Kennedy was outraged at what appeared to him to be their complete callousness.[77] His questioning in March 1973 finally pushed the CDC to draft a letter offering to pay for treatment and to send public health advisers out to the survivors' homes to deliver it.

Even after this, however, it remained to be seen exactly how much medical care the CDC was willing to pay for and for whom, and who in the Tuskegee area would provide the services. Dr. Cornelius L. Hopper, John A. Andrew Memorial Hospital's medical director, argued that the program had to be comprehensive and well funded. Otherwise, he underlined in his letter to CDC officials, his institution would not be involved. With a prescient sense, Hopper concluded that "our society will be judged—by these patients and by history—as much on the basis of our constructive response to these individuals in their remaining years as on the fact of the forty year experiment."[78] The CDC was aware of this too, and of the fact that the costs could become very high.[79]

While the negotiations went on, Fred Gray was beginning to locate the plaintiffs among the men and their heirs for what would become the lawsuit. Gray and Kennedy had decades-old civil rights connections. Gray came before the committee twice to explain what had happened and to bring four of the men—Charlie Wesley Pollard and Lester Scott in March and Herman Shaw and Carter Howard in April—to provide testimony. Gray had begun his legal case against the government and was concerned that if the men accepted an offer of payment for treatment they might not receive anything else. Aware that the legal basis for a suit would be difficult, Gray was hoping that Kennedy would push through a compensation package for the men, or at least that political pressure to settle the case would be created. His testimony emphasized his sense of the men's exploitation and provided the outlines of what could have been the opening statement for his lawsuit.[80]

In their testimony, Pollard, Scott, Shaw, and Howard all made it clear that they had been misled by the government: they were never told they had syphilis and never thought they were not being treated for "bad blood." Both Pollard and Shaw told stories of being kept from treatment in Birmingham by a nurse.[81] These statements would be repeated again and again as the story of the Study continued.

Each of the men made the case for the need to be compensated for what had happened to him. What the men did not need was government payment for their medical care. This was not merely a result of distrust. As Shaw stated after a public health worker showed up at his home in April to offer him care: "I told the man that I have Medicare. I have medication and hospital insurance. I can walk. I do not see any need for anybody holding my arm. I can stand on my own feet and walk. I had everything they offered me and so compensation is what I need now." Howard concurred: "Everything he [public health worker offering care] promised me I already had, Medicaid and Medicare, and private insurance. . . . I told him I did not need that because I already had it. . . . I need some money, that is what I need."[82]

The men's statements were part of a reasonable legal strategy to gain compensation for their suffering and for that of the heirs of those who had died. But it also made clear that they were not all illiterate, trusting sharecroppers without access to physicians and reflected the fact that at least some of them could and did get to private doctors. Whether, despite this, they were still being kept from treatment for their syphilitic complications if they had them, as the official story would have it, was never addressed.

When panel members Vernal Cave and Jay Katz and syphilis-tracker Peter Buxtun came to give their testimony, their frustrations with the limitations of the HEW Ad Hoc Advisory Panel and the CDC's response were aired. Cave denounced the "sinister climate of racism" that surrounded the Study and the HEW panel's failure to hear from the men, Nurse Rivers, or Buxtun. He focused on justice. He wanted both decent compensation for the families and what he called a "Little Marshall Plan for Macon County" so that health care facilities could be improved. His testimony—that "fortunately the information shows that most of the participants in this study received antibiotic treatment at some point in their lives either for syphilis by some doctor who was not aware of the study or for some other illness"—was never followed by questions of how successfully the PHS had actually kept some men, and which men, and when, from treatment. No one asked whether the penicillin and antibiotics given some of the men would have made a difference.[83] No one asked who made this treatment possible.

Katz came to the panel twice. With his Einstein-like appearance and German accent (he had fled Germany as a teenager in 1938), he carried great moral authority and was a reminder of the Nazis' horrific medical experiments on the vulnerable. He argued for the need for a National Human Investigation Board to formulate research policies and restrictions on the research community, which he thought was incapable of policing itself. Buxtun, in turn, was his usual rambling and indignant self. He retold his story of the 1960s encounters with the CDC, placing into the record the letter he had gotten from them explaining that the physicians knew what they were doing.[84]

The Study was now on its way to being enshrined as *the* case of medical researchers' racist indifference and federal foot-dragging. The racial aspects had been played down, to near invisibility in the official HEW panel report, but they underlay the outrage at the Kennedy hearings. Fred Gray's appearance, and the knowledge that he had been the lawyer in the Montgomery bus boycotts for both Rosa Parks and Martin Luther King Jr., tied the Study forever to one of the civil rights movement's greatest moments and one of the South's legal heroes. The appearance of the men sitting ramrod straight in their chairs and thoughtfully answering Kennedy's probing was an indelible picture of wrongdoing to men who had trusted their government and its doctors.

Aware that it would have to make amends, the CDC finally made the arrangements for medical treatment. Elizabeth Kennebrew, the nurse who had replaced Eunice Rivers Laurie, was given a position that would, as the CDC put it, "expand . . . the scope of [her] job . . . considerably," and she stayed on as the liaison between the men and the CDC.[85] Arrangements were now made for the men to receive free medical care.

As the hearings concluded, Kennedy proposed a National Commission for the Protection of Human Subjects of Biomedical and Behavioral Research. After Senate negotiators wrangled with a House of Representatives' version of the bill, where concern for "undesirable curtailment of research" was deeper, the National Research Act was passed in July 1974, which began the *requirement* for institutional review boards that had to rule on protocols of federally funded medical research. A commission was set up that would eventually be responsible for what became known as the Belmont Report. It articulated principles of informed consent and patient autonomy and was particularly forceful on the need for protection of vulnerable populations.[86]

Kennedy's hearings allowed the men's views to be articulated but could not provide the compensation they now thought necessary. A lawsuit would become a crucial step toward a formal acknowledgment that something had happened and someone would pay. Suing the U.S. government and the State of Alabama for a forty-year study in which so many of the men were already dead turned out to be a complicated endeavor.

The Lawsuit

Legal questions abounded for a civil action. Who would have standing and be the plaintiffs? Was there a statute of limitations? Did sovereign immunity protect state officials from being sued in federal court? What legal theory could be used? Wrongful death, as the 1964 killings of the civil rights workers in Mississippi had shown, was not an offense under federal statutes. Even more critically, who would be sued and in what court? Legal theory aside, who would pay for what could prove to be an expensive and possibly long drawn-out effort.[87]

While the HEW panel was doing its work and Kennedy was proceeding with hearings, Gray sought assistance to develop the legal theory, to finance the case, and to find the plaintiffs. Support came from his civil rights contacts. Through the NAACP Legal Defense Fund, Gray received assistance from Columbia Law School dean Michael L. Sovern and professor Harold Edgar. Gray and his wife agreed to remortgage their home to cover some of the legal expenses.[88]

Gray had brought class actions before, but this one proved difficult. Plaintiffs had to be found who were either survivors in the syphilitic and control arms of the Study or heirs of those who had died. The heirs had to prove their connections to the Study's participants, no easy task when few of the men had died with probated wills and widows and children often could not produce records. The effort moved slowly. It took a year before Gray filed the suit, in July 1973, in U.S. District Court in Montgomery, representing 41 of the 112 men who were still alive and 48 of the heirs of those who had died.[89] Gray believed that the suit was the men's only chance for justice: "If we hadn't filed a lawsuit," he said, "it all would probably been pushed under the rug."[90] Although Gray was probably correct in terms of compensation for the men, he was certainly wrong in terms of how knowledge of the Study would continue.

The plaintiffs asked for $1.8 billion ($3 million for each man or his heirs) and sued the federal and state governments, as well as individual doctors and the Milbank Memorial Fund. As interrogatories were sent out to the government doctors as part of the suit's discovery process, Gray was told what the HEW panel had thought was true: there were no records of the Study's earliest years.

But Gray was trying the case in the public arena as well as in the courts. With Gray's "knowledge and consent," Charlie Pollard spoke to a reporter from *Ebony* magazine. The result was a long article entitled "Condemned to Die for Science," which would also be put into the record at the Kennedy hearings.[91] Discussions of compensation began to surface in the Kennedy hearings in 1973 and before the press. The Allan and Sparkman Senate bill had died in the Judiciary Committee, but a month after the suit was filed a study committee from the National Medical Association called for "reparations," receiving national coverage.[92]

The news coverage brought Gray some serendipitous assistance. Historian James H. Jones read an article buried in a back page of his newspaper about Gray's difficulties gathering the evidence. Jones called Gray (whom he had never met) to tell him that he had the documents Gray needed from his research in the National Archives, where he had found the PHS's 1930s records. Gray realized from the phone call that what Jones had was critical to his case, and he was on a plane to Jones's house outside Washington the next morning to collect the information the CDC and the HEW panel thought did not exist.[93]

Gray and Jones, with the assistance of lawyer Harold Edgar, met on weekends in an Atlanta airport hotel, to sort through documents retrieved from the archives to prepare to depose the PHS doctors.[94] With this evidence and the men's affidavits about their experiences, Gray built his case. The new information helped to fight the statute of limitations under the Federal Tort Claims Act, because it persuaded the judge that, because of the government's actions, the men and their families could not have known what they had and how they died. With this evidence, Gray could argue that the clock on the case should start ticking in 1972, not 1932.[95]

More important, race could become central to the legal argument and the pressure for settlement. The claim of racial discrimination, the lawyers advising Gray argued, would "virtually guarantee federal jurisdiction." The federal government, they predicted, could possibly argue "that race was accidentally rather than determinately involved."[96]

The men, Gray wrote in an initial brief, had been chosen because they were primarily poor African Americans.[97] Their government and its doctors had been negligent and had violated Alabama state law concerning reporting syphilis and the men's constitutional rights to equal protection. The men had been left to suffer and die and had been lied to and could not have known what disease they had. This had been, Gray claimed, "controlled genocide."[98] Although Gray acknowledged that the men had received some treatment, most of his argument was about the failure to provide proper drugs, the callous danger to the families who might have been infected, and the efforts made to keep the men from treatment.

Frank M. Johnson Jr., the federal judge presiding over the case in Montgomery, Alabama, understood the importance of racial justice. Gray had appeared before him many times in civil rights cases, sometimes winning, sometimes not. Johnson was known for the courageous stand he had taken against Alabama's governor, George Wallace. He had made favorable rulings against the state for its inadequate medical treatment of prisoners and mental patients and had supported claims against the federal government in racial discrimination cases.[99]

Gray focused his case on the need for racial justice. Nurse Rivers, the Tuskegee Institute, and the Tuskegee VA Hospital were considered possible defendants in the original legal memorandum, but they were all dropped.[100] When queried about this, Gray argued that Tuskegee Institute had not set policy and that Rivers was herself "powerless" to do anything.[101]

One could hardly imagine Fred Gray doing anything else. Gray did not need anyone to tell him how race, class, and power worked in Alabama. He had lived it. His own connections to Tuskegee Institute, where he served as legal counsel at the time, may have been part of his decision, but he also had to make the best argument he could for his clients.[102]

Gray's argument of victimization based on race kept Rivers, the Tuskegee Institute, and even the local black physicians who may or may not have been treating the men from ever being part of the case. As law professor Larry I. Palmer has argued, "Gray's theory of racial selection" kept him away from any analysis of structural arrangements and any thought that the institute and the VA Hospital physicians had been, in Palmer's words, "co-investigators." It thwarted any possibility that the men might sue local physicians for malpractice for not providing penicillin to the patients they saw.[103] What Palmer does not point out is that involving these physicians might have hurt Gray's case. If the physicians had been treating the men, the case of the men as "pure victims" would have been even harder to make.

The PHS doctors made their stand on the medical science. Their lawyers argued that experts disagreed about the advisability of using penicillin in cases of late syphilis. Sidney Olansky, the physician who had run the Study in the 1950s, continued to state in his depositions that it was "not beneficial" to treat late latent patients and that "no treatment is 'risk-less.'" The state officials were adamant that by the time they were involved in the Study the men were no longer contagious and thus their "public health" responsibilities had ended.[104] Vernal Cave, the venereal disease specialist who had served on the HEW panel, was outraged that the men and their families had to go to trial to get compensation, and he swore an affidavit countering the government doctors' analysis.[105] Judge Johnson was not persuaded by the government's pretrial arguments.[106]

Gray's legal advisers, however, knew they had a problem when the patient records and reports showed that many of the men who had lived into the antibiotic era had managed to get to treatment.[107] The lawyers advising Gray wrote in their memorandum: "The fact that all but one of the surviving syphilitics received treatment unauthorized by the government which removed them from the 'pure' class of untreated syphilitics" could be a problem for the lawsuit. But the government, they argued, would be "estopped" from making such an argument, since the very reason the men were alive to file the suit may have been the unauthorized treatment.[108]

The legal maneuvering on all sides continued. Judge Johnson ruled in July 1974 that only those affected physically by the disease could sue. Gray would have to add more affidavits as to the harm, from survivors and their families and from other doctors.[109] By October, the state of Alabama and the U.S. government were differentiating their cases. The Alabama public health officials used the 1930s documents to claim that it was the PHS, not them, who had not fulfilled their obligation to treat. It was not them but the nearly all black Macon County Medical Society that had agreed not to treat in 1969.

The U.S. government went on to claim that the Study had been a "research project," and therefore the "usual physician-patient relationship did not exist." The PHS doctors, they contended, did not have a "duty to treat," and they did "advise patients to see private doctors." Vernal Cave's testimony at the HEW hearings had stressed the need to treat; the CDC's own records and the very fact that the government was now offering to treat the men undermined these arguments. There was "no medical doubt on this question," Gray contended. But, at a trial, there would have been dueling medical experts on this "doubt."[110]

With lists of witnesses drawn up and the judge pushing for a speedy trial, the court date was set for December 1974. But settlement negotiations were also going on. Pressures were building on the CDC to get this over with. There was no way, attorney Harold Edgar recalled, that the government would not look "horrible" in court. After a particularly powerful set of depositions, Jones remembered reminding the government's attorney that at trial the case would not pass the "nose test," once Gray and his team presented a picture of a man with an untreated aortic aneurysm sticking out of his chest.[111]

Trying the case in the federal courthouse in Montgomery, only forty miles away from Tuskegee, Gray had the possibility of a sympathetic jury—but, then again, his own experiences in Alabama always put this in question, especially when the plaintiffs were black. Gray knew that the arguments could go on for a very long time, and his aging plaintiffs wanted the case settled. The CDC considered settling. Their offers made to Gray and his clients were larger than what had first been proposed before the case filings had happened and more than the Sparkman/Allan bill had proposed.

On November 27, 1974, the parties settled, the case ended, and no trial was ever held. The judge ruled that the surviving men in the syphilis arm were entitled to $37,500; the heirs of those who had died were to receive $15,000; the living controls would receive $16,000; and the heirs of deceased controls would get $5,000. All survivors and some of the families would also get continued medical treatment paid for by the federal government.

The legal work, however, did not end in 1974. All those entitled to compensation had to be found. There were often tensions between Gray and the CDC over the monumental task of finding these individuals. For more than two decades, Gray's office oversaw compensation to more than 6,000 people. They negotiated back and forth with the CDC, attended hearings to adjudicate whether the claims of heirs were legitimate, and searched for descendants, until they finally gave out the last of the funds held in escrow and interest-bearing accounts by the court.[112]

The lawsuit became a black-and-white story in which justice was to be found in legal proceedings through financial compensation to a victimized group. Such a lawsuit could not provide the "institutional analysis," as law professor Larry Palmer labeled it, of how to think about medical experimentation. "Accusation," one former CDC physician mused in the end, "exceeded what was known."[113] It could not, and did not, provide a sense of reparations or a sophisticated understanding of how race, medicine, research, and racism fit together.

The public exposure of the Study took it out of the hands of the doctors who organized and perpetuated it and of the men and their families who experienced it. It would begin a decades-long process of being fully transformed into metaphor and symbol. To the public, the testimony had seemingly been gathered and exposed by 1974. Next, the testifying and traveling deep into the American soul began. But not before those involved in the Study morphed into iconic figures whose motives and experiences would be implied and whose contexts would be stripped away.

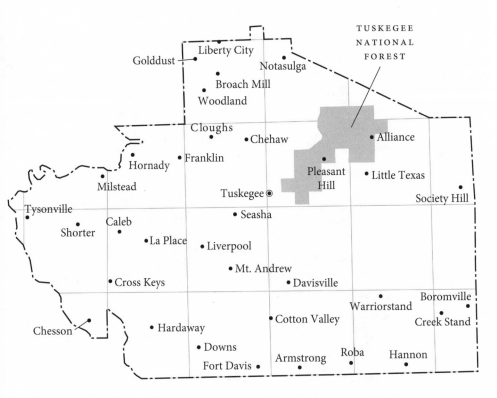

TUSKEGEE
NATIONAL
FOREST

Golddust

Liberty City

Notasulga

Broach Mill
Woodland

Cloughs

Chehaw

Alliance

Hornady • Franklin

Pleasant
Hill

Little Texas

Milstead

Tuskegee ◉

Society Hill

Tysonville

Seasha

Caleb

Shorter

• La Place

• Liverpool

Cross Keys

• Mt. Andrew

• Davisville

Chesson

• Hardaway

• Cotton Valley

Warriorstand

Boromville

Creek Stand

• Downs

Fort Davis •

Armstrong

Roba

Hannon

Map of Macon County, 1936.
(WPA Property Map, Cartog-
raphy Laboratory, Department
of Geography, University of
Alabama, Tuscaloosa)

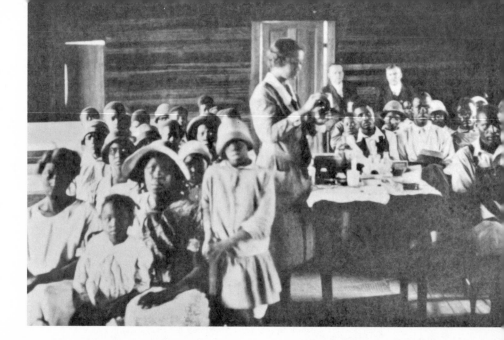

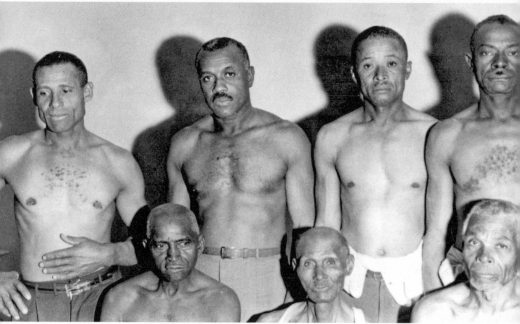

Seven men from the Study, 1953. In the original photograph (available in the National Archives), the PHS identified them by name and put an S (syphilitic) or C (control) next to them. In the interest of preserving some semblance of privacy, their names and their presumed disease status have been obscured. (National Archives, Morrow, Georgia)

ildren, women, and men in a Rosenwald Fund/PHS syphilis control demonstration project

atment clinic at a church in Hardaway, Alabama, circa 1930, *before* the Study began. (Taliaferro

rk, *The Control of Syphilis in Southern Rural Areas*, 1932)

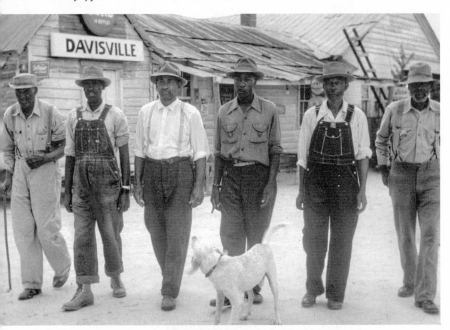

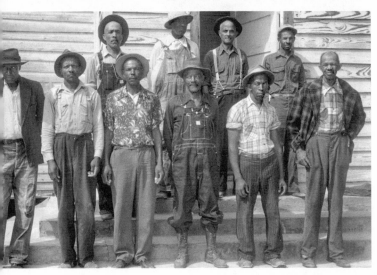

ABOVE
Men from the Study
in Davisville, Ma-
con County, 1953.
(National Archives,
Morrow, Georgia)

LEFT
Ten men from the
Study outside a
church in Macon
County, 1953.
(National Archives,
Morrow, Georgia)

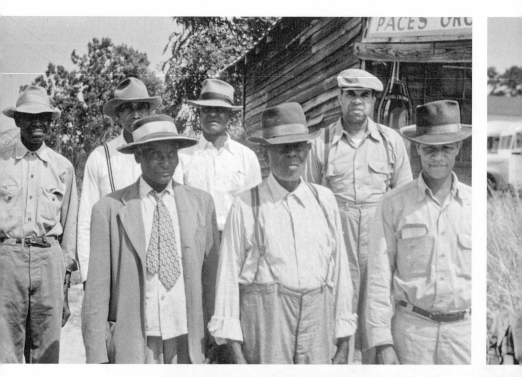

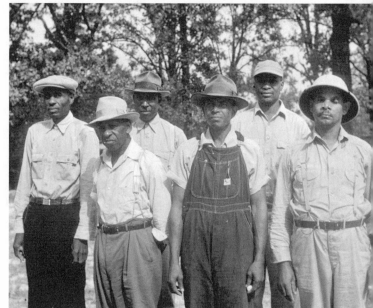

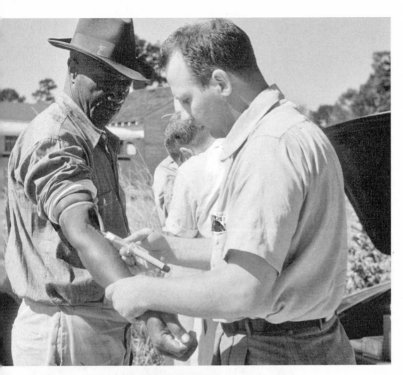

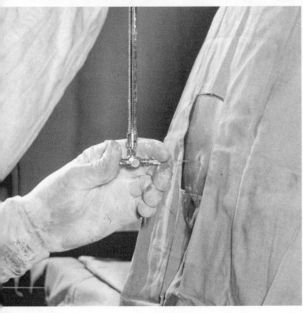

ABOVE

The PHS's Dr. Walter Edmondson (foreground) and Dr. David Albritton (background) taking blood from Study men in Milstead, Macon County, 1953. (National Archives, Morrow, Georgia)

LEFT

Spinal tap of a man in the Study, 1953. (National Archives, Morrow, Georgia)

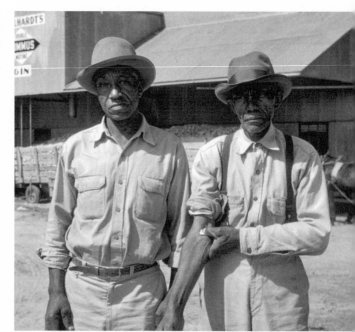

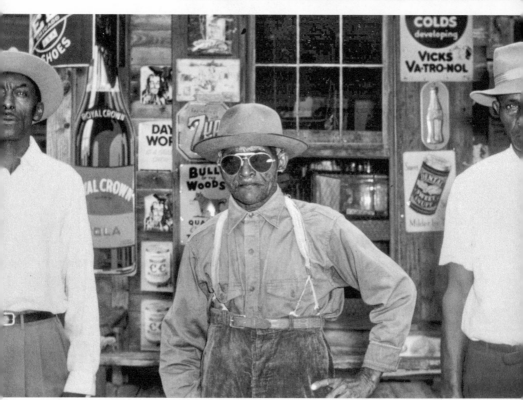

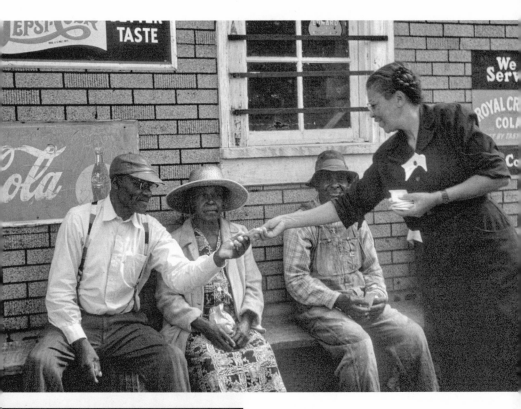

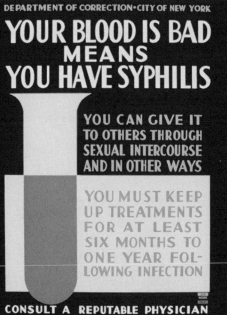

ABOVE

Nurse Rivers handing out vitamin and/or aspirin packets outside a store in Davisville, Macon County, 1953. (National Archives, Morrow, Georgia)

LEFT

"Your Blood Is Bad Means You Have Syphilis," WPA poster, 1937. (Works Progress Administration Poster Collection, Library of Congress)

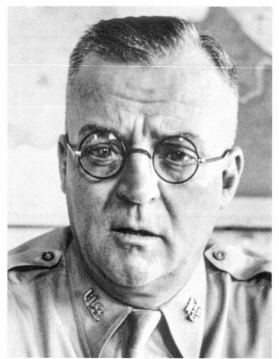

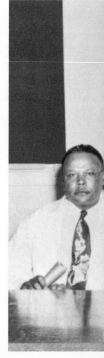

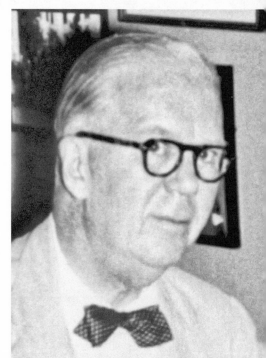

ABOVE
The PHS's Oliver Clar-
ence (O. C.) Wenger,
1941. (National Li-
brary of Medicine)

RIGHT
Johns Hopkins syphi-
lologist Joseph Earle
Moore, 1955. (National
Library of Medicine)

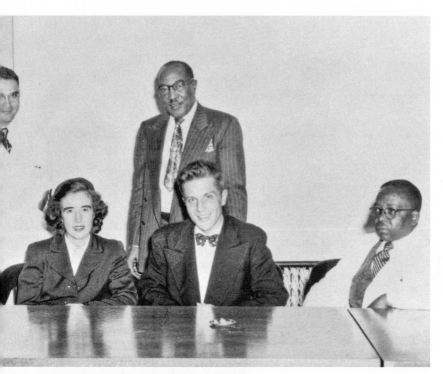

Group of Study and Tuskegee VA Hospital physicians. *Left to right, standing*: unidentified doctor and Dr. Branche (VA Hospital); *seated*: Dr. Odum (VA Hospital), unidentified woman, Dr. Olansky of the PHS/Study, and Dr. Peters (VA Hospital, John A. Andrew Memorial Hospital, and the Study), circa 1950s. (National Archives, Morrow, Georgia)

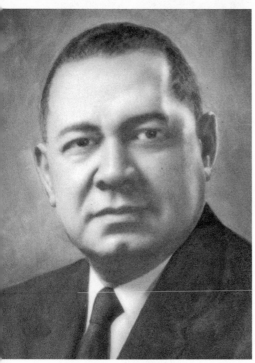

Eugene H. Dibble Jr. portrait. (Tuskegee University Libraries and Archives)

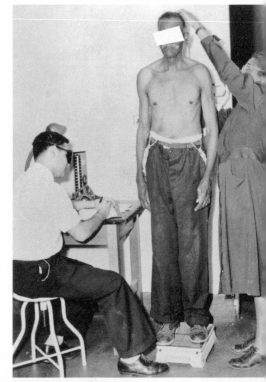

BELOW
Eunice Verdell Rivers
Laurie, photograph for
the "Women of Courage"
exhibit, photographer, Judith
Sedwick, 1984. (Schlesinger
Library, Radcliffe Institute,
Harvard University)

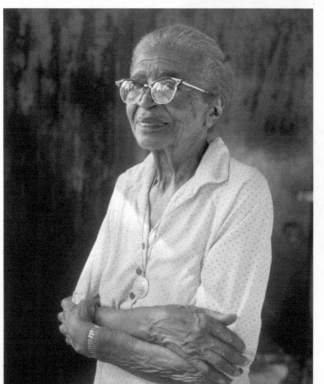

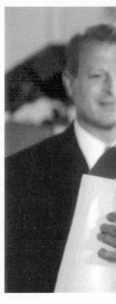

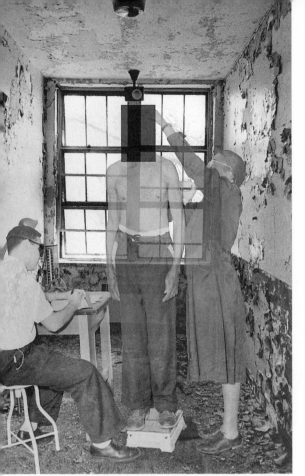

Nurse Rivers measuring a man on a scale before a Study physician takes a fluoroscope, 1953. (National Archives, Morrow, Georgia)

Nurse Rivers measuring a man on a scale superimposed on a photograph taken of the John A. Andrew Memorial Hospital, more than ten years after it closed. Photomontage by Tony Hooker for the exhibit "The Greater Good." (Tony Hooker)

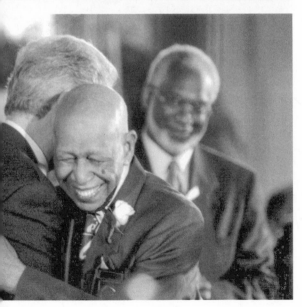

Herman Shaw with President Bill Clinton, with Vice President Al Gore and CDC Director David Satcher in the background, at the White House for the federal apology, May 16, 1997. (Paul Hosefros, *New York Times*, Redux)

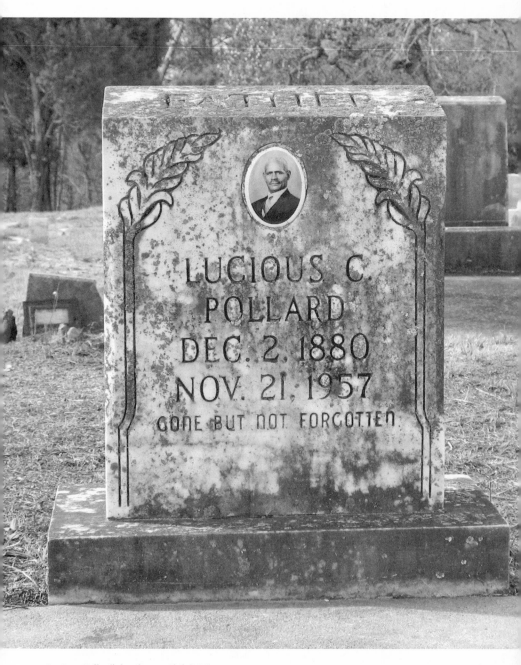

Lucious Pollard's headstone, Shiloh Missionary Baptist Church graveyard, Notasulga, Alabama. (Susan M. Reverby)

PART II

Testifying

6

What Happened to the
Men and Their Families?

For Herman Shaw, it actually started with the rocks in Plano, Texas. Maybe if the Texas soil had been as good as the dirt in the Alabama Black Belt, his father would have kept the family there. In 1922, however, it became too hard to plow around the rocks. So as a young man and without the help of a map, Herman Shaw drove the family car for over four days back to his birthplace in Tallapoosa County, just north of Tuskegee. On a farm just outside of a town called Tallasee, they could grow cotton, corn, oats, and the greens admired by the neighbors. If his family had stayed in Plano, he would not have become what he called one of the Study's "guinea hogs."[1]

Herman Shaw pushed his father's mule and then his own tractor along those rows. After his father died in 1931 and the Depression settled more deeply in the Alabama fields, the crops earned little on the open market. He took a second job as the first black man to run a cord machine in the Tallassee textile mill. When his mill job proved sporadic and he had so little cash that he could not afford to buy the license tags to be able to drive his car off his farmland, Shaw's family stayed closer and closer to home.[2] Nurse Rivers and the county's public health doctor, Murray Smith, came calling in 1932 to say that there would be "free treatment" for men who allowed themselves to be tested for bad blood. Herman Shaw did what any man would do to help his family manage in those days. He agreed to what he thought was free care.

After 1972, Herman Shaw became one of the most visible men in the Study. In interviews, whether on television from his Alabama farmland or in a Senate hearing in Washington, he became *the* southern black man, a reminder of the humanity the PHS had ignored.[3] With his beautiful eyes, dignified bearing, soft southern cadences, and carefully articulated sense of what had happened, he lived until 1999, an individual memorial to all that had been done wrong.

Herman Shaw stands out, but most of the men recruited for the Study remain undifferentiated except to their families, friends, and communities.[4] The power of the Study hinges, in part, on this sense that we can imagine somehow that we know them all. It is as if "600AfricanAmericanilliterate-sharecroppers" was all we needed to know, as if there were no individual differences to their literacy, economic status, families, or health experiences. And the ability of the Study to shock us comes as much from where they come from and what happened. We think we know this place Tuskegee, this southern town and its surrounding farmlands that embodied both hope and despair in the African American odyssey. The Study and the men have become, as historian Edward Ayers has written about much of the South, "a formula . . . that is easily pegged, easily caricatured, easily explained."[5]

In trying to "testify" to the communal truths of the Study, I had to look behind these images and words. In attempting to understand how the men and their families experienced the Study, I have balanced statistical data about them as a group with the individual stories the records reveal. Interviews of some of the men and family members, even if all done after the story of the Study entered public and media space, reveal some of their memories and experiences.[6] The opening of their medical records in 2004 allows me to peer into their bodies in a different way, I hope, than those who examined them or measured their tissue samples.[7] I am well aware that medical records can be prevarications as much as can any interview.[8] Yet using what is available, and having been written up before the Study went so public, provides another mode of understanding.

As I entered the medical records, I faced an ethical dilemma of how to use them. Here were more than 600 men whose illnesses, vital data, and even secrets I was privy to.[9] I did not want a family member to find out about their grandfather here, even though the records are now in the National Archives and their names are available in print, in museums, and on the Internet. After discussions with some family members in Tuskegee, I made a decision: when I present information from the medical records, I provide invented pseudonyms linked to the men's actual record numbers. When I use these, I will put the names in quotes. I give the men's real names and records if they or their families had been public about being in the Study or had put their names on the legal affidavits.

I am aware that this may still be for some near an ethical line and may raise privacy concerns. But I did all of this to attempt to answer key questions. What really do we know about what happened to the men, and how do they explain it? Were the men all the same? And what happened to their wives and children? However problematic it may be to still explore these documents, I decided that it was crucial to understand this part of the story.[10]

Numbers, Names, and Lives

We will never know exactly how many men were involved in the maltreatment that occurred. The PHS recruited nearly all of the men (81 percent) between 1932 and 1934. Others were found over the years, with the largest group of approximately 18 added in 1938 and 1939.[11] The published reports give conflicting numbers, from a high of 634 to the usually quoted figure of 399 subjects and 201 controls, giving a total of 600 as a round and memorable number. The CDC's final count in 1974, based on the medical records, is 427 with the disease and 185 controls, plus 12 controls switched to the syphilitic arm, for a total of 624.[12]

Although Ernest Hendon, the Study's last survivor, remembered, "I was really young then" when the Study started, in reality most of the men were in middle age.[13] Hendon was in his early 30s, but the average age for both controls and syphilitics was 43. The youngest man in the Study, labeled a control, was 16 when it started, and the oldest, a 90-year-old man, was placed in the syphilitic category.[14]

The PHS thought the Study's men were similar to other southern rural African Americans, and in many ways they were right. Some of the men were old enough to have been born into slavery, and others were only one or two generations out. The majority of those who survived to be part of the lawsuit never left the small hamlets surrounding Tuskegee, but at least 20 percent had joined the great black migration out of the rural South to the industrial centers of Detroit, Cleveland, Gary, and Chicago or to the warmer climes of Florida. They had spread to fourteen different states in search of work or the company of their relatives and friends.[15] Fred Simmons, whose wry wit never deserted him, survived till he was 102, worked a range of jobs, and raised nineteen children, of whom nine were still living in 2000. Ernest Hendon, the last of the men in the Study, who died at 96 in 2004, had tended his family's farm in Roba. In the early 1940s, the family moved to Cleveland, where he worked in a chemical plant. He served in the army during World War II and then moved back to Alabama after he retired. A control in the Study, he never married.[16]

Most of the men raised their families on what they made farming—either their own land or someone else's—or in tough laboring jobs. Less than 20 percent had been schooled beyond the sixth grade, often all that was available to black children. Most spent their Sundays in the rural churches, sang in the choirs, joined lodges, hunted, and spent time with their friends.[17] The phrase still used in the county that a family "stayed here" rather than "lived here" reflects the movement from farm to farm and house to house that characterized a common inability to hold on to space or jobs for very long.[18]

The men were primarily farmers who owned land or worked on shares; others did a range of blue-collar jobs, from elevator operators to lumber mill worker to fruit picker to day laborer. One man reported that he was a retired schoolteacher with a college degree.[19] Another had been a trucker in a fertilizer plant in Hurtsboro in the 1930s, making $1.25 a day. In the 1940s and 1950s, he worked in a small mill for 35 cents an hour and then farmed, bringing in an income of about a $1,000 a year in the 1960s. In the 1930s, a man at the Tuskegee Lumber Company received the same 35 cents; by 1972, his wages had gone up to $1.80 an hour. Another man found employment at the Tuskegee air base, then as garbage collector and farmer, never making more than 75 cents an hour.[20]

In 1931, the year before the Study started, conditions in the county deepened the difficulties for its residents. The *Tuskegee News* reported that the "cotton yields" were way below production costs; a year later the crop throughout the state was the "smallest in ten years," as boll weevils and drought took their tolls. Under such dire circumstances, the Red Cross brought in 125 barrels of flour for "the white people . . . who are in distress" and who would sign an affidavit that they were not receiving "a pension or compensation from the government or [had] means of support." Nothing was set aside for the county's overwhelmingly black population. By November 1932, when an income tax and bond amendment failed at the polls, the public schools were closed indefinitely, and soon after the banks began to close and savings were lost.[21] Yet many of the men worked their land through the Depression years and managed to make good for their children.

"It was rough, it was rough," Herman Shaw said about the low prices the cotton brought and the difficulties in the 1930s. "It has been some furious times here. . . . 1600 pounds of cotton [a little more than 3 bales] only bought seventy seven dollars and some few cents." New Deal racism kept funds out of the hands of black farmers. Nearly sixty years later, Herman Shaw still had that receipt from what the bales ginned out for in 1936, and he remembered remorsefully how little cash it brought. He farmed his acres for his entire adult life and continued to work in that nearby textile mill until he was 74. While he kept his old tractor going on his land, he remembered his history lessons that had taken him through the eighth grade in Texas. He sent his two children to Tuskegee for lectures—even when he and his wife did not go—and then on to college. A deacon in the New Adka Baptist Church with a clear biblical sensibility, Herman Shaw was a courtly man and a skilled and dedicated farmer.

Shaw remembered the violence in 1932 when the Sharecroppers' Union was organizing in nearby Reeltown and their leader shot back at the sheriff. As with most rural men, Shaw had owned a gun since he was 12. A local white man told him to give it to someone else as the tensions rose over the Sharecroppers' Union's organizing and rebellion. "They [authorities] were going into every house and if you had a gun they broke it," Shaw recalled. "I learned that thinking supersedes action." Using a long metaphorical story about baseball, he chuckled and said, "You may be able to get someone out at second, but it['s] better [to think] and get the double play." He learned too, as did every black southerner who survived the Jim Crow era, how to do what was needed to stay alive.[22]

Charlie Wesley Pollard inherited his farm in Notasulga, just outside of Tuskegee, from his family and continued to buy land until he had more than 160 acres. He recalled making money from his farming, being able to bargain for the cotton that he harvested with the "the first mechanical cotton picker in the county owned by a black man," and always thinking about buying more cows and horses.[23] As good at carpentry as at farming, Charlie Pollard built his own house and helped build the Shiloh Missionary Baptist Church, where he was a member, on land his family had owned. A generous man, he was remembered for his easy smile and for making sure that the children at his church received a gift of money on their birthdays. He was an officer in the Macon County Democratic Club and district captain for the civil rights organization the Tuskegee Civic Association. Loquacious and thoughtful, he too had a deeply developed sense of the racial dangers of Alabama.[24]

When the sociologists came to study the county and Surgeon General Thomas Parran wrote about them in the 1930s, it was assumed that the men were almost entirely trusting.[25] But much of the deception that the PHS went through would have not been necessary if the men had been as compliant as they had supposed. Nurse Rivers certainly knew the men were not as unquestioning as the PHS assumed.[26] Over the years, she saw their considerable resistance to the "medical care" of the PHS doctors—from disappearing when she came to call and refusing procedures to speaking back to the physicians about what they were doing and the pain they were causing. One man, his medical file noted, "used to hide in corn fields to avoid exam." Another even brought his lawyer with him in 1971, a year before the Study was made public, and refused to see the government doctors.[27] Some families lost track of their relatives in the Study over the years, but surely others concealed where they had gone.

The men's willingness to participate was *not* because they were compliant or knew nothing; they were expecting treatment. Even with little education and experience outside the world of farming and manual labor, they thought they were doing the right thing. An examination of their medical records offers a way to understand how "right"—or not—this was, and how more complex their experiences were than the usual narrative of the Study allows.

Confusing the Categories: What Do We Know?

If trust and deception were the only issues, the Study would not have the power it does to evoke such anger and fear. It is the foreboding and morbid sense that the PHS watched, year after year, as the men died, their bodies brought to autopsy in Tuskegee, their tissue samples sent off to labs at the National Institutes of Health. In using the medical records and reports, I am trying to determine as best I can how much the men were harmed and how many died. Even if it were just one (and clearly there were more), it would matter. But the wild estimates often made of the Study's effect on their health also need as much clarification as it is possible to provide.

The reports and medical files reveal the damage. Up until the last years of the Study, those who were assumed to have syphilis did much worse than the controls. Life tables created in 1955 showed that, at least for the younger men in the Study, ages 20 to 50, those assumed to have syphilis had a 17 percent shorter life expectancy.[28] They became sicker and died sooner (the controls on average at age 70 and the untreated and inadequately treated syphilitics at age 65). The PHS physicians were surprised by the extent of cardiovascular disease, even in the younger men, and the overwhelmingly greater illness in the men with syphilis.[29] John Stokes, a leading mid-twentieth-century syphilologist, summed up the general problems succinctly. "The high points of syphilis of the cardiovascular system may be touched in three words: ubiquitous, insidious, disastrous."[30] And, as the PHS should have known from finding the men in the segregated public asylums in Alabama, black men could end their days in madness due to the neurological complications.[31]

This conclusion—that syphilis in any form made the Study's men worse—

depends of course on accurate diagnosis and correct grouping. Some subjects had their categories switched, from control to syphilitic, when they were found to be positive on the blood tests or autopsies showed syphilitic lesions. The numbers moved are not totally clear and run from 23 in one report to 12 in another.[32]

Although the records also show that a number of the men were probably not syphilitic at all (although how many cannot be easily determined), their category was never switched in the formal analysis.[33] The switching in the formal record only went one way: from control to syphilitic. And the only men added to the Study after 1934 were those the PHS thought were syphilitic. "Henry Monroe" died in 1957 from hypertensive cardiovascular renal disease. Although listed as one of the syphilitics, he was negative on all the serologies and should probably have been a control. As J. Jerome Peters, the Tuskegee radiologist/pathologist who did the autopsies, noted on another man's case: "'Fred Fox' was a syphilitic, but shows none of the evidence commonly seen in syphilitic vascular disease." Peters thought that control "Jonathan Hamilton" had "luetic aortitis" on x-ray in 1958. His category was then switched to syphilitic, but his data up until then had been used in the control category.[34] Given this violation of what are now standard experimental protocols, it is statistically difficult to treat the two groups (controls and syphilitics) as discrete categories for the entire time of the Study.

Even though the men were assumed to be in the latent stage (and at least five years out from their initial infections), the amount of time they lived with the infection ranged more widely than their ages. From sampling the dates that 143 of the men reported for their first lesions of the disease, the median was 19 years from their first infection, with a range as wide as 1 year to 47, even including one man whose infection had started 72 years before the Study began. But at least 19 in this group, and in all probability many more of all the men who were syphilitic, were probably not yet in latency, since they were less than five years out from an initial lesion and could still have been contagious.[35] These were the men, along with their families and partners, whom above all the PHS should or may have been treating if there had been more concern about the disease's spread.

Yet, even with the autopsies, medical records, death certificates, published articles, and stories told within the families, we will never know for sure how many of the men actually died from their syphilis directly, as opposed to "with syphilis," and how much damage it actually did.[36] The initial news stories, based on the published articles, estimated that at least 28 of the men and as many as 100 "died as a direct result of untreated syphilis," while other accounts circulate that make it appear as if all the men died from the disease.[37] Given the shift in categories for how to report cause of death over the years, the failure to have records on the men who passed away after the Study closed, and the differences between the autopsy reports and tissue data, we will never know this number exactly. At best, a CDC study done by cardiologist Dick Bruce in 1974 concluded, after reading the autopsy records, that without treatment the men "would have [had] roughly a 50–50 chance of demonstrating syphilitic cardiovascular involvement at autopsy."[38]

Three-quarters of the men who died before 1973 ended up on the autopsy table. Yet, despite the assumption that Rivers was able to get *all* the autopsies, this means that 97 of the 419 men who died and left records before 1973 when the Study finally closed down were not autopsied. Another way to consider this requires thinking about all the men in the Study, not just those who died before 1973. There were no reported autopsy findings on the men who passed away during the next three decades after 1973. Of the total number of men in the Study, only 36.5 percent of the men had their bodies examined by pathologists with results sent to the PHS.[39]

While the Study was ongoing, Rivers tried her best to reach the families to get them to agree to autopsies. She was not always successful, and she wrote to the CDC to admit in 1953 that "it seems as if the odds are against me. I have lost another autopsy."[40] The man whose record is number one in the Study died in 1958 in Montgomery, only forty miles from Tuskegee, but his "family would not give permission for an autopsy."[41] The medical files make it clear that more than one family turned her down and that others refused to have their relative's brain examined for neurosyphilis, even if they agreed to the autopsy. Nearly 100 never had their cause of death determined by the PHS before the Study closed.[42]

Trying to establish why the men died is even more difficult. Those with untreated syphilis died younger, and from more widely differing ills, than did the controls, although by the end of the Study their numbers evened out. This is clear from the published reports and records. Most of the men showed the signs of arteriosclerosis and hypertension as they aged, and they wore their lives of hard labor on their bodies: shortness of breath, severe pains in their chests, aneurysms, and an inability to work to support their families.

Physicians at the time thought there was a relationship between arteriosclerosis and syphilitic cardiovascular complications but agreed that even with autopsy it was difficult to tell which disease had been more aggressive in causing the deaths and how they interacted.[43] There was disagreement between the pathologists who looked at the organs and those who examined the tissues. Other men clearly had co-morbidities, such as diabetes. Even after the Study ended, the physicians from outside the PHS who examined the men were unsure what had caused their ills. "Rare was the heart," as one researcher on another study noted, "in which one process was the only operative factor."[44]

The records show the story of this confusion. "David Founders" was a control shifted to the syphilitic category. His blood tests were negative, but his diagnosis by 1958 was "luetic aortitis," a syphilis-related cardiovascular problem. Because he died after the Study ended, we do not know whether this proved to be true or not, or whether it caused his death. Another physician wrote "no evidence of venereal disease" on his record. "Fred Pendleton," born a year after slavery ended, entered the Study as a control in 1933 and died of "old age" from arteriosclerosis and edema. Peters wrote "luetic aortitis" in his autopsy findings, but another physician wrote "NO!!" in green pencil on the record.[45] As one leading syphilologist had noted, "The more one looks for cardiovascular material of whatever type, the more one finds."[46]

Autopsy did not always mean clarity. As Peters noted on one record of a control, "Only the enormous size of the heart suggests the possibility of syphilis. There are no other findings."[47] In 1938, "Ryan Clark" died from "syphilis" when he was only 52.[48] When he entered the Study in 1933, he was already 27 years out from his initial infection. His physical exams and autopsy showed the complications of "marked arteriosclerosis, hypertension," and "syphilitic involvement of all his arteries," yet the pathologist who examined his tissues at the National Institutes of Health concluded that there were "no microscopic findings in this case particularly indicative of syphilis."[49] For many others, the causes of death appeared to be clearer. Aortitis, aneurysm, and other heart diseases were much more common in those men labeled as syphilitics than the controls, and at least 16 of the men had syphilis listed as their cause of death.[50]

Although we will never know for sure how many of the men died because of the PHS's callousness or even what they all had, the Study matters in understanding how racial assumptions are central to medicine and how easily medical uncertainty masks ethical blindness. The men's reports to the PHS doctors make this clear. "Senility from history," one report said, in a double entendre that probably escaped the physician who wrote it.[51] The men reported over and over that they suffered from "misery," a term that seemed to reflect their aches, pains, and ills. The diagnostic and painful spinal taps added to this general misery. "I laid in the bed a whole week," Charlie Pollard remembered.[52] Another man told the PHS, although there is no supporting evidence, that in 1932 the "fellow before him died on table—needle broke."[53]

Knowing what really happened, as much as possible, to all the men and their families matters if we are to understand this Study. The PHS makes clear it provided some treatment in the first year. Yet another crucial question hangs over all the records and over all of the Study: was it ever possible for the men in the Study to get other treatment and would it have helped?

Possibilities for Treatment

Because of the treatments at the beginning of the Study, more than half of the men (54.4 percent) who were the subjects had some amount of metals treatment that could have rendered some of them noninfectious, if they were not already. Yet only 25 of them (5.7 percent) had more than 10 injections of the metals pre-penicillin—an amount considered adequate to stop contagion but not to cure an individual.

Treatment pre-penicillin might, however, have stopped some of the syphilitic complications for some of the younger men whose infections were newer, even if their blood tests continued to show signs of the disease.[54] Joseph Earle Moore, the Johns Hopkins syphilologist, made it clear in 1943 what the pre-penicillin beliefs were even when there was full treatment. "The radical 'cure' of late syphilis . . . is rarely if ever obtainable with our present methods. . . . Late syphilis in human beings is not curable in the biologic sense," he argued.[55]

Penicillin, when it became widely available in the later 1940s, made it possible to cure individuals with the disease in its earlier stages. For those in late latency, the use of penicillin became more common by the 1950s. If severe organ damage was already present, providing penicillin would have been of little help. When the Study finally closed, all the men still alive were offered penicillin. But without their medical and death records after 1973 (and the archives do not have them), we cannot really know if it made a difference or not.[56]

During the Study, the PHS's efforts—talking to the local physicians, providing names to other providers, tracking the men down when they left the area, keeping them from the army—all clearly affected whether or not the men were seen and treated by anyone else. But Macon County was not a concentration camp, not all the local doctors cooperated forever if at all, and the Depression ended even if severe rural poverty in Alabama continued. Local physicians, even those who worked at the John A. Andrew Memorial Hospital, maintained private practices in their homes in the surrounding communities, and we will never know what they did there.[57] Rivers was good at her job but not always that good. The possibility that men were getting treatment, either intentionally or by serendipity when other ills occurred, has to be considered.

Even the PHS knew that follow-up was never as complete as it wanted. O. C. Wenger admitted that by 1948 "26% of the syphilitics and . . . 35% of the controls . . . had been lost from observation," although an attempt was made in 1970 to find anyone still alive.[58] We will never know if these men died without ever finding treatment. None of this changes the PHS's intentionality, but it does change our understanding of what actually happened.

The assumption is usually made that *none* of the men could have gotten individual attention. Both the historical record and the extant medical records complicate this picture. In 1938, the Rosenwald Fund began operating its "bad blood" wagon, and the letters back and forth and James's testimony in the Senate hearings are evidence that the men in the Study were deliberately kept from treatment by Nurse Rivers's presence. This assumes, of course, that Rivers was doing precisely that: keeping the men from treatment. But Rivers did not always do what she was told. The Tuskegee hospital's medical director after Dibble, Dr. C. A. Walwyn, described her as a "most conscientious worker." The county health department's Murray Smith did not agree. As the PHS's Austin Deibert reported to his boss, Smith was "rather disgruntled at his lack of administrative supervision of Rivers. Smith related that frequently she failed to make appearances in his office for several weeks at a time and did not turn in reports of her activities."[59]

If Rivers was not reporting regularly, what else might she have been doing? We only have James's word that Rivers was screening all the men of the Study who might have shown up at the mobile clinics for treatment. Nor was she the only nurse—at least four others worked on the mobile clinic project. The medical records support the possibility that, at a minimum, the physicians on the mobile bus treated some of the men in the late 1930s. The medical record for "Bill Walsh" reports "shots in hip for over one month, from mobile bus," for example.[60]

Reginald James, who staffed the mobile bus in 1940 and who claimed that Rivers stopped the Study's men from getting his help, was treating others across the county. As he had explained to the HEW panel, he gave talks in schools and churches, showed movies about syphilis where there was electricity, handed out pamphlets, and sent letters to his syphilitic patients that said in capital letters "you have a disease called 'syphilis.'"[61] It is possible that this educational and treating work reached at least some the men in the Study or perhaps their more literate children. Without the names of the mobile bus's patients (which do not seem to exist) to compare to the names of the men in the Study, we will never really know.[62]

The World War II era presented another possibility for treatment, beyond Murray Smith's efforts to keep the men from the draft and treatment.[63] As part of the campaign to make syphilis care more available, the PHS developed "rapid treatment centers." The centers were based at first on a model developed by the PHS in Hot Springs, Arkansas, for a shortened treatment of neoarsphenamine and bismuth (down to "one day to eight weeks as contrasted with 18 months required by standard methods"). During the World War II era, the PHS set up these centers near "military training facilities or important war industry cities," primarily at first as a way to contain prostitutes and "camp followers," who were seen as the major "vectors" for venereal disease. As penicillin became more widely available, they dispensed this as well.[64]

The PHS established such a center in Birmingham (about 130 miles north of Tuskegee) at the local Army Air Force Base and at other clinics. In 1945, following the passage of a 1943 state law requiring blood testing for syphilis, Birmingham became the site for a huge 42-day effort for mass venereal disease control. Using hundreds of blood testing sites, the state health department and the PHS worked together to get a massive publicity campaign out to both the white and the black communities. As local health officials reported: "Posters appeared in store windows, in street cars. . . . Ten thousand cards were displayed at one time. More than 500,000 pieces of printed literature were distributed. Milk-bottle collars carried a blood test message on 175,000 bottles. . . . Four radio stations gave full support and much time through numerous spot announcements." More than 200,000 people were tested.[65]

Herman Shaw and Charlie Pollard both remembered the treatment center in Birmingham. Their stories, told in their affidavits in the lawsuit, before the senators at the 1973 hearings, and in subsequent interviews, all testify to the fact that both of them at one time were supposed to get to Birmingham for some kind of treatment. Mr. Pollard recalled that he never got out of Tuskegee to go "to Birmingham to receive treatment for syphilis by the use of penicillin," but "was told by a nurse that because I was in this study I could not go."[66]

Mr. Shaw's memory of what happened is even more dramatic. In front of the senators at the 1973 hearings, he related his story in detail:

In the late 1940's—I do not remember the exact date—they sent me to Birmingham. We left about 2 o'clock and we got to Birmingham before dark. They gave us our supper and put us to bed. The next morning they gave us breakfast. I saw a nurse roaming through the crowd. She said she had been worried all night. She said that she had been looking for a man that was not supposed to be here and his name is Herman Shaw. Naturally I stood up. She said come here.

She said, "what are you doing here?" I said, "I do not know, they sent me here." They got me a bus and sent me back home. When I notified the nurse of what happened in Macon County, I did not get any response.[67]

In all the interviews and writing about the Study, however, no one seems to have asked Mr. Shaw who sent him to the Rapid Treatment Center and why. With interviewers so focused upon the horror of his coming close to treatment and then being denied it at the last moment, these questions were not asked: How did he get there in the first place? Was it merely a mistake? Was the "they" of his words "they sent me to Birmingham" someone from the Study in Tuskegee or some other family member or health professional? Had the publicity from the Birmingham campaign made it into Macon County?

I tried to ask him about some of these matters in 1998 when he was 95 years old. By then, the story was intertwined with so many other events in his life that it was impossible to distinguish when he learned what. He talked about the "state conscripting him to Birmingham," but I was not clear what this meant. It may be that he understood that under the 1943 state law there was this effort to get everyone tested. He did say, "The only remorse I have about it is in [19]47 the rumors came out that they were treating us for bad blood; and they had found the medicine that alleviated the pain and withheld it and didn't give it to us." But there was no way to tell when he found out about the penicillin and what he knew and when.[68]

In his original telling, Herman Shaw becomes almost a twentieth-century medical runaway slave, who tries to escape but gets caught and returned to enslavement. In the context of the PHS's efforts to keep the men from treatment, Mr. Shaw's denial of care is taken as one more tragic example of the PHS's deadly callousness. And it may indeed be that he was sent back home because the center in Birmingham had a list of the names of the men in the Study, as his statement implies.

There is, however, another possible explanation. At least in Birmingham during the mass campaign the drugs were only being given to those with *early* cases of syphilis. The state health officials stated this clearly in their 1940s news accounts: "Unfortunately, some inferred that all cases of syphilis were eligible for penicillin treatment, when actually its use was limited to early cases. This inaccuracy was never completely corrected. Many chronic cases demanded penicillin treatment of practicing physicians and public clinics and were not always satisfied as to the reasons for its refusal."[69] Was Mr. Shaw sent back to Tallasee because he was in the Study or because it was presumed that he was not an early case?

Mr. Shaw's story becomes even more complicated once the medical records are examined. Mr. Shaw was originally a control who was switched into the syphilitic category after 1945 when his tests turned positive. There is no way to know whether he had been positive before and just did not register on an earlier blood test or whether this was a new infection. Thus it is possible that he should have been treated in Birmingham since he could have been in the early stage and infectious. But if it was not early and if it was known he was in the Study, his rejection could have been because of the stage of his disease. The irony is that even though he was turned away in Birmingham, Mr. Shaw actually got to penicillin in the 1950s.

This part of Herman Shaw's story gives us another clue as to what might have happened to others. Many did get to doctors more often than the focus on the Depression years makes us think. In 1953 and in 1956, Mr. Shaw was hospitalized in Tallasee for a total of 20 days for pneumonia. And the treatment: penicillin every 3 hours for 9 of those 20 days. His status in the Study did not affect his care. Did this make a difference in his syphilitic illness? We will never know.[70]

Others, the records show, actually were treated in Birmingham at the Rapid Treatment Center or at the local health department. "May 1951[—]Penicillin 5,000,000 units R.T.C." report the records in one man's case; his wife was treated at the Macon County Health Department. Another 49-year-old man in the Study had a similar experience: both he and his wife were treated at the same time in 1949 at the "Rapid Treatment Center, Birmingham." Still another man, who died from a stroke, perhaps a complication of neuro-syphilis, remained a syphilitic in the Study even though he too had penicillin in 1949 in Birmingham, supposedly 27 years after his first infection.[71] It is not clear why some men who were clearly in latency also were treated. Mr. Shaw remembers being turned away, and there is no reason to doubt him. What about these other men? Why were they not turned away?

Most likely those who did make it to some kind of treatment did so because doctors, either in Macon County or elsewhere, did not know they were in the Study or did not remember, or treated them for their syphilis before penicillin, or treated them for other ills with penicillin after the late 1940s. One man received "IVs" for his syphilis at the John A. Andrew Memorial Hospital at Tuskegee Institute every two weeks for three months in 1937, even though he was in the syphilitic category. Another reported to the PHS that he was given bicillin (a form of penicillin used specifically for syphilis) and arsenic injections there in 1955. A Cleveland physician diagnosed a man in the Study with early and late syphilis and treated him with appropriate amounts of heavy metals from 1944 to 1950 until his serology was negative. Another, who had moved to Clewiston, Florida, was treated by his physician, who, it was reported, "was unaware he was a research patient."[72]

This went on in and outside of Macon County. Fred Simmons declared in his affidavit for the lawsuit: "I was told by a private doctor whose name I do not recall that I had syphilis. This occurred in the 1950s in Macon County. He informed me he was treating me for my condition." But then, later in the statement, he said: "I only learned it was syphilis in the spring of 1972 when told by government representatives." Did Mr. Simmons really know with what he was treated? Or was he lied to? His records show that he received penicillin for other ills in the late 1950s and early 1960s, some of it even from health officer Murray Smith. His wife was treated too in the 1950s. Or what should we think of the case of a man listed as a control who developed syphilis in 1941 and then was given a "course of [penicillin] shots at Health Dept, Tuskegee, [around] 1945." Most important, would any of this treatment, especially for those who had long-standing cases, have made any difference? We cannot really know.[73]

Despite claims by the PHS that antibiotics had not "defeated" the Study, its own reports tell a more complex tale. By 1961, it knew, and stated in a published report, that "approximately 96% of those examined had received some therapy other than an incidental antibiotic injection and perhaps as many as 33% [had] had curative therapy."[74] In 1971, its published report again stated that "all but one of the syphilitic survivors have received some amount of medicine considered anti-luetic."[75] Indeed, just before the Study made the newspapers, an observant Maryland medical school physician and his student wrote an article using the published reports that argued that the Oslo Study and the Study could not be compared because of the "treating" in Alabama.[76]

The medical records bear this out. By 1945, as penicillin became widely available, 114 of the men in the syphilitic category were still alive. The records report that over the next decades at least 58 of them, or 51 percent (a lower figure than the 1961 report) had been given penicillin. It is possible that the penicillin might have positively affected the course of their syphilitic complications *if* their cardiovascular or neurological complications were not too developed to be beyond repair and the amounts of the drug were high enough to kill off the spirochetes. For those whose deaths are recorded, it appears that the men who received penicillin died at a later age (69.5 versus 56.3), although the numbers are too small to be statistically significant. Nor can we tell if the penicillin changed the cause of death, again because of the small numbers.[77]

Doctors clearly treated some of the men where they lived. Others, as with Mr. Shaw, were given penicillin by physicians because of its widespread use in the postwar years.[78] Dr. Robert Story, a Tuskegee physician, remembers being told in the 1960s by a nurse at a local hospital not to give his patient penicillin because he was in the "government" program. She asked him to check with the local health department. It was after 5 P.M., and the health department was closed. Story claims he gave the man penicillin. We cannot know if it made any difference, or why the local nurse knew about his status.[79] The aspect of this tale emphasized—in this case, that the local nurse knew but the doctor treated anyway—depends on what kind of story we want to tell.

Physicians, unlike in the Depression years, were more available to at least some of the men over the years. The men's records report penicillin from a "company doctor" or in Birmingham or from a range of county and city health departments.[80] Dr. Dibble treated another three of the men, including one who reported that he "told Doc that he needed some shots" in 1956. In Gary, Indiana, a man in the Study received penicillin five times in 1958 for his prostate and gonorrheal infection. Although an earlier x-ray exam in 1952 had shown "a slight cardiac enlargement" but no neurosyphilis, by 1963 his heart was declared "normal."[81]

"Treated adequately in 1968 in Birmingham" the records for one man reported, as did the records of another who was referred to the Birmingham Rapid Treatment Center in 1951 by the Macon County Health Department. Another man, a control who was then switched to the syphilitic category by 1948, nevertheless told the PHS that two years later he had received "penicillin administered every two hours for 14 days at Rapid Treatment Center, Birmingham, Alabama, March 1950."[82] The PHS's Joseph Caldwell and his team wrote in the last published report on the Study, in 1973: "In this age of widespread penicillin and antibiotic usage, it is seldom that a person can live 25 [years] without receiving one of these effective drugs. Following the introduction of penicillin, *only one of the Tuskegee syphilitics has apparently received no treatment* [italics mine]."

The question remains, as Caldwell noted, as to whether those who were treated by what he labeled "nonstudy physicians" received enough to be considered "curative for syphilis," although he also concluded that the two subjects with "aortic valvular disease" were showing either "stability" or "improvement . . . follow[ing] administration of penicillin." Both age and "antimicrobial therapy," he concluded, "accounted for the lack of morbidity." It was the controls who seemed to be doing worse in this final survey in 1968–70.[83]

The PHS was vague in its descriptions of the Study to other health care providers. Caldwell wrote to a doctor in Lima, Ohio, in 1970, that "through the years we have been following the health of 'Mr. Jones' of Lima," without explaining why. The form sent to the Chicago Health Department in 1952 calls the project "Syphilis Research Study (Macon County)." In other places it is referred to as "the Tuskegee project," and another form labels it "Macon County Untreated Syphilis Study." All of this suggests that other physicians and health departments may, or may not, have actually known that treatment was to be withheld.[84]

It was not just men who left the Tuskegee area who might have received treatment. Dr. Stanley Schuman, one of the PHS physicians who worked on the Study in 1952, treated with 15.6 million units of penicillin a 64-year-old man in the Study whose first lesion dated to 1910 and who was diagnosed with central nervous system lues. The man lived another 12 years, and whether the penicillin helped is not certain.[85] Dr. Murray Smith's name comes up numerous times in the records as giving treatment. In 1936, for example, a man reported getting "bismuth and neo[arsphenamine]" from him at the health department before penicillin was available.[86]

Once penicillin became available, other men list ills—colds, pneumonias, flu, back pain, urinary infections—for which they were given penicillin in amounts that might have affected their syphilitic infections. One man's record notes "10 shots one every other day of penicillin for general weakness and water trouble and again in 1952 by Dr. Murray Smith Tuskegee" or "a series of penicillin injections [amount not given] over four consecutive days in Feb. 1952 for influenza" from a doctor in Union Springs. Another man's record states that "for past three or four years patient has been going to Dr. Murray Smith in Tuskegee, each month for check up, usually gets a $5 shot on each visit, sometimes returns at weekly intervals for additional shots. Pt. was told these are penicillin shots."[87] All of this suggests that Smith was treating intentionally or without recognizing that the men were in the Study, or that he was lying to the men that what he gave was penicillin.

When the PHS doctors claimed they were referring men for treatment, they may have also meant nonsyphilitic related care. Records show referrals for heart disease, tuberculosis, and other ills.[88] In 1970, the PHS's William Brown wrote to the Macon County Health Department regarding a 66-year-old man in the Study who had developed what appeared to be anemia and possible prostate cancer. "In keeping with previous customs in our Tuskegee surveys, I wish to report to you the ill health of one of patients seen by us during this present survey," he told the health department. Brown concluded: "We shall continue to report to you on patients who need medical care but have no private physician at the time they are seen."[89]

Macon County physicians were still seeing the men. Dr. Luther McRae received reports in 1970, at the patient's request, on a man in the Study and his problems, "dyspnea, anemia and chest pains."[90] A man examined in 1972 was "found to have heart murmur and mitral insufficiency. To follow-up and consult [with] pt's pvt. physician Re: CDC findings." Two months later, the man was taken to John A. Andrew Memorial Hospital for x-rays and then admitted four months later by Dr. Robert Story to the Macon County Hospital. Despite surgery and being followed by "Health Dept. as Medicare referral," the man died of "stomach cancer" just after the Study became news in July 1973. The local pathologist, the report concluded, "will not perform autopsy due to present controversy surrounding the program, although the family was given a check for the 'family allotment.'"[91]

The records reveal that the PHS could not always control what happened. Even within the county, Murray Smith gave penicillin to some of the men; the clinics at the John A. Andrew Memorial Hospital at Tuskegee Institute provided the earlier drugs and penicillin to others. Other local doctors or those in faraway cities, even when apprised of the Study, provided a range of medicines and treatments to cover syphilis's possible complications. Even with all the rural poverty and the difficulties of paying for care, it was possible for those who survived into the antibiotic era to get help that may or may not have made a difference.

That many of the men suffered and died of the complications of the disease is indisputable. It would matter if it was even just one, and it is clear that the number is at least 16. Most of the men thought they were being treated and most never really knew in a meaningful way what they had.[92]

Some, however, clearly by intention or by serendipity, received treatment for their syphilis and for other ills. This causes us to ask, What happened to the women and children who were the partners, wives, and offspring of the men in the Study? Did any of them get syphilis? Did any of them get to treatment before the Study ended?

Women and Children

When the story of the Study first broke, the news focused on the men and on what the disease had done to them. The differences among the stages of syphilis and what it might mean for them and their families was rarely addressed. The men chosen for the Study were supposed to be in latency, during which time the possible health threats were to their bodies, not to someone else's.[93] Yet we know from the dates of initial infection that some of the untreated men were clearly still contagious and could have passed the disease on to their wives/partners—and then perhaps through the women to their children. This, of course, begs the question of whether or not the men had already infected others or been infected by them, or whether the diagnosis of the stage of their disease was accurate, or if their partners were always women.

If, as likely, some of the men were still contagious (because they were in earlier stages of the disease and had not been treated), then the failure to notify their sexual partners allowed the infection to spread.[94] This becomes a "truth" of the assumption that the PHS was infecting the community. Alabama began requiring blood tests for syphilis before marriage in 1919, but there is no evidence of whether such tests were given to all the wives or of how many were common-law as opposed to legal wives. The PHS was clearly haphazard in checking to see what happened to the women. There is no evidence to assess if the wives might have found treatment even if the tests were positive, or whether they became positive after marriage.[95]

Whether some of these women and children did have the disease and were later treated, either through the Rosenwald Fund program, at health departments, or by private physicians, will never be known. The men's records are of little help because the women's names and disease status are blacked out. This could have been done for confidentiality reasons after the women were treated (as the PHS's letters seem to suggest). Because of this covering up of their names, only 62 of the 624 records had information on the examination and treatment of the wives before the Study ended. Of these, 28, or 45 percent, of those for whom there are records showed that their wives had been treated. Nor do we know whether any of the men passed the disease on to other sexual partners or in subsequent marriages, if they were still infectious.

As with the men, the treating that did happen was in Tuskegee, in Birmingham, and in other cities when the families moved. The Rapid Treatment Center in Birmingham provided treatment for "Robert Jones's" wife, in 1949. "David Houston's" wife received treatment from a doctor in Lima, Ohio. But the wife of "Theodore Harrison" was not tested. "William Green's" wife was treated at the Macon County Health Department (he was counted as a syphilitic, but the record suggests that he may not have been).[96] Charlie Pollard asserted, "You know some of them thought the wives got something but the wives didn't get nothing."[97] But the medical records contradict this view. In 1952, Charlie Pollard's first wife was reported to have been treated at the same Rapid Treatment Center in Birmingham that he never got to.[98]

The medical records reveal the hardship of living and birth—miscarriages and deaths of children abound (whether from syphilis is not clear). If women were treated, as the PHS claimed, they could have become reinfected if the men were still contagious. After the Study ended, the government admitted that "there is ample proof that a sizable percentage of wives became infected after their husbands entered the study."[99] Even then Nurse Rivers maintained that "it was always the policy of the V.D. Control program in Macon County to treat any infected wife or child of the study participants."[100] By the time the CDC finally counted, 89 out of the 180 wives who were still alive and were tested were positive on the serologies, although some of them could also have been treated and remained seropositive.[101] Nevertheless, this number is sobering to consider.

The effect on the children is even more complicated. The CDC "guestimated" that the syphilitic participants "had a total of 1035 children," averaging 3.13 living children for each man.[102] Of the 68 records that indicated examination of the children, only 4 were treated before the Study ended. This does not tell us how many of these acquired the disease through their mothers, however, or whether their mothers became infected through their fathers.

Some of the physical and emotional toll for the families emerged after 1972, as did the pain of even discussing it. In September 1973, more than a year after the Study became public and the "initial examinations and treatment of the consenting participants . . . [had been] nearly completed," the CDC turned its attention to "identify[ing] any spouses or children who might have been infected as a result of not treating infected study participants." In the lawsuit, Gray collected affidavits from at least one wife who claimed her syphilis and that of her child came from the lack of treatment of her husband.[103]

As the lawsuit was playing out in 1973, the CDC realized that it was impossible to gain "adequate medical history" from the wives and children of what the CDC believed were "439 syphilitic study participants (whether now dead or alive)" so as "to distinguish a congenital infection in a 'child,' attributable to withholding treatment from a father, from an acquired infection having no relationship whatsoever to the infected father." Sencer, the CDC's director, recommended that anyone positive (regardless of how they acquired the infection) be treated and provided with comprehensive lifetime medical care, given all the complications that syphilis could cause, a policy he believed would possibly mean federal responsibility for "75 spouses and 150 children" for the rest of their lives.[104] In trying to argue its side in the lawsuit a year later, however, the CDC's lawyer claimed that "how and when they had contracted or discovered they had it" would have to be considered on a case-by-case basis.[105] Sencer's promise to treat every wife and child who was positive prevailed. In the end, this "lifetime benefit" of medical and then health benefits went to "22 wives, 17 children and 2 grandchildren."[106]

Confusion over what happened to the women continued. Three years after the Study ended, a prisoners' rights group in Philadelphia was querying why the Study had been done *only* on "black women." Once again, Sencer explained that women "were excluded [from the original Study] . . . to prevent occurrence of congenital syphilis." And he declared that "the women . . . found to be infected were offered treatment, as were all the males with recently acquired infections."[107] Bill Jenkins, the CDC epidemiologist who tried to have the Study stopped in the late 1960s and who then ran the medical care program for the survivors and their families, more openly stated twenty years later that "some family members became so distrustful of the Government that they refused to be tested for syphilis." And, as a reporter looking into what happened to the families found, "no effort was ever made to track down sexual partners of the men, other than their wives."[108]

Being caught up in the Study's vise became part of narrative explanations for illnesses. Children of infected wives who developed chronic ills sometimes blamed the Study. Men and women who had been to the Rapid Treatment Center in Birmingham thought they had been given syphilis rather than treated for it. Individuals who had lived in Macon County at some point between 1932 and 1972 wondered whether they had been involved in it. Until the actual names became public in the late 1990s, and even after that, the Study functioned as an explanation for a wide variety of health problems.[109]

Victims to Survivors with "Quiet Courage"

"We are all full, red-blood American citizens, full grown men," Herman Shaw declared. "They should have told us." Albert Julkes Jr., the son of one of the men and the nephew of two others, recalled, "I listened to my father talk about this . . . and what sticks out is the falsehoods that they were told."[110] His Uncle Warren, Julkes remembered, "spoke very little" about the Study. But he knew "he was cheated through trickery and [hurt] for others to know that. Uncle Ephrom didn't feel as tainted."[111]

In listening to what the men said, one senses that the assault on their sense of self was almost worse than what might have happened to them physically, a betrayal that was deep and abiding. It did not matter whether they were controls or syphilitics: they all felt that they had been "had" and harmed. On a video documentary, even decades after it ended, Ernest Hendon, a control and the last man in the Study to die, captured this sense when he said, "I never could understand what it was about," as the camera panned his fingers moving achingly back and forth against one another.[112] For these churchgoing, aging, and primarily married men, it was clearly difficult to answer these strangers who descended upon them to ask the most personal of questions and to tell them that they had been lied to and deceived for decades.

Searching for men to make the story real, the reporters wanted to know what it *felt* like. The initial media blitz was a shock, and the individual men who had been identified were mortified by the attention. Who would want to fit either stereotype—of a sexualized black man or of an innocent who had been taken advantage of by his government? Johnny Ford, Tuskegee's first black mayor, who had risen out of the community's working class, decried the Study as an issue in his first campaign in 1972.[113] As writer Tom Junod found by 1993, "It is hard to meet a person in Tuskegee who did not have some acquaintance, by friendship or lineage or simple proximity, with one of the men involved in the Study."[114] Their community, their Tuskegee—with its proud history of the institute, the science of George Washington Carver, the World War II airmen, and as the site of the gerrymandering Supreme Court case, a major fight over school desegregation, and the birthplace of civil rights icon Rosa Parks—began to mean something very different in the American vernacular.

It was not easy to acknowledge involvement. It would take several years before all the survivors could be found and even longer to find the nearly 6,000 heirs who would receive some of the settlement money.[115] Not everyone wanted to be part of the lawsuit, however, nor wanted to have the free treatment that the CDC finally began to offer.[116] Even in 1972, decades after the campaigns to make it at least acceptable to discuss syphilis, this was not personal information anyone wanted discussed.

Asked if there was a negative reception to the men in their communities, attorney Fred Gray wrote: "Few adverse reactions were reported to me. . . . The men themselves were generally accepted without stigma."[117] But Dr. Howard Settler, a Tuskegee ophthalmologist who had been seeing men with the ocular complications of syphilis, reported in 1972 that "his patients have great personal pride and consider the diagnosis of syphilis stigmatizing." In setting up a treatment program, Settler argued, "any program . . . must be structured in a manner such as not to make apparent to the community any distinctions of persons clearly identifiable as part of the Tuskegee Study."[118] They developed, in taking on the lawsuit, what Tuskegee's mayor, Johnny Ford, labeled "quiet courage."[119]

Others remained angry or made their peace. Interviews with the men's families provided example after example of how the men had been harmed, even if their stories did not match up to the medical records. Their relatives' participation explained to them why a man could "no longer hold his water" or became blind or short of breath.[120] Albert Julkes Jr. admitted that members of his family did not accept the attention his public discussion of the Study had brought.[121] Others wanted to know if their homes could become historical sites because of what had happened or saw this as fitting with other racist experiences, as they came to terms with the past.[122]

There was anger over deaths and illnesses that might have been prevented, but there was also the sense of betrayal by a government that had failed them. Herman Shaw talked about how they had thought that they were being treated and were being of service to something bigger than themselves. Charlie Pollard, having spent years in the civil rights struggle, understood what had happened in racial terms: "The white people worked against Tuskegee all their lives, all their lives you know about it, you know."[123] As the story then spun out, the men became every southern black man, their individuality lost and the crimes against them a measure of the depth of American racism.

As the story was told over and over, only the numbers kept being repeated. Any complexity of what might have happened—how some of the men might have gotten to treatment, the stages of their disease, the medical debate over penicillin for late syphilis, or whether they even had the disease—dropped away. "Tuskegee" became a metaphor, not an individual experience.[124] As aging victims of the Study, their sexuality became hidden and their agency denied. As Albert Julkes Jr. would claim, "We can no more forget this than we can forget slavery because it was just an atrocity in these United States."[125] And as historian Walter Johnson has argued for slavery, there was the "willful incapacity . . . to imagine a world in which enslaved people were anything other than the often fragile, sometimes resistant, but ultimately disposable vessels of slaveholders' [or in this case the doctors'] desires."[126]

Only with the documentaries that began to appear in the 1990s did some of the men resurface. Only with the federal apology in 1997 and the publication by lawyer Fred Gray a year later of all their names did they become individuals. When the state of Alabama expressed its regret for the Study in 2001, a reporter asked Ernest Hendon, then 94, "how he felt about being a victim of the study." He replied, "I survived. That's good."[127] By then, as in any group recovering from historical and political trauma, the men—both living and dead—had stopped being victims and had become survivors or participants. Only when what happened to them could be discussed did parts of the trauma begin to heal. But the pain and anger never really went away.[128]

No matter what the truths, the story of the men's "use and abuse" was spread widely, and the men would become linked to the larger story of black experiences in America. Herman Shaw put it clearly: "We want to be remembered."[129] The question became, however, in what way? Meanwhile, the doctors would only be remembered as monsters whose moral compasses had failed.

7

Why and Wherefore

The Public Health Service Doctors

If the Study's subjects and controls meld into one seemingly abject black man, the doctors become one amoral white man. Their military outlook and willingness to condemn others to death and debility is underscored by their formality in photographs, whether they are dressed in PHS uniforms with epaulets and brass buttons or are standing ramrod straight in business suits. Knowing about the Study, it is easy to read into their faces and stances an ethical myopia and a distance from the lives of the black men in work jeans whom they dealt with.[1]

With so many different doctors in and out of Macon County over the Study's forty years, it is hard to keep track of who came when, what they did, and why. All of them were focused on public health, not just medical research. Their culture required constant triage, political maneuverings, and the reality of limited funds. Rendering syphilis patients "noninfectious" and then cured if possible was the public health mission transferred from the realm of treatment to shape the questions for research. The ways in which "race" was read into the data, the research and treatment questions that syphilis posed, and the available treatment and resources changed over the Study's forty years.

Simply thinking of these doctors as following orders from the state and as blinded by the demands of science keeps us at a distance. It stops us from delving into how racial beliefs, medical uncertainty, and public health imperatives rationalize and transform one another. Exploring the meaning of research for public health, not just as dedication to science, gives us more insight into the doctors' thinking and the construction of their ethical sensibilities.

The increased findings from outside the Study that inadequate treatment could limit contagion and that sometimes not treating made sense affected their judgment. As the Study was beginning, a leading syphilologist reminded his colleagues: "The great ailment of modern syphilological practice is a lack of comprehension of the why and wherefore rather than the 'what to do.'"[2] It was this "why and wherefore" that was supposed to be answered by the Study.

The Hopkins Imprimatur

If the Study required the thinking of the "best men," then Joseph Earle Moore at Johns Hopkins University Medical School was one of the best of the best. Born in 1892 and trained at Hopkins, he became a close friend of Surgeon General Thomas Parran and a leading syphilologist. Moore's World War I army experiences turned his interests from psychiatry to venereal disease, and he gave his life to the study of syphilis.[3] He reflected: "But syphilis! — here was an infectious disease of most fascinating interest. . . . Its exquisite chronicity made it a problem . . . from womb to tomb, or from sperm to worm."[4] From 1929 to 1954 he headed Hopkins's famed "Department L," the euphemistic name, which he hated, that had been given the syphilis clinic on the assumption that the scientific name "lues venerea" would be known only to medical professionals and would thus hide its purpose from embarrassed patients.[5] Moore was considered, historian Harry Marks writes, a scientific "taskmaster" focused on studies whose "methodology" was above reproach. Anything less than the strictest research standards to Moore "was morally unacceptable."[6] His colleagues recognized his love of research and sent out a list of his publications, "in lieu of cards," when he died in 1957.[7]

A respected, exceptionally productive, and competitive academic researcher, Earle Moore, as he was known, was also remembered for his successful efforts to integrate Hopkins medical elite by supporting the granting of staff privileges to black physicians.[8] He was convinced from his research that, as he so famously wrote the PHS's Taliaferro Clark in 1932, "syphilis in the negro is in many respects almost a different disease from syphilis in the white."[9] He was relying on his own research as well as on a massive analysis in 1930 by colleague Thomas B. Turner of 10,000 cases from the Department L data, which concluded that racial and sex differences were visible in the disease.[10] The Hopkins numbers argued for greater cardiovascular complications in blacks, but Moore was also part of a debate on what might cause the various neurological symptoms in whites or blacks. He wanted more data.

Moore's focus was on latent syphilis, and he believed that those at this stage did not always do "so badly." Decades after he began his research and clinical practice, he declared: "At best, it is probably that he [the latent syphilitic] has only 1 chance in 4 of developing any serious trouble; at wors[t], not more than 3 chances in 10."[11] In the late 1940s, he supported a reanalysis of the Oslo Study data. It led to the conclusions published in 1955 that it might be closer to 4 chances in 10, but that nearly 60 percent of "*untreated syphilitics went through life with little or no inconvenience as a result of the disease* [italics in original]."[12]

Moore became concerned that all the heavy metals might make things worse. In a study of "long-term results" in his own clinic, he and his colleagues argued that in both black and white men and women "prognosis of truly latent syphilis is exceptionally good with relatively small amounts of treatment" and that perhaps all the drugs they gave were overwhelming their patients' bodies. Moore thought, before penicillin became available, that "a long standing infection in man cannot be eradicated, biologic cure cannot be achieved, by means of any form of treatment so far developed."[13] He shared fellow syphilologist John R. Stokes's concern over the importance of finding out "when and under what conditions inadequate treatment produces the strikingly satisfactory effects that it sometimes does."[14]

Moore believed wholeheartedly in treatment but wanted to make sure that it was the right kind and amount. As one of his memorialists described him, "Earle became a skeptic . . . early in his career" and always looked for evidence, even if it countered orthodoxy.[15] He began to be concerned that there was overtreatment, not undertreatment, especially for those in the latency stage, and that even small amounts of the arsenical drugs taken at the earliest stages could both stop infection and protect individuals later. He was aware of how differently individuals reacted to the drugs—cured in one case and not in another.

Even before the Study, Moore knew syphilis had to be a "life work," because researchers had to follow their "clinical material" through death and autopsy. This was the only way a researcher could escape the problem of "too many philosophical papers and not enough facts."[16] He knew it was difficult to keep patients coming back to the urban clinics for months at a time for treatment, let alone for years of follow-up, yet he seemed somewhat oblivious to the question of why. He expressed annoyance, for example, when a man in his clinic with neurosyphilis who kept vomiting from the drugs and who had had his skull drilled into on both sides chose not to stay in treatment.[17] Only a study that would "follow over a period of many years a large series of patients who have never received treatment," he thought, would tell them the disease's natural history, what was reinfection or relapse, and what could safely be left alone.[18] Although the textbooks repeated the early Oslo information as medical gospel, leading syphilologists were aware that the data were more muddled. And, as Moore declared in 1944, "only with a knowledge of the natural evolution of any disease process if untreated can one be sure that any type of treatment is successful in ameliorating the condition."[19]

The PHS's offer to provide "more facts" through the Study must have intrigued Moore's research mind and captured his great desire for more information.[20] In advice to the PHS's Taliaferro Clark, Moore laid out the elements of a good study, from sample size to demographics to specifics of the examinations and tests.[21]

Moore continued to be intrigued by the Study, even if there is some evidence that he doubted its scientific rigor. He assisted in the reading of the x-rays on the cardiovascular complications, adding his expertise to their analysis and questioning the findings. He continued to train some of the PHS men who were sent to Tuskegee. Despite serious misgivings on the scientific validity—in particular of the Tuskegee VA Hospital's J. Jerome Peters's paper on the autopsy results and his reading of the x-rays—Moore eventually published several of the 1950s Study reports in the medical journal he edited.[22] He must have had his doubts about the "morality" of the research methods, however, since he never cited any of the Study articles in his major textbooks.[23]

The issue of not treating or of lack of consent did not seem to have troubled Moore, since it was assumed that good researchers would know best at the time. During World War II and as the chair of the National Research Council's Committee on Venereal Disease, Moore supported *giving* gonorrhea to prison volunteers to study "chemical and chemotherapeutic prophylaxis" of the disease, in part because he and his committee did not think "inmates of 'institutions for the feeble-minded or insane' could offer meaningful consent to such a study." The debates he was part of during World War II thus make clear that the medical researchers knew this kind of deliberately infecting study could be "potential dynamite for those sponsoring it." They did think about what would count as "meaningful consent." But, as historian Harry Marks makes clear, they saw the politics of doing it a "public policy" issue but that it was up to the scientists to decide if it was "necessary."[24]

Moore, too, was tentative at first about penicillin and was probably aware that the Study was indeed what the PHS called "the last chance" to follow this many undertreated men, however flawed the work.[25] Penicillin posed a problem for Moore's life work. His skill as a diagnostician and researcher was wedded to syphilis as a chronic and complicated disease. The PHS researchers noted to one another a decade after his death that Moore had tried to stop the publication of the major paper on the seemingly miraculous killing effect penicillin had on the spirochetes that caused syphilis. But he did finally write about penicillin and syphilis as he revised his major text and turned his research attentions to other chronic illnesses.[26]

Even in 1956, as penicillin use became widespread and the year before he died, Moore waxed nostalgic over what was never learned about syphilis as the debate over the specifics of treatment continued in the literature.[27] He told a group of British physicians: "The biologically minded clinician regrets, however, that syphilis seems to be vanishing with most of its fascinating and more fundamental riddles still unsolved." Among the concerns Moore listed was "why do race and sex modify the course of the infection?"[28] Even with penicillin, Moore believed there still was "the impending loss of a partly won war against venereal disease."[29] The link between the need for scientific inquiry on a complex disease that posited such seeming differences intrigued Moore through his entire lifetime. In turn, his interest gave the PHS connections to the country's major medical school and support, even if not always positive, to the Study's continuation.

"The Boss and General": O. C. Wenger

If Moore's fascination with syphilis was with the facts and research, Oliver Clarence (O. C., as he signed his letters) Wenger of the PHS was concerned with more practical matters: how to deal with syphilis in the field. Although he was never actually in charge of the Study, Wenger provided it experienced leadership and medical expertise throughout the 1930s. Wenger was a logical choice to do this, as he was the PHS's most knowledgeable and "very conscientious and hard working" syphilologist on what he once described as "the regulation and control of the venereal menace."[30] Wenger would be sent numerous places during his career—Mississippi, Alabama, Arkansas, Illinois, Colorado, Puerto Rico, and Trinidad—to do battle on the PHS's behest against syphilis.

It is Wenger's words about the Study, "as I see it, we have no further interest in these patients *until they die* [underlining in original letter]," that symbolize the PHS's callousness.[31] Wenger's toughness and use of racist and derogatory language ("darkey," "colored," "ignorant," "unmoral and prodigal," "sex appetite") creates a sense of a coarse man who would not have cared whether or not black people were treated.[32] It is his brusqueness, for which he was well known, that epitomizes the hardened verbal racism of the PHS physicians. But such language does not capture his concern to eradicate syphilis in black communities.[33]

Wenger was born one of seven children, to a German American family in St. Louis on September 2, 1884. He went to medical school at St. Louis University in 1904 with the support of a doctor uncle and "much against the wishes of his father, who proposed that all his sons would follow in the machinery manufacturing business." After a few years in hospitals and the health department in St. Louis, he took the U.S. Civil Service examination and became a medical inspector in the Philippines Constabulary between 1912 and 1915. He learned early to work in conditions that were "primitive" and with people who did not share his view of medicine, as he was part of what was described by a fellow officer as "a unique and successful application of the principle of employing native infantry, officered by white men, in the subjugation of their own tribesman."[34] When he married upon returning to St. Louis, he tried private practice but clearly had neither the temperament nor the interest for what he thought of as "too tame . . . too confining."[35]

While in the army during World War I, as did Moore, he worked on issues of control of venereal disease in military bases in the United States and Europe. Joining the PHS after the war to continue the work on such diseases was a natural next step. Wenger had worked in conditions that would make the rural South seem tame. By the time he was sent to the South, he had already survived amoebic dysentery and malaria.

His PHS superiors, noting his stutter, "rough manners," and less than average rating on "tact," detailed him to a national survey in 1919 and then sent him to set up a clinic for indigent venereal disease sufferers in Hot Springs, Arkansas. Known as "the boss" or "the general" at the Hot Springs clinic, Wenger arrived at 5 A.M. and worked continuously, knew how to get tables built from lumber scrounged from other sources, and barked at patients and workers alike when, his daughter remembered, "things went against his direction." Patients were kept in nearby institutions, segregated by race, or found themselves on the streets or in "leased hotels and rooming houses" as they waited out what were initially yearlong treatments.[36]

Wenger knew how hard it was for the poor to get the drugs and care they needed. Over the fifteen years he spent in Hot Springs (1921–1936), he saw over "36,000 cases of syphilis." He began by "mixing the arsphen[a]mine in a wash basin and boasting of only one ten c.c. syringe," but by the mid-1930s he had worked with local physicians to build what became a "modern" center for venereal disease care.[37] Wenger had seen both the demand for treatment and the difficulties and expense of providing it. Like generations of physicians who have worked in under-resourced parts of the world, he was constantly making do and trying to determine who to help and how.[38] It was under Wenger's direction that the rapid treatment model, of providing drugs on a daily basis for a few months, came to be used.[39] And the PHS brought him into Mississippi in 1927 to survey syphilis in black communities. It taught him how to "march . . . into Negro churches" and to offer "FREE BLOOD TEST BY GOVERNMENT DOCTORS AND FREE ICE WATER" to obtain his patients.[40]

When the Rosenwald Fund money came through in 1930, Wenger was the obvious man for the PHS to call to begin the mass serological surveys and treatments throughout the six southern counties. He understood the necessity of using epidemiological findings to prove that there was even a problem. He knew how to draw blood under an oak tree and get it stored on ice until it could be shipped properly and how to make those who worked with him do what he wanted. He shared a belief, as one physician called it, in the "ritualistic orgy of bloodletting," which was a hallmark of mass testing.[41] "My idea of heaven," he is supposed to have said, "is unlimited syphilis and unlimited facilities to treat it."[42]

As a public health man, he came to the campaigns against syphilis with enormous energy and the faith of a true believer on a crusade. If Moore's dedication was to the god of medical research, then Wenger's was to the public health deities. Writing about Wenger in the late 1930s, the president of the Chicago Board of Health declared: "He has . . . what amounts to a feeling of evangelism and belief in his work for humanity, giving him that dynamic power and inspiration which we must have to carry out our work to a successful conclusion. Without that spirit all of the knowledge in the world is of no avail."[43] In the flamboyant language of microbiologist and popular writer Paul de Kruif, Wenger is supposed to have called the disease the "back-stabbing gangster among human pestilences."[44]

Wenger's primary focus was making sure the PHS treated those who could spread syphilis. As Surgeon General Thomas Parran had argued in 1938, a few shots of neoarsphenamine could stop infections but not cure an individual, serving as "a method of chemical quarantine which is as effective in preventing spread from person to person as is the physical isolation of a smallpox patient in a quarantine hospital."[45] But Wenger, Parran noted, understood the politics of treating: "Public health theory said, 'yes. The old syphilitic can't hurt anyone but himself. Concentrate on the infectious cases and try to slow up the spread.'" But Parran deferred to what he labeled "the practical psychology of Wenger," who told him, "No. Treat the old syphilitic with 'rheumatism,' give him the painless mercury rubs. He will feel better and will bring in the whole family for the treatment they need. Don't forget, they listen to their granddaddies."[46]

Thus, when Wenger was helping to organize treatment, he held the opinion that giving mercury rubs to the older patients was a public health "loss leader" to get to the real problem of those with infection.[47] Even when the Rosenwald Fund Demonstration Project was treating in Macon County, the workers did not provide intravenous heavy metals to everyone; they used only the old mercury rubs for those over 50 or with a 20-year history of the disease. Parran noted, "It was not good enough but even so, many infectious cases were eliminated and many person-to-person epidemics stopped."[48] As with the urban clinics and in campaigns in both Chicago and Baltimore, the focus was on the spread of the disease, not the treatment of someone who had lived with syphilis for years.[49] Even though there was an understanding that treated individuals might have reinfection or relapse, the focus was primarily on those in the early stages and keeping them in treatment.[50]

Wenger's understandings of syphilis were steeped in his racial beliefs about the prevalence of the disease. With more than a decade of experience of both treating and field research before he came to Macon County, Wenger saw syphilis as almost endemic to black lives.[51] It was this sense of "saturation" that provided the rationale that made the research seem ethical and necessary in the face of what we would now call "disparities."[52] It is not clear if Wenger also shared in the eugenic beliefs that African Americans had a racial propensity for the disease "located in the germ plasm" and that there was a biological basis for the supposed inability to control sexual urges.[53] He clearly assumed, however, that sexual pathology was part of black communities. Such understandings would help to ground his experiential sense of the disease's inevitability in poor African Americans.

As a public health physician with a venereal disease specialty, such ideas would not have kept Wenger from thinking that control and treatment in black communities were necessary. Making a triage decision to jump from public health treating of syphilis to a long-term experiment that denied treatment would not be such a big step. He agreed with the way Vonderlehr subsequently explained the Study to a local Alabama physician: "The Public Health Service already has on hand records of a fairly large number of Negroes who have been both adequately and inadequately treated for syphilis and it is our desire to use the untreated group now being examined in Macon County as a comparison to indicate the value of treatment."[54] He knew, as he would tell other PHS officials in 1950, that they were "not yet finding and treating all of the cases" of syphilis in the country. The Study, he felt, would let the "medical profession . . . 'Know for Sure' what happens if the disease is not treated."[55] At the same time, he was well aware that in Macon County they might have misdiagnosed some of the men. Writing to Raymond Vonderlehr from his stationing in Puerto Rico in 1941, he told him, "You will recall that while working together in Tuskegee we frequently found false positives" because other diseases affected the blood tests.[56]

His racist language and disdain, however, did not mean he fought to deny care in every situation, as his later work on massive treating programs in both Chicago and Trinidad attests. When he ran the PHS's treatment campaign in 1937 in Chicago he made sure that black people were treated for syphilis, since he assumed that African Americans could not be relied upon to use any form of prophylaxis. His "uncover and treat" Chicago campaign in black communities would be based on the assumption of the need to instill fear in the populace and power in the medical professionals to be allowed to treat. Wenger exuded moralizing, as historian Suzanne Poirier noted in her book on the Chicago effort, rather than acceptance of sexual behaviors and prevention.[57]

Wenger clearly saw that the Study would provide needed knowledge. He argued continually for more thorough follow-up and new ways to track the men. And, as a later report would document, he had every reason to believe that those in the Study with "acute syphilis and younger patients [were] treated and omitted at the start of study."[58] The Study was not an ethical dilemma for him since it was on a continuum of seemingly good public health practice.[59]

Although historians have debated whether or not there existed a sense of "truth-telling and consent seeking" in the medical tradition at the time that should have given the Study researchers pause, there were no structures that required it when Wenger was involved in these pre–World War II years. Although grand statements from major medical figures such as William Osler and Richard Cabot had declared truth telling a central requirement in nontherapeutic settings, the practice depended upon the researcher and institutional practices. As historian Susan Lederer has argued, there was talk of, but not regulation of, ethics in medical research.[60]

There were, in addition, legal precedents that gave the state the power to do what it thought necessary to preserve the public's health, even against the will of individuals.[61] Within the history of research overseen by the surgeon general, most famously Walter Reed's yellow fever experiments in Cuba at the turn of the century, there was a written consent and an outcry when several of those in the Cuban studies died after being deliberately infected.[62] But by the time the Study was organized, this knowledge had passed into lore, but not policy.

Wenger clearly saw the work of the Study as part of his service to public health and the men not as "citizen patients" but as citizen subjects who could be drafted into these roles by the state.[63] In doing so, Wenger and the other PHS researchers were allowing what historian Rebecca Herzig calls the "imagination of science as a sovereign subject" to "reorganize . . . time—a submerging of the individual's present life for the sake of the envisioned future of the collective body."[64] Wenger knew he was hiding the nature of the disease and the need for autopsies from the men in Alabama. Lumbar punctures were not, he knew, "the special treatment" he had promised them, and he understood the fear of autopsy in the community.[65]

The trust that was set up was among the doctors on a mission for the state, not between the physicians and the men. As in other national contexts, "useless bodies were rendered useful by being made usable in the national project of regeneration."[66] Wenger, ever the public health man doing battle against syphilis as a bacterial foe, never seems to have doubted the importance of what was being done, even when he knew how flawed it had become. Deception, when needed, could be harnessed to this cause.

The Post-Penicillin Explanations

When the PHS's John Mahoney and his colleagues made their announcement at an American Public Health Association meeting in October 1943 that penicillin could cure early syphilis, excitement that a few injections might end such a centuries-old scourge was "overwhelming" and "the audience burst into cheering applause."[67] But many of the older syphilologists were not so sure. What about reinfection? Could penicillin be used as a prophylactic? What about the dangers of the Herxheimer reaction, when the dying spirochetes produced toxins that might prove more dangerous than the dormant disease? "A decade or more [would be required] to know what penicillin does in syphilis," because the disease's "chronicity" meant that "longer periods of experimentation and observation" were needed.[68]

The Study's leadership in the search for facts in the post-penicillin era fell to two men—John C. Cutler and Sidney Olansky—men with differing temperaments and backgrounds. Born in Cleveland in 1915, Cutler trained at Western Reserve University Medical School, graduated in 1941, and joined the PHS a year later during the war. Sent first to the PHS's Venereal Disease Research Laboratory, he went on to do research in Guatemala and then in India. He completed his career as an international health expert on sterilization and family planning and as professor of population studies at the University of Pittsburgh's Public Health School. As Cutler aged, he developed white hair, a pinched visage to go with his piercing blue eyes, and a matter-of-fact doctor voice.[69]

Olansky, the son of Ukrainian immigrants and two years older than Cutler, did not so easily find his way to medical school after his undergraduate days at New York University. Turned down by Columbia because of its Jewish quota system, he went to medical school in Glasgow, worked for the PHS in Panama during World War II, and then in the rapid treatment centers. By 1950, when he was tapped to lead the Study in Tuskegee, he was running the Venereal Disease Research Laboratory for the PHS. Olansky remained in charge of the Study until 1955, although he recalled that he actually went to Tuskegee only twice. He went on to teach at Duke University and then to a major professorship at Emory in dermatology. He served for two terms as president of the American Venereal Disease Association and retired into private practice with his doctor sons until he died at age 94 in 2007.[70] Olansky looked more the genial family doctor, with wide cheeks, a boyish giggle, and a bowtie.[71]

Olansky's name appears on half of the Study's thirteen published reports; Cutler's appears on two. Their articles provide a narrative that hid the Study's fault lines. In one article, they documented that half of those in the Study who were assumed to have syphilitic aortitis before autopsy proved not to have it once their bodies were examined, but this did not lead to questioning of the analysis.[72] In other research, Olansky concluded that it was very possible to misdiagnose syphilitic cardiovascular disease.[73]

Despite written claims that the Study had not been changed by the "antibiotic era," Olansky and Cutler knew by 1955 that 7.5 percent of the men had been "adequately" treated and that another 22.5 percent were "inadequately treated."[74] They argued that the treating really did not "defeat" their data, although it was obvious that it already had.[75] Although their data could have supported a narrative of defeat and confusion, they refused to read it that way. Instead, they manipulated the statistics, leaving out the undertreated and treated men to claim that nothing had changed.

Olansky's reports reveal the commitment to timelessness. Charles Johnson's 1930 sociological survey provided the explanation for conditions in Macon County, even though it was now twenty-four years later, and Olansky would argue, after just short visits, that the men lived their lives in the same conditions with the same views of health care. To be sure, the poverty was still widespread and access to medical care was still difficult. Yet he did not analyze the difference made when the younger men moved to urban centers and when doctors treated others.[76] The PHS needed for time to stand still in the Study, and Olansky's reports emphasized this understanding.

Olansky assumed that the men in the Study were not being harmed. He explained in his articles and told the worried Count Gibson in his letters that he believed that the men were being cared for by Nurse Rivers and were sent to treatment when they needed it (just not for syphilis) and that they were better off than other African Americans.[77] Olansky labeled them "volunteers with social incentives," suggesting that he was ignoring what the incentives meant or that he did not know how they were recruited.

Difference was always the desideratum. When the Norwegian physician who reexamined the Oslo data was brought to Tuskegee, in 1955, Olansky wrote, "He saw, first hand, the remarkable socioeconomic and racial difference between the rural Alabama Negro farmers and the fair-skinned Norwegians whom he has been studying."[78]

Research mattered to both Cutler and Olansky, and their other medical research provides a way to view their commitment to the Study. "Research is the root from which effective control springs," Cutler told a group of public health nurses.[79] Olansky and Cutler, both of whom spent more time at the Venereal Disease Research Laboratory and on other research than in Tuskegee, seemed comfortable letting the men become data to measure against all the other research being done on penicillin, reinfection, and necessary treatment.[80]

Their knowledge of the debates over penicillin's usefulness in latent cases, especially in older patients, must have allowed them to believe that continuing the Study was acceptable. Discussions of studies done elsewhere, including their own, showed that the spirochetes persisted even in the face of "massive doses" of penicillin. Such research gave scientific validity to arguments that treatment at this point would not matter, even when the findings of their own studies often argued for treating.[81]

Cutler and Olansky were part of another infamous study, at New York's Sing Sing prison in 1955.[82] Concerned with examining both the problem of reinfection and penicillin's power, the Sing Sing researchers inoculated their "prison volunteers," some of whom had previously been treated for syphilis, with a very high level of the disease's spirochetes, watched for four months, and then provided penicillin. Other inmates, who had syphilis but had not been treated while in latency, were also watched to see if they reacted to the new disease challenge.

The Sing Sing study concluded that men who were left untreated with low levels of infection in latency could not become reinfected with contagious forms of the disease and were "resistant to superinfection."[83] The Sing Sing findings were meaningful: not treating during latency could protect new infections from occurring and preserve an individual's immunity to another bout of the contagious stage. Nontreatment could be a cure, not a problem. Explaining these findings ten years later, Olansky would write, "If treatment is given after latency is well established or *if the patient remains untreated*, considerable immunity to reinfection may remain [italics added]."[84] Even now, the Sing Sing data is used to show that "latent syphilis is associated with a strong and long lasting state of immunity and that active infection helps to maintain such resistance."[85]

Olansky's and Cutler's other research made it possible to carry these kinds of dual thoughts: 1) treatment would cure neurosyphilis or stave off cardiovascular disease; and 2) no treatment could prevent reinfection. Other research begun to study penicillin's limits, after the initial excitement in the 1940s, allowed this kind of duality of thinking to persist. Cutler did work on the Herxheimer reaction after the discovery of penicillin and was aware of the dangers of treatment.[86]

At an international conference in 1962 in Washington sponsored by the PHS, researchers were startled to learn "on the basis of these experimental findings that any amount of a penicillin treatment is unable to destroy all treponema if administered at a late stage of the infection."[87] In 1969, just before the discussion on continuing the Study took place at the CDC, yet another study on black patients in Alabama concluded that "there is good reason to believe that even sub-curative doses of treponemicidal drugs administered in the early phase of the disease will prevent serious cardiovascular aftermath."[88] In the face of these debates and research and their knowledge of how long the men had been infected, it was possible for them to have believed that penicillin would do little good.

Cutler's and Olansky's commitment was to the Study as a scientific endeavor. Olansky expressed this almost romantically in 1955 when he declared: "A quality of dedication to the ideal of a long-term study based upon love of and respect for the dignity of the individual within the group, and upon the satisfaction of making a single, valuable contribution to the increment of knowledge, without concern for credit, is fundamental and must exist in the research team."[89] Faced with strong group dynamics and a sense of importance, medical uncertainty allowed the Study to seem critical.

The Defense Continues

It is painful but possible to understand why these doctors defended their views in the 1970s after the Study was made a media spectacle. But how could they take the same positions twenty and thirty years later?[90] In the 1970s, most of the defenses these doctors mounted focused on how hard it was to keep patients in the treatment programs before penicillin and then on the view that penicillin would have made no difference to *most* of the men with cardiovascular complications by the time it was available.[91] Although some of the remaining PHS researchers continued to defend the Study when historian James H. Jones interviewed them in 1977, most of them had been silenced by the clamor against them.[92]

The twentieth anniversary of the Study arrived in the early 1990s, amid growing discussion about the distrust of medicine and the widening AIDS epidemic in the black community. ABC's *Primetime Live* and PBS's *Nova* revisited the story. Reporters went out to find both the surviving participants and the doctors. ABC's Jay Schadler first found the congenial "Dr. Sid," with his smiles and bowtie, still in practice in Atlanta with his sons. Then George Strait interviewed the cheerful Olansky and the more dour Cutler for PBS. "We're dying off, and we've borne this burden for years," Cutler told an Atlanta newsman, explaining why he agreed to the interviews. "We have an obligation to tell our story. Tuskegee was undertaken for the highest ethical reasons."[93]

In the *Nova* film, Cutler seemed angry that the Study had been, as he put it, "grossly misunderstood" and that providing penicillin would have "interfered" with it. He believed that the Study would have "improved care for the black community." He deeply opposed stopping it in the 1960s and kept to this position into the 1990s.[94] For Cutler, as with Wenger before him, it was the war against syphilis. And in war, he told a reporter, you know "some will die. It's in the interest of the total society. These men in Tuskegee helped us learn how to treat syphilis among blacks. They were serving their race." The men served, he said directly, as "controls for the entire race."[95]

Olansky, in "one nervous close-up after another," was straightforward in the *Primetime Live* segment. He told the millions of viewers that he had no "moral doubt" about the conduct of the Study. Most of the questions focused on how he saw the men, however, not the medical science. He recalled that they were "nice people" who were "not dumb just uneducated." Their "illiteracy," he commented, meant they "couldn't read newspapers" and did not know what was happening. But, he thought, "the rural black fears not being buried decently," so they "got what they wanted." When pushed by Schadler to admit that the Study was racist, he refused and noted that if there had been this much syphilis in a group of "hillbillies in West Virginia" they would have done the Study there.

When Schadler demanded to know why Study doctors did not provide penicillin when it became available, Olansky argued the science and that the Study would have been "negated." Schadler asked, "Wouldn't you have treated yourselves?" Looking more and more like a deer in the headlights, Olansky replied, "I don't know. . . . It is a trick question." The program, as edited, switched between interviews with participants Herman Shaw, Charlie Pollard, and Price Johnson, with a quick cameo by attorney Fred Gray, and then back to Olansky. After Herman Shaw talked about the pain and lack of respect, Schadler asked Olansky what had been learned. "Syphilis isn't too bad a disease," he replied.[96]

Olansky seems to have been unable to explain any of the medical reasoning behind the Study's failure to provide the men with penicillin, although these thoughts may have been cut from the film as too complicated for a lay audience. Six months after the show aired, Olansky told an Atlanta reporter: "Penicillin was not considered because it would not have helped these men." But the ABC audience never heard this. What they saw was a seemingly cheerful white doctor completely indifferent to suffering and without any sense of how racist and callous his remarks appeared. Olansky knew he had made mistakes on the show. "They made me look like a mad scientist and a bigot," he complained.

It did not stop there. Journalist Tom Junod profiled Olansky for an article titled "Deadly Medicine" in the magazine *Gentleman's Quarterly*, which was published after the ABC segment. By then, Olansky had received "hate mail, a bomb threat and angry phone calls." Fliers about his role in the Study were posted outside his office, and his name was taken off the Dermatology library in the department he had built up at Emory's medical school. "When I die," he told Junod, "my death certificate will say 'KILLED BY TUSKEGEE STUDY.'"[97] To Junod, Olansky tried to explain that, for the participants, "the damage was done" by the time penicillin came along. But Junod, too, made his medical explanation seem a cold rationalization.

Only after Olansky and his family watched the *Nova* segment on the Study did Olansky begin to put the pieces together about the deceptions. What he had ignored and thought was only a result of medical uncertainty became more real. His son Alan then wrote a letter to Emory's dermatologists explaining that Dr. Sid "finally realized that the patients in the study were deliberately and systematically deceived . . . [and] that the patients should have been given penicillin." It is not at all clear that Olansky changed his mind *because* he understood that the medical thinking in the Study was shaped by racial assumptions. But he did understand the deceptions, and he thought they mattered. As the blurb on his practice website stated, with no little irony, "Dr. Sid has many years of experience. He believes that patient education is a vital part of therapy, and that an informed patient is most likely to have the best outcome."[98]

Some of the younger PHS researchers involved in the Study did learn that medicine and race had not been separated. Don Millar, a white southerner, had come back to the CDC from the smallpox eradication projects in West Africa because he wanted to be part of the civil rights movement. He headed the CDC's Venereal Disease Division when the Study went public in 1972. He believed that the men had "burned out on syphilis and that the penicillin would not have been helpful." He also feared the possibility of Herxheimer reactions. He had seen a fellow resident when he was in training in Utah get into what he described as a "heap of trouble" when he gave penicillin to an asymptomatic syphilis patient, who then died in the emergency room.

Millar began to perceive, right after the story of the Study broke, why this kind of medical understanding would be buried in a racial uproar. He was taken aside by colleagues in the Atlanta area who explained to him how the Study was being seen in local black communities. He went to an event at Atlanta University to discuss the Study as a representative of the CDC. He "got" that it would be impossible to get the story "right" just on medical grounds.[99] Millar came to see that the interconnections among biological assumptions about race, cultural assumptions about race-based behaviors, and medical exploitation could not be separated from medical ideas and practices.

David Sencer, the CDC's director, understood what had happened. "No one wanted to treat from a medical standpoint since there was no hard and fast rule about treating those with inactive tertiary disease," he recalled in 2005, decades after the Study ended. "But if we stopped it [the Study] they would not have been helped, they would have gotten none of the death benefits." But Sencer agreed that the PHS had not thought about the rights of the men to make this decision, and once the story broke, he advocated saying what the doctors really thought and not just "spin."[100]

Medicine and Race, Racism and Medicine

"The Tuskegee Study" connected race, medicine, and racism. A belief that the disease needed to be understood—and that it was different in whites and blacks—began the Study. The public health practice of focusing primarily on the infectious blinded the researchers to the problems of those in latency. Questions about whether treatment was needed in late latent syphilis were debated. Moore, who was sure they were overtreating, even before penicillin, clearly influenced the thinking of those at the PHS.[101] And the many studies that came in as penicillin became more widespread brought a number of concerns about whether giving penicillin mattered once the spirochetes had buried themselves into various organs and tissues of the body.

Penicillin—in policy and in practice—was given out. But the PHS researchers wanted to really understand the disease. The spirochetes they saw swimming in their microscopes, even after penicillin was given to rabbits and humans alike in numerous other studies, mattered to them as scientists. This allowed them to rationalize the lack of continued treating in the Study.

The doctors failed to consider that assumptions about race had made the Study seem both needed and "natural" to do in Macon County. Their distance from the concerns of racism and mistreatment within the black community blinded them to the ways that their medicine would be read. They saw politics as something completely separate from medicine. Their policies and the ways they thought about race's seemingly biological impact were built into their science, and their actions and public health perspective kept them from thinking about the individual men. In the face of their continued belief in the Study's medical necessity, they seared the image of the amoral white doctor when faced with a black patient or subject into collective memory.

8

———

Triage and "Powerful Sympathizing"

Eugene H. Dibble Jr.

"The results of this study will be sought after[,] the world over," Tuskegee's medical director, Dr. Eugene H. Dibble Jr., promised Tuskegee Institute leader Robert Russa Moton in 1932. Dibble's words were to be prescient in ways he could not have imagined.[1] Certainly he did not expect the name of his beloved institution to be forever linked with ethical failure and racism in research. Dibble understood the ways of Tuskegee Institute to his core, and he used his position to cajole, organize, and provide for those under his care. As an indefatigable race man, Dibble devoted his life to improving health care for all African Americans. Why then would he agree to the Study?

No one ever asked Dibble this question publicly, because he died in 1968, four years before the Study made national news.[2] Those who have tried to explain Dibble's position either fall back on the assumption that he knew nothing—another duped innocent in a clear black-and-white story— or else paint him as a race traitor or accommodationist willing to sell out his patients for professional advancement or misguided values. In reality, Dibble's motives remain a mystery. Was he, as Tuskegee Institute's founder is seen, "both 'sage' and 'wizard'; shrewd and candid; selfless and self-centered; race man and race traitor?"[3] A naïf he was not: the surviving letters make it clear that Dibble understood what the Study was about and supported it until his death. The PHS wrote to him, and to Nurse Rivers through him, for nearly four decades. His "why and wherefores" for participation in the Study demonstrate the tie between racial politics of the seemingly possible and medicine.

Son of the South

Eugene Heriot Dibble Jr. spent his entire career at either the Tuskegee Institute hospital or the VA Hospital where the men of the Study were examined and autopsied. He arrived in 1920 when he was 27 years old, following his internship at Freedmen's Hospital in Washington, D.C., to become the assistant to medical director John Kenney Sr. at Tuskegee Institute's John A. Andrew Memorial Hospital. He left "John A.," as it was known in the community, to spend two years at the VA Hospital in the early 1920s. When Kenney departed in the mid-1920s, Dibble returned to John A. to replace Kenney as the medical director. Dibble stayed until 1936, when he left to run the VA Hospital for ten years. In 1946, he returned finally to John A.'s leadership, keeping this position for nearly two decades, until shortly before his death, when his worsening cancer forced him to retire. He saw the hospital through the depths of the Depression and into the civil rights era.

This "son of the South," as Howard University labeled him when he was given their Alumni Award in medicine, was born in Camden, South Carolina, in 1893, educated at Atlanta University and then at Howard's medical school, and took postgraduate courses at Harvard.[4] Dibble came from a distinguished and prosperous black family with a history of several generations of literacy and education.[5] In 1926, Dibble married Helen Taylor, the daughter of MIT's first black graduate who was also the illustrious architect of many of the Tuskegee campus buildings.[6] This wedding linked Dibble to the faculty aristocracy.

A chain-smoking, tall man with a determined face and tired eyes, Dibble was a force to be reckoned with in the medical world, both in and outside of Tuskegee. Striding around his hospital, he was "affectionately known as the doctor who each night puts to bed all patients at the hospital . . . and returns the next morning to greet patients with a cheerful smile."[7] His was an esteemed presence, hard to ignore, and he inspired deference and respect. "Dr Dibble is a wonderful man—just the kind of doctor I like—he's powerful sympathizing," Macon County resident Irving Harris told an interviewer in 1930. Three decades later, a former patient sent a few dollars to his hospital as a contribution and wrote: "We just love Dr. Dibble. One indeed has to be very human to earn that phrase."[8] He could also be difficult, but he respected those who could argue clearly with him.[9]

As with all the other Tuskegee faculty and staff of his time, Dibble spent his life within the confines of a strict segregation system. Lynching was the starkest reminder of the danger. Just months before Dibble came to Tuskegee, two black men were lynched in nearby Montgomery County, another just after Dibble took the institute position. There were thirteen recorded lynchings in Alabama in the years between Dibble's arrival in 1920 and the beginning of the Study.[10] Dibble was on the campus when the fight over the VA Hospital erupted and the Ku Klux Klan marched.[11] When the Reeltown shootout between sheriff's deputies and the organizers of the Sharecroppers' Union occurred, Dibble treated one of the injured sharecroppers and was then quoted in the local paper as explaining the man's actions. It was to be just one example of Dibble's role as a racial spokesman, translating actions of the black working class to the white world.[12]

Despite his education and authority, Dibble, as with every other African American in the county, dealt daily with the culture of humiliation that sought to keep whites in power. A drive around Tuskegee's main square would bring him into contact with the Daughters of the Confederacy's statue built to honor their "War between the States" dead.[13] Because it was segregated, he would not have been allowed to walk across the square.[14] Just a few months before the Study began, the Tuskegee News reported on the local entertainment: the "Moonlight Cabaret Minstrels . . . played to a capacity house" as "Cliff Stewart Jr. of Opelika gave an impersonation of Al Jolson that was very credible indeed." To finish off the evening, "Plantation Melodies were sung by Miss Elna's Black Boys."[15] In 1958, when Dibble was about to go on a medical vaccination project to Liberia, the funds were almost pulled because it was assumed by the trip's funders that Dibble "was not fit to carry the banner of American goodwill to the people of Africa."[16] To survive this, Dibble practiced with precision the "politics of deference" and stood his ground when needed.[17]

On the campus, dominated by the statue of Booker T. Washington and the impressive buildings designed by Dibble's father-in-law, however, it was possible to create a separate existence. Within the institute's confines and that of the black doctor world, this medical "wizard" focused on doing whatever he could to improve the lives of those he cared for and to break down the walls of segregation. His massive correspondence reflects the work of a man devoted to cajoling, arguing, and organizing for change and respect. He worked ceaselessly to bring federal programs, research, and health care programs to his community. With his connections and contacts, he could have left Tuskegee for other black hospitals and medical schools. But he stayed in Alabama and did what he thought possible.

Dibble practiced his careful politicking inside and outside of the institute. He continually nudged its presidents to improve conditions in the hospital and to direct scarce funds his way. In keeping with Booker T. Washington's requirements for hands-on control, Dibble sent Moton and his successors daily reports on the hospital census, the condition of patients, and the lists of what needed to be fixed. He kept Moton apprised of the white physicians who came to the John A. Andrew Clinics and told him which ones had useful political connections.[18] His correspondence shows the ways he tried to make white physicians see the immorality of segregation and its effect on black lives.[19]

The endless search for funds became even more difficult as the Depression deepened and demands on the hospital increased. Conditions in Macon County were calamitous by the 1930s, and not much better at Tuskegee Institute. In 1933, Dibble told Moton that if they didn't fix the floors in John A. a "serious accident may happen."[20] That year Moton had to cut the school's annual budget by more than 20 percent.[21] Dibble was clearly worried about how he was going to provide care as more and more indigent patients showed up at his door. The hospital was a private institution set up to care for the institute's faculty, staff, and students, but it was now serving a wider and wider swath of Alabama's black population, caring for patients from nearly half of the state's counties.[22]

The Tuskegee Institute, as well as its hospital, lived on the largesse of white philanthropy and carefully cultivated connections to the federal and state governments. Its leaders had to scrimp and continually search for support and funds. Given the overwhelming needs of the community, Dibble focused on finding ways to pay for improved clinical care. In the 1930s, a high-risk-pregnancy program for indigent women was created. With support from the National Foundation for Infantile Paralysis, a special center for the rehabilitation of polio patients was built and expanded into a multipurpose adult rehabilitation center two decades later.[23] By the 1940s, the pregnancy program had been expanded into a special obstetrical wing of the hospital, and a decade later a mental health center would be added.[24]

Even when the Depression ended, the demands did not.[25] Dibble would tell a national commission in 1953 that there were "almost a million Negroes" in Alabama and "less than 85 Negro doctors in the whole State."[26] Writing to the director of the Alabama Health Department's Maternal and Child Health division in 1961, Dibble cited a case of a severely ill pregnant woman from a nearby county who was refused admittance to a hospital that was nearer to her home because "the local hospital would not admit colored patients." He recounted, "Of course, while we have no money, we rather felt that we had to take her, and it just points up the problem that exists." Dibble wrote that when he told a local health official that he would take the young woman everyone involved with the case cried.[27]

As Dibble administered his hospital and served his patients, he was always conscious of the ways the hospital had to relate to the white community and to white physicians in particular. Writing to the institute's president, Frederick D. Patterson, in 1936, as he prepared to leave to become the medical director at the VA Hospital, he reminded Patterson of the skills a new leader at John A. would need: "Our hospital," he wrote, "is just a little different from most any other hospital in America because most of the cases that are referred to us are referred by white doctors; so that, the man who takes this place, if you are not to be embarrassed, must be one who can work with the rural white physician and put the program over, and, at the same time, maintain the respect and confidence that is necessary in the administration of this work."[28] Dibble was right about the difficulties at John A. Less than two decades after he died, the institute could no longer continue to subsidize the care, as demand also decreased. The hospital closed and to this day has not been replaced.[29]

The Clinical Society and Backwaters

Dibble witnessed what one historian described as the "numbing and often destructive impact" of medical and social segregation, which left many black doctors in backwaters without a "sense of professionalism and settled into careers marked by sloth, factiousness and in some cases, outright exploitation of patients."[30] Since the AMA did not officially desegregate until 1968, the year that Dibble died, providing a place for black physician camaraderie and continuing education fell to the National Medical Association, to Howard and Meharry medical schools, to some northern medical schools, and to what became the John A. Andrew Clinical Society.[31] In the early 1920s, Dibble worked with John A. Kenney Sr. to build up the Clinical Society and to bring both black and white physicians to Tuskegee for clinics and teaching. As his Howard alumni citation noted, "Long since[,] you discovered how quickly in medicine the certain knowledge of today can become the outmoded practice of tomorrow. You knew, because you had seen with your own eyes how rapidly a man of promise in the field of medicine can die professionally, a victim to segregation in a small town of the South."[32] To avoid this, Dibble remained committed to the training and retraining of black physicians through the Clinical Society.

At the annual events, black physicians became apprised of the latest findings, and specialists were provided for black patients who otherwise would not be seen. The numbers reflected his labors. At the twenty-fifth anniversary meeting, 181 doctors and surgeons were on hand for eleven daily clinics that led to the hospitalization of 102 patients and "52 major and 83 minor operations." The scientific meeting attracted nearly 1,800 people, and the public health portion brought in 2,000.[33]

Dibble believed in scientific progress and its link to what was then called "racial betterment." As he explained the role of the Clinical Society in a confidential letter to the institute's president in 1935: "I think we can say without flattering ourselves, that it is conceded by all concerned that this is the outstanding scientific development that we have in Negro medicine. . . . It gives the Negro doctor an opportunity for Post Graduate Work with these high type men whom he could probably not get an opportunity to see work in any other place. Then too, it gives the white surgeon an opportunity to see Negro surgeons operate[,] which Negro surgeons he would probably not see otherwise. This makes for mutual good will and makes, also, for very fine inter-racial cooperation."[34]

In its first decades, the Clinical Society concentrated on providing clinics for treating "unusual" cases and on showcasing the talents of black doctors. By the late 1930s, the focus had shifted toward what Dibble labeled a more "didactic program involving exchange of the latest ideas and developments in the field of health."[35] "He knew everybody," John A.'s administrator Mike Rabb remembered. Dibble arranged for famous white physicians to come to the institute for the meetings and clinics.[36] As part of his effort, he let the PHS explain to the Clinical Society what it was doing in the Study or give talks on syphilis.[37]

Dibble also tried to ensure that presentations at the Clinical Society meetings were of high enough caliber to warrant publication. W. Montague Cobb, Howard University professor, president of the National Medical Association, and editor of its journal, appreciated Dibble's endeavors. In nominating him for a National Medical Association award, he wrote: "Through Dr. Dibble's unceasing effort the scientific quality of the John A. Andrew Clinical Society meetings has been so steadily improved that nearly all presentations made there come to be submitted in manuscript form to the Journal. This represents colossal effort."[38] Without the Clinical Society, the skills and knowledge of many rural black physicians would have been even more limited.[39]

The Institute and Research

Dibble understood that his hospital and Tuskegee Institute needed to provide research opportunities as well as clinical care and up-to-date education. Agricultural research had been central to the institute's work, especially under the auspices of George Washington Carver and later the Carver Research Foundation. Dibble carried this tradition into medicine and his hospital. The institute was the site in the mid-1950s of a cell culture lab to produce massive amounts of HeLa cells to be used in field-testing the Salk polio vaccine.[40] Dibble's cooperation made blood serum from a number of the students available in 1957 for a study on human gamma globulin to be used to cure rabies. In 1963, he arranged to work with the Population Council to provide patients for a study on intrauterine devices (IUDS).[41] From early in the institute's history, Tuskegee's leaders based their efforts on the concept that research, improvement of conditions for African Americans, and contributions to science were linked.

When the offer came from the PHS to work on the Study, especially in its first stage, when some treatment was being provided, it would have been understandable for Dibble to sign Tuskegee Institute up. In circumstances in which every penny counted, the need for medical care was overwhelming, and the economic crisis and racism was limiting everything, Dibble agreed to research in order to gain resources for his underserved population.[42]

He most likely assumed that the men were no longer contagious, and thus this kind of triage to get help must have seemed appropriate to him. Dibble knew that syphilis stigmatized and labeled the black community. He kept copies of important studies on syphilis, stayed abreast of treatment options, and gave talks on the problems of venereal disease throughout his career.[43] It would have been in his hospital's interest to understand it and to see what kind of treatment would really be needed.

This was one more way to bring education to his interns, residents, and attending physicians. It would get the federal government to pay for identifying other illnesses in the men as Rivers brought them in or took them to the health department. The Study provided specialists for the people Dibble had to care for, a continuation of what he had been doing through the Clinical Society each year.[44] When a member of the institute's staff was diagnosed with a syphilis-caused heart complication, for example, Dibble had the PHS's Vonderlehr look in on him.[45]

Through his national contacts, Dibble continued to find ways to bring treatment to Tuskegee in the forms of research. He made this clear when he wrote to Alabama's head of hospital planning in 1960 to argue that his hospital's connection to various state agencies "has the possibility of being expanded in the future, in not only serving a real purpose in developing the health needs of the people but in using this clinical material as a source of teaching."[46] His connection to John R. Heller, one of the PHS physicians in Tuskegee in the 1930s, continued long after Heller left the Study. In 1957, Dibble worked with Heller, by then the director of the federal National Cancer Institute, to develop a cancer center at Tuskegee. As he told a friend in a letter: "Of course, I understand from Dr. Heller that the only funds that can be obtained from the American Cancer Society and the National Institute of Health are for research. He is in hopes, however, that we can get some private firms who would be willing to provide the necessary funds for hospitalization of the cases that we would need to hospitalize. A similar situation was worked out when he and I together with Dr. Vonderlehr worked out the syphilis control problem."[47]

Cooperation with the PHS research meant working with the Macon County Health Department as well. In 1934, when it appeared that the state would stop funding Macon County's public health unit, public health officer Murray Smith appealed to Dibble for help from the institute. Every dollar mattered. Dibble concurred, explaining to the institute's Robert Moton that the health unit "has done all of our Wassermann tests, all of our malarial slides and our sputum's. . . . It has furnished us the supplies, such as test tubes, culture tubes for Diphtheria smears, materials, such as vaccines for use in inoculations against Diphtheria and typhoid and Smallpox . . . and just now, has approved of a plan by which all of our leaching ditches from our sewage disposal plant will be drained. . . . It has saved us many dollars in the eradication of epidemics and the saving of lives." Tuskegee should be willing to contribute $25 a month to keep it going, Dibble concluded in his argument.[48]

Not everyone knew about the Study at John A., but Dibble was not alone. When he left for the VA Hospital in 1936, John A.'s acting medical director, Joshua W. Williams, discussed the Study in his report to institute president Patterson. Williams, who later spoke with AP reporters and testified in front of the federal panel investigating the Study to denounce it, clearly understood the significance of the Study then. He called it "the study of untreated Syphilis in Macon County." He explained how the Study had been discussed at an American Medical Association meeting and in its journal, with "due credit . . . to the John A. Andrew Memorial Hospital as well as its staff, for its collaboration in this work."[49] Dibble's colleague J. Jerome Peters performed men's x-rays and autopsies until he retired in 1965; at that time, Dibble helped find his replacement.[50]

By the 1950s, when Dibble reported on the Study as part of the work of John A., however, the title was more circumspect: "the U.S. Public Health

Service study of syphilis in the Negro male in Macon County." Dibble added that the hospital's cooperation meant that the "600 patients [are given] a complete physical examination, including chest X-rays, electrocardiograms ... and repeat serologic testing."[51] Although the existence of the Study was never hidden in this report, the word "untreated" was now left omitted. By the 1950s, it is possible that Dibble was trying to keep the true nature of the Study from the institute's authorities, even though the checks for the autopsies kept arriving in the comptroller's office at the institute.[52] By including the Study in this report, he demonstrates his commitment to it and to the process of research.

A Race/Science Man

Dibble was a race man—committed to the improvement of conditions for African Americans. But he was also a science man—dedicated to research to cure the multiple ills he saw around him. For Dibble—as a doctor, Tuskegee stalwart, and administrator—race and science were not separate concerns. As with other African American scientists in this period, Dibble wanted the social and economic factors that led to what we would now call racial disparities in disease incidence acknowledged. He shared the beliefs of other black leaders that empirical information was needed to disprove racist assumptions.[53]

He certainly understood the impact of racism on health. During World War II, a disturbed soldier was sent to his VA Hospital. In a news story, the reporter noted that the man "had become very upset as a result of the Army forcing him to do menial work, including 'picking up papers' at the white officers' quarters. The Tuskegee doctors prescribed a simple and effective treatment: His transfer to radio work. Quickly, he improved."[54]

Dibble may have been a race/science man, but he was not a researcher. His name appears on only one research article (and that one not about the Study). He did not write about his understandings of racialism, that is, the belief in racial differences.[55] We can only guess at some of his understandings—from the articles he clipped, his correspondence, and his links to others who did research. As with his close colleague and friend, Howard University's W. Montague Cobb, and as with Chicago's Provident Hospital's Julian Herman Lewis (the first black Ph.D. in physiology), Dibble understood that there was a different "racial susceptibility" to disease, although whether he thought there was something that could be labeled "Negro blood," which Cobb disputed but Lewis thought possible, is not clear. While Dibble never went as far as Lewis, who called for an "anthropathology" to link disease and racial groupings, he did see difference—but not deviance—along racial lines.[56] Given what Dibble was reading and concerned about, it is clear that he believed that research on the response of African Americans to disease was critically important.[57] He was struggling to understand what might be different disease patterns in African Americans.

Dibble's support for research on neurosyphilis done at the Tuskegee VA Hospital demonstrates his concerns. Syphilis was believed to be one of the causes of the neurological disorders that led black veterans to seek care. Three years before the Study began, the VA Hospital pathologist at the time, H. A. Callis, argued that the assumption that syphilis was more prevalent in "Negroes" was false. He thought, rather, that darker skin pigmentation only marked some lesions more visibly. He did not believe that the disease distinctions between blacks (of any skin tone) and whites were caused by any underlying biological differences.[58]

Dibble supported research done by physicians at the Tuskegee VA Hospital on the use of malarial fevers as a cure for neurosyphilis to see if this standard cure of the time worked as well with black patients.[59] It was the current medical wisdom that African Americans were already either genetically immune to malaria or carried a heavy load of the parasites because the disease was endemic in southern black communities.[60] Major textbooks repeated the belief, based on observational studies, that the more commonly used tertian strain of malaria would thus not be effective on black patients. The only caveat, the medical wisdom repeated, was the patient's skin pigment. As one key 1932 textbook's authors explained, this resistance to tertian malaria could be overcome "the lighter or closer to the Caucasian the particular Negro is."[61]

Dibble clearly thought that finding appropriate treatment for black neurosyphilitics was of grave import, even if the PHS doctors were assuming there was less neurosyphilis of any kind in African Americans. At the Tuskegee VA Hospital, with nearly 1,500 patients, with both general medical and neuropsychiatric illnesses by 1940, 30 percent of those in the latter category suffered from what he labeled "organic disorders, such as brain syphilis and chronic encephalitis."[62] In a 1940 address to VA hospital administrators, Dibble expressed his focus on this problem and his hospital's role in finding a solution.

Dibble was disturbed that for many years they had been unable to help those with "syphilis of the brain and spinal cord . . . by means of the modern and accepted method—malaric therapy—as Negro patients did not respond to the tertian strain of malaria fever." He believed that there were differences between whites and blacks in the disease, although he never stated clearly *why* he thought this.[63] Given that many black physician researchers who were his professional colleagues thought that differences were probably due to differences in historical exposures of different racial groupings to disease, it can be surmised that Dibble understood biological difference but not whiteness as the "norm"—as a natural reality. Research on this topic would not be anathema to a physician like Dibble, one so focused on finding the right cures for African Americans.

Dibble reported in 1932, the same year that the Study began, that "through the exhaustive study and research of our Assistant Clinical Director, it was found that by the use of the quartan strain of malaria—a foreign strain to which the Negro patient had not developed an immunity—gratifying results could be obtained . . . and beneficial results began to be achieved." The hospital, he concluded, had since "treated more than five hundred cases, with a large proportion of complete recoveries and returns to gainful employment." This success was recognized within the VA system, and the Tuskegee hospital "furnished blood to many other Veterans Administration Facilities and to numerous State institutions. The development of the quartan strain for use in treating neurosyphilis among Negroes," Dibble concluded, "is one of our most interesting accomplishments; and we are just proud that we have been able to rehabilitate so many patients through this more modern method of therapy."[64]

In these studies, the differing malarial strains were compared to the older use of the arsenical drugs.[65] His support for this kind of research suggests that Dibble was deeply concerned with finding treatment for syphilis and very aware of the limitations of the arsenicals. He had seen in the wards of the VA Hospital the dangers of neurosyphilis and the failure of the older treatment forms. It seems reasonable that the PHS's suggestions that studying the "natural" history of the disease in African Americans might lead to ideas that would eventually make new treatments possible would have appealed to him.

Dibble's commitment to research into finding better treatments is made even clearer in a speech to VA administrators after penicillin had begun to be used for syphilis in 1945. While he again applauded the use of the quartan strain in malaria therapy, he acknowledged that "constant research is still going on to solve some of the other mysteries of the body." This form of malarial treatment still required patients to remain hospitalized, he noted, for one and a half to two years, at best, and longer "in the less favorable cases." Penicillin, he reminded his audience, was changing this, "but very little had been done in treating the later stages which included the various forms of neurosyphilis, especially with the Negro patient group."

What follows next in this narrative represents an extraordinary contrast to the Study: an explanation of a research program at the Tuskegee VA Hospital that *treated* 70 syphilitic patients with malaria and penicillin. Dibble was heartened by the research but clear that there was still uncertainty. He told his audience: "Of this group many have been discharged after a period of from two to four months as compared with one and [a] half or more years formerly required when the heavy metals were used with malaria as follow-up treatment. Even though we have had gratifying success, penicillin combined with malaria is still under study and a final absolute opinion as to its effectiveness in modifying the positivity of the blood and preventing relapses of neurosyphilis cannot be given at this time."[66]

How did he oversee this kind of research at the Tuskegee VA Hospital and at the same time allow the Study to continue? Was he still so committed to research that he thought the "natural history" was needed? Is it possible that Dibble was enough of a science man that he was willing to sacrifice men to the research needs, justifying the greater good that would hopefully come from the research? Perhaps he accepted that there were "natural" differences between blacks and whites and that the Study would be useful in showing this. He was never asked.

There are only hints that suggest Dibble remained committed to such medical research. Reuben L. Kahn, the Michigan immunologist who developed one of the more accurate tests used to identify syphilis in the blood, became one of Dibble's correspondents and friends. Kahn sent him his articles, even the typescript report of his funding by the Wenner-Gren Foundation in 1953 to explore with European colleagues whether ethnicity or race affected the serological reactions to syphilis.[67]

Dibble's "consenting" to the Study on behalf of others would not have been unusual when it started. As ideas about consent changed, however, Dibble's position did not. Certainly by the 1960s, Dibble understood that patients in a research study needed, at the very least, to indemnify their physicians in writing against complications. In 1964, Dibble was working with University of Chicago demographer Donald Bogue, in conjunction with the Population Council, on a study at John A. on the use of IUDs to prevent pregnancy. Bogue was very concerned that it be a well-conducted scientific study and that the women who accepted the coils were followed properly. Dibble saw it as a way to get family-planning services for the women who came through his clinics, while his staff would also be involved in collecting and analyzing the data. But most important, Bogue told him: "All patients who accept the coil are to sign the medical waiver that is standard procedure in experimental programs, to protect you and the Hospital from fraudulent claims. I do not know whether this requires the patient to sign a waiver, but recommend you follow the same procedure being followed in other experiments around the nation."[68]

This came nearly thirty years after the Study had started. Nothing in the records suggests that Dibble paused to reconsider the meaning this kind of waiver might have for the lack of consent in the Study. Perhaps he might have said something had he been alive to attend the 1969 CDC meeting, where the Study was reconsidered. But by then, cancer had taken him, and there is no evidence that he ever changed his mind about the Study's importance.

What Was He Doing?

Nothing in Dibble's correspondence directly hints that he ever had any questions about the Study or its science, morality, or procedures. His experiences with neurosyphilis research at the VA Hospital suggest he had his doubts about the arsenicals as treatment, but he never wrote whether his doubts extended to the disease's cardiovascular complications.

The men's medical records provide a possible hint of what might have gone on. A handful of the men reported that they had received penicillin from Dibble.[69] It is possible that either Dibble did not remember their names when they showed up at his hospital or that he changed his mind and started to provide treatment when the men had other medical needs. Rivers noted in her deposition that most of the men saw Dibble. She did not say what he did.[70]

Dibble did have supplies of penicillin at his hospitals. He was constantly asking for more from the state health department, especially when he headed John A., where his major responsibility would have been to treat students or staff from Tuskegee Institute. As he was to tell a state health department official in 1955, the student body was a "fine, healthy looking group. . . . Of course, as you know, the percentage of positives each year has declined greatly. Certainly this is the result of the fine work of the State Health Department and U.S. Public Health Service."[71] It must be assumed that he meant the PHS's work in venereal disease control, not the Study.

The easy answer is sometimes the correct answer, or at least part of it. Dibble could have accepted the PHS's medical reasoning in both the pre-penicillin and post-penicillin eras, supported it, and turned away from the problems of these poorer men. The easiest way to view Dibble is as an elite black man, willing to go along to get what he thought was needed, operating out of an older model for racial justice.[72] In Dibble's case, the commitment to science and the fight against racism together are stronger arguments, however, for what he must have been balancing.

Nor would Dibble have probably heard criticisms from his friends. Historian Susan Smith interviewed famed Howard University public health physician Paul B. Cornely about the Study in 1989. Cornely knew about the Study through the decades before 1972, taught it in his classes to future black physicians, and never questioned it or heard his students raise concerns. "I considered myself to be an activist," he told Smith. "I used to get hot and bothered about injustice and inequity, yet here right under my nose something is happening and I'm blind." As he admitted to her, "It shows you how we looked at human beings, especially blacks who were expendable." Smith concluded that, for Cornely, the need for attention to black health care overrode any ethical concerns.[73] It is not difficult to imagine that Dibble felt the same way.

Change came to Alabama by the mid-1950s as the civil rights movement exploded. The Montgomery Bus Boycott, the Tuskegee Civic Association's fight against the racial gerrymandering of voting districts and efforts to desegregate the schools, the integration of the University of Alabama, the police battles in Birmingham, and the Selma-to-Montgomery March were in the forefront of the revolution. By the end of Dibble's life, voting by African Americans became really possible. He lived to see Sammy Younge, a civil rights organizer and Tuskegee native, gunned down in 1966 near the downtown square. When Younge's white killer was acquitted at trial, protesters painted the Confederate soldier statue in the main square black (with a yellow stripe down its back) and marched in the streets. Black power in a form different from what had been counseled for decades at Tuskegee Institute had finally arrived.[74]

Dibble was part of this change, in the quiet organizing that went on, even if he never planned or participated in the protests.[75] His reports and letters show his efforts time and again to desegregate the county and state medical societies and to have membership based on character and training, not on race. Dibble continued to believe in the necessity of desegregation, but he never pushed for it to come quickly. In 1946, for example, when major black organizations were arguing for desegregated veterans' hospitals, not the building of another southern VA hospital just for blacks, Dibble was one of only two black physicians who favored the segregated plan.[76] He wrote continually to businessmen who gave money to Tuskegee Institute to point out what was being accomplished and how change was coming. But by the 1950s, the town in many ways had become more of a rural backwater than it had been in the 1920s. Dibble was directing a local regional but private hospital that tried to serve a wider community. He was not in the forefront of research nor even any longer in the struggle for black rights. Even the John A. Andrew Clinical Society was becoming less important, as other options for black physicians were opening across the country.

Johnny Ford, Tuskegee's mayor at the time the Study ended, remembered Dibble and thought that he had become "locked into a situation. I guess it is kind of hard to explain why they didn't protest more vigorously. They found themselves in an embarrassing situation and didn't want to publicize it that much. Or tried to fight it quietly," he surmised.[77] Dibble was a proud man who gives no evidence of being either intimidated or flattered by whites, and his connection to the PHS was in getting recognition for the enormous health problems of African Americans and help where he could.[78]

Seen in retrospect, the Study seems to take on a larger role in the life of John A. Andrew Memorial Hospital than it probably had occupied on a day-to-day basis at the time.[79] Even the PHS's blood draws and roundups were sporadic, taking place in the Macon County hamlets rather than at the hospital itself. For his part, Dibble accepted what he could change and provide—and triaged the rest. He might have developed what a critic of this careful Tuskegee Institute strategy labeled a kind of existential "mauvaise foi," or "culpable self deception involved in declining to accept responsibility for one's choices," which shaped an existentialist worldview that made survival possible.[80] Perhaps his sense of the needs of black communities overrode his concerns for the individual men. In any case, the why questions could not be asked of Eugene H. Dibble Jr., because he was no longer alive in 1972. Instead, they came to be directed at the Study's one seemingly visible woman: Nurse Eunice Verdell Rivers Laurie.

9

The Best Care

Eunice Verdell Rivers Laurie

In the photograph, a dignified elderly woman stares out at the camera, her church-lady glasses framing a small face, her graying hair pulled back into a neat bun. Her arms are wrapped in front of her frail body; a gold medal rests comfortably on her chest.[1] Her "caring hands," as the photographer labeled them, are long-fingered, veined, soft, and wrinkled. In 1984, twelve years after the Study entered national infamy, this photograph of Eunice Rivers (after her marriage she became Eunice Rivers Laurie, although many still called her "Nurse Rivers"), the Study's public health nurse, was chosen for the poster and cover for a nationally touring photography exhibit and book on older African American women.[2] For this portrait, she chose to wear the Oveta Culp Hobby medal, which was given to her in 1958 by the federal government for her meritorious service in the Study. This public portrait of her private self, taken just a few years before her death, is a clue to how she wanted to be seen.[3] Yet her own presentation is as constructed as the stories that swirl around her and purport to explain her actions and motives.[4] The shadows in the background of her photograph are as telling as her braced body and hands.[5]

No one seemed to doubt that Eunice Rivers Laurie cared for the men she recruited and helped to keep in the Study. She evinced trust and respect. "Oh my God, she was their mama," Emma Cooper, the daughter of one of the men in the Study, remembered.[6] Indeed, this is what seems so troubling in her legacy. When asked if the men became her friends, Rivers told the lawyers at her deposition, "They did and still are, those that are living."[7] Study survivor Herman Shaw agreed and said, "We loved her and she loved us."[8]

The Rivers part of the Study is often seen as simple: she was either a middle-class race traitor or a powerless nurse. One scholar has even named a specific "Nurse Rivers syndrome"—a willingness to sell out her poorer charges to keep her position or to perpetuate a paternalistic use of the "folk" for what she perceived as racial betterment.[9] For others, she was—like the men who "did not fully understand the dangers of the experiment"—a powerless victim.[10] For those who conveniently forget the forty-year history of the Study and see it as a still photograph, she was the nurse who had to follow doctors' orders and could not have understood what was going on.[11]

As the hypervisible black nurse whose caring appears to have been deadly, it is Eunice Rivers Laurie herself who absorbs the moral complexities of the Study. Somehow she is expected to have done nothing—or everything—to stop it. It is upon her body and motives that many of the emotional reactions to the Study are written and her caring fictionalized in poems, plays, and music.[12] Yet she was interviewed just once by the federal investigating committee and she never came to Washington to give testimony, nor did she ever appear before the Kennedy hearings.[13] She was not a defendant, although she was deposed, in the Study lawsuit. Attorney Fred Gray labeled her "a victim just like the men."[14]

When reporters came knocking at her Brown Street door in Tuskegee in 1972, she turned them away. Indeed, as her actions were questioned she withdrew more and more from her community and her beloved church and was even hospitalized for stress after the questioning began.[15] Her only defense of her role publicly available is in three oral history interviews done in the late 1970s and in her deposition from the lawsuit.[16] As historian/physician Vanessa Northington Gamble has noted, "The real Nurse Rivers did not leave us a lot to understand if she was conflicted."[17]

Reading her letters, published article, and interviews, we must attempt to see what the silences mean, to explore the coded language used, and to understand what she faced. Her various forms of testimony are convoluted, and the testifying she was doing to communal truths becomes speculative or fictional. Her untended gravestone in Tuskegee is becoming covered with grass, but her story grows.[18]

From Jakin to Tuskegee

Eunice Verdell Rivers was not a Tuskegee native.[19] She was born in Jakin, a small farming community in southwest Georgia, on what appears to be November 12, 1899. "Appears," because this was the date given in her funeral program and in one interview. The year 1901 is on her gravestone, on PHS employment records, and in the deposition she gave in the Study's lawsuit.[20] Those who came to her family's home when the census was enumerated recorded her "color" differently as well: in 1900 she was black, she became a mulatto in 1910, and she was back to being black by 1920. Those who saw her, whether in the census or in history, imagined who she was.

Jakin lay on the Alabama Midland Railroad line amid sawmills and farmlands full of cotton, corn, and peanuts.[21] Her father, Albert, listed as black in the census, farmed his own land, thought of himself as "independent," and worked as a laborer in one of the sawmills whose logs were floated down the Chattahoochee River to be made into paper in Apalachicola. Her somewhat sickly mother, Henrietta (whose "color" changed in the census in the same ways as her daughter's), mostly stayed at home to care for the children, spending little time in the fields. Her parents were both born after emancipation. Despite a dearth of schooling, her father could both read and write and could easily calculate in his head how much he was supposed to get for his cotton crop. The family lived with her maternal grandmother, Kittie Harvin, who was born "abt 1851," although it appears that she died before Rivers could have remembered her stories of slavery.

Eunice was the first Rivers child to survive; two others died in infancy. Two younger sisters, Alma and Maude, followed her into adulthood.[22] Among Rivers's crucial childhood memories were her mother's early death at age 45 and her commandment for education so that her daughter would not have to work in the fields.[23] Albert Rivers shared his wife's concern. School in Early County for black children at the time consisted of meeting in one room in a church for about three months a year. Her father worked extra hours and jobs and bucked criticism about sending his young daughter away so that she could go to mission boarding schools in Fort Gaines, and then in Thomasville, Georgia, after sixth grade. Concerned that whites were her only teachers, he pulled her out before her last year of high school and sent her to Tuskegee Institute.[24]

Eunice Rivers grew up within a culture of white violence. In detail, she recalled what happened when the "white people rioted" because a black man in Jakin had shot a policeman in self-defense. "Riot" for her meant a parade of white people from surrounding communities on "great big mules . . . with the shotgun riding across their backs." Because her father was rumored to have helped the man get away, the family was in danger. "And one night, they came by and they shot in our house," she told an interviewer, "and the bullet—you're sitting there, I'm sitting here—the bullet didn't hit him, didn't hit any of us, but it hit the chair, right under there, right between us." Her father moved the family into safer space and protected his home.[25]

Rivers arrived at the Tuskegee Institute in 1918 and began in handicrafts, making baskets and mattresses. Her father thought this wasted her previous education and suggested nursing. After much discussion about her fears of people dying on her, she "made up my mind myself" and switched to the nursing program. Even as a student, her skills were recognized. She was given the toughest cases, remembering that she got over her fears, prepared bodies, and accompanied them to the morgue.[26]

Rivers graduated from the institute in 1922. In her first position, she traveled into rural Macon County to teach basic sanitation and health, for the Movable School wagon program, which had state funding. She explained to women and midwives basic safe birthing procedures—how to put newspapers and clean rags on beds to prepare for deliveries and not to grease up a baby after birth, for example. She taught toothbrushing as well as "social hygiene," the coded term for information on sexually transmitted diseases.[27] She went on to work throughout Alabama, registering births and deaths for the state, while continuing to teach midwives. When cutbacks at the beginning of the Depression pushed her out of these positions, she was hired as a night supervisor at the Tuskegee Institute hospital. She did the job for ten months but hated it. She thought about leaving for hospital work in New York, and then the Study came along.

Caring as Treatment, Working for Science

In 1932, at the time Rivers was recommended for the "scientific assistant" position by Eugene Dibble, she was one of the best nurses the institute had produced. She knew the back roads and byways of Alabama and had mastered the racial politics of dealing with white doctors and the state health department.[28] She explained to Dibble when he told her about the Study and syphilis, "You know I don't know a thing about that."[29] Her modesty belied the fact that she had already been teaching about syphilis in the Movable School program.

Macon County health officer Murray Smith agreed that she would be the right person to do the work. It had to do, she said, with her ability to handle difficult white doctors. As she later recalled, the PHS's O. C. Wenger was, she thought, "one of those fussy folks, just fussy, just plain fussy." She told Smith, "Well, he don't make me no difference. I know what I'm doing, and I hope he know what he is doing. . . . He can yell all he wants. I don't even hear him. . . . He'll be the one dying of high blood pressure not me."[30]

When the Study was in its early stage, her duties were simple. She recalled getting "the syringes sterilized, washed and boiled" for the blood draws by "keeping the alcohol stove going and little things like that." At that time, she stated, "I had very little contact with the patient." For the first months of the Study, she watched as the doctors took the blood, retested the positives, and then began treatment with the heavy metals and mercury. She remained concerned with the men's reactions to the mercury, the "salivation . . . sores," and the "terrible reactions" that they had to these drugs.[31]

As the Study progressed, Rivers was given more responsibility. She drove the men into Tuskegee for examinations and x-rays, did the follow-ups, drew blood in the field, took in the urine specimens, helped in their assessment and in the provision of tonics and analgesics, assisted at the spinal taps, created the camaraderie that kept them in the Study, and encouraged the families to allow autopsies by promising and providing money for burials.[32] As this extra inducement, she helped set up what was called "Miss Rivers' Lodge," the insurance scheme with the Milbank Memorial Fund that guaranteed a decent burial in exchange for the autopsy agreements.[33] Although the doctors involved in the Study changed regularly, Nurse Rivers was the constant.

Rivers knew how to get compliance, although not always. She was nonjudgmental with the men and their families. "I accepted them as they were. And they accepted me. . . . I tried to accept them as they were, see, not as what I wanted them to be," she asserted. The men also trusted her to protect them from the harshness of the PHS doctors, she argued. One man told her, "'Mrs. Rivers, go in there and tell that white man to stop talking to us like that.' I had two white doctors who apologized. They said, 'Miz Laurie, I didn't mean it like it sounded. I guess I was kind of upset.' I said, 'Well, you sounded terrible. I hope you don't do it any more, 'cause they are all human.' . . . 'These are grown men; some of them are old men. Don't holler at them.'"[34]

Rivers knew how to listen to the joshing that went on among the men and thought they understood what "bad blood" meant and how it was transferred. She recalled: "You could hear them teasing each other about where they been and who, [laughs] they were just having a good time. Uh huh. 'Don't it catch up with ya. Un huh. I know it catch up with ya. Un huh. I know it catch up with ya. Uh hun, yes sir, uh hun. What you done in the dark sure come to the light,' ah ah. I sure loved the expressions of those folks. So they knew. So they knew. But the word 'syphilis' was not used."[35]

She continually reassured the PHS that the Study could continue. She wrote to a colleague after the men were given a certificate and $25 for their years of participation: "I don't think there is any fear of their quitting now."[36] Elizabeth M. Kennebrew replaced her in 1965, but Rivers still assisted when the PHS physicians came to town, and she stayed in contact with the men.

Rivers never worked full time on the Study. She continued to be employed by "the health department in the maternity service, with the pregnant mamas and the midwives in the clinics," assisted in the venereal disease control projects, and taught in the Tuskegee nursing school.[37] She was remembered as the school nurse who gave out vaccinations, standing tall with her hair in a bun and her sturdy black nursing shoes covering her feet.[38] She served a term as president of Tuskegee's Nursing Alumnae Association and fought when the school was threatened with closure.

For Eunice Rivers, the men were both patients and subjects. Future bioethicists would become concerned with what has been called the "therapeutic misconception," the idea that if an individual is in a study or clinical trial of a new drug or procedure he or she will get the best care for themselves and will benefit.[39] Since the men thought they were being treated, they had no "misconception." Rivers, however, may have held this kind of view.

Her focus was on caring, but the science, too, seemed to intrigue her. She knew what the men had and learned about the disease.[40] She understood that the purpose of the Study was "to find out the effects of syphilis on the Negro." She spoke of the comparison to the study on whites in Oslo several times, suggesting that this mitigated some of her concern and normalized the research.[41] She hung the Nightingale Pledge of nursing on her living room wall, but she also took the idea of being the "scientific assistant" seriously.

So did the PHS. When she won the 1958 award, Study physician John C. Cutler wrote her a note of congratulations and linked her caring to science's travails: "The type of work that you have done is often lonely and at times must seem almost futile," he told her. "But it is only this kind of dedication that makes possible the acquisition of the knowledge needed to provide better treatment or prevention of many of the diseases which now afflict mankind."[42] She listened carefully to what the doctors told her and wrote to the state health department's head nurse to ask for books on venereal disease. In the 1940s, she taught venereal disease and public health to Tuskegee Institute's nursing students.[43]

Describing the dangers of the 1930s treatment regimes, she claimed they were "really worse than the disease if it was not early syphilis." Again she said, "If syphilis was *not* active the treatment was worse than the disease."[44] She viewed treatment from a nursing perspective and was aware of the pain and the suffering at the very moment of caregiving. She took pride in trying to mitigate the spinal taps. They were "very crude" in those days, she recalled, and the pain they caused troubled her. She seemed relieved when they were stopped, and she added, "So if they had continued with the spinal shots the study would not have been."[45]

If at moments she thought of herself as a "scientific assistant," above all she was doing the professional nursing work of caring. As an African American woman and member of the Tuskegee community she was also healing — seeing that the men and their families got attention, bringing them baskets of food and clothing — being as much social worker as nurse. Although she maintained adamantly that as a nurse she never diagnosed, she equally argued that she cared.[46]

Knowing how little medical treatment was available and how little attention was paid to black ills, she shifted resources to the men. She knew at the beginning that few had family physicians.[47] But her letters make it clear that she was helping them get attention, as the PHS physicians had claimed. Writing to one of the men in the Study in 1952 who had developed lung cancer, she told him: "The results of your recent examination at the Veterans' Hospital have been checked. The x-ray of your lungs shows a large 'spot' on the right side. The government doctor would like to see you this Saturday at your home (February 29, 1952) and explain the x-ray to you. He will bring with him some medicine to start your treatment."[48] A decade later she was writing to the CDC's Dr. Anne R. Yobs about a subject whose blood levels had gone up and who might have had syphilitic reinfection. Yobs assured her that the man had been given 5 million "units of penicillin and has been considered adequately treated." If the physical examination showed no new disease, Yobs concluded, "I would continue to see no reason for retreating this patient at this time."[49]

She knew there had been treatment. She declared: "Now a lot of those patients that were in the Study did get some treatment. There were very few who did not get any treatment."[50] She knew that the "iron tonics, aspirin tablets and vitamin pills" that she gave out were not treatments for syphilis. But she described these drugs, as well as the physical exams, as being part of treatment. She knew the aspirins helped with the pains of arthritis and that the iron tonics gave the men "pep" in the spring. She said: "This was part of our medication that they got and sometimes they really took it and enjoyed it very much. And these vitamins did them a lot of good. They just loved those and they enjoyed that very very much." To emphasize her construction of these medications as "treatment," she pointed out that there were others who tried to get into the Study in order to get these "treatments." Her words suggested that she was choosing to emphasize the problems with the available drug regimens for the disease, the men's ability to be seen by a physician, and the provision of simple medications. Protecting herself from the idea that they were not directly treated for their syphilis, her sense of healing focused on her own caregiving role, the medical consulting for other ills, and the providing of minor medications.[51]

For Rivers, the work of the public health nurse was, above all, to care for those in her community. "I think if I had wanted to take medicine, I could have gone into medicine. . . . I never was interested in medicine as such," she explained. "I was interested in the person, and it just never occurred to me that I wanted to be a doctor. I always felt that the nurse got closer to the patient than the doctor did, that was the way I felt about it."[52]

She found a way to solve what continued to be a dilemma for many public health nurses: she saw herself as providing both preventive health nursing and "sick" nursing at the same time.[53] Well aware of the great needs around her, she said, "These people were given good attention for their particular time." In her narratives she emphasized how much the men got out of being examined or even fluoroscoped so they could see their own hearts or old buckshot still lodged in their chests. It was, she thought, the kind of attention they had never been given.[54]

Caring brought power and spiritual satisfaction to Nurse Rivers.[55] She acknowledged her role in bringing the men in and showing them around Tuskegee, driving her small Chevrolet with its rumble seat and later a government-provided station wagon. Laughingly, she reflected on how the men called their experience "Miss Rivers' project." Her chuckle underlay her sense that it was not hers, and yet it was hers in some real way.[56] Her nursing gave her status, purpose, and a connection to the community she adopted as her own. She stayed single most of her life, giving her time outside of work for the church, the institute, the Red Cross, and her garden. In her 50s, in 1952, she married Julius Laurie, a nursing worker at the hospital whom she met at church. She was a "woman deeply rooted in faith," her pastor said. Rivers must have seen her power to help as part of God's work.[57]

Between 1938 and 1940, Rivers also worked with the "bad blood wagon," which brought treatment into Macon County. Even in the lawsuit when she was deposed, she hedged on whether her naming the men in the Study to the physicians in this treatment program meant that they received no treatment. She said both "not that I know of" and "I don't know" when asked this. This is either the language of denial in a deposition or the ways she protected her knowing.[58] It may be that she allowed the differences between early and contagious syphilis (in the treatment program) and late syphilis (in the Study) to let her imagine that she was just doing the right thing in a world of unmet need.

Rivers was listed as the first author in the 1953 published report on the Study, which explained its "nonmedical aspects." Some of the language and internal mistakes in the article suggest she may have been interviewed but did not write the actual piece. This article directly called the men "patients" and reported that anyone in early syphilis was "treated." It emphasized her work as the "bridge" between the doctors and "patients." The paternalistic tones used in the telling of the anecdotes of the "patients'" strange home remedies and failures to understand modern medicine were similar to other contemporary reports on uneducated people. It was assumed that the men could not be appealed to "from a purely scientific approach" and had to have inducements and "persuasion." The claims were also overreaching: she actually did lose more than one autopsy in the Study's first twenty years. It was her job, the article concluded, "to help in the most ethical way to see that they get the best care."[59]

The Nursing Voices

Nurse Rivers seemed more troubled when she talked in her interviews about what penicillin had meant for the treatment of syphilis after the 1940s. When this topic came up, her voice shifted and she spoke more slowly and directly about what the doctors had told her. She communicated in a "just following orders" nursing voice, and then she moved back into discussion of the early days.[60] This suggests that when she spoke about penicillin she was more troubled about the moral implications of withholding it. But, as with many of the doctors, she also emphasized the dangers of the Herxheimer reactions and her memory of someone dying from anaphylactic shock from a penicillin allergy. She also misremembered the extent of syphilis in the county, stating both in interviews and in her deposition that the rate was 80 percent, more than doubling what was actually found in the initial Rosenwald Fund Demonstration Project and much more than in the Study itself.[61] This factual slippage suggests she thought syphilis was ubiquitous in the county.

Rivers may have lost the nursing voice that gave her professional authority (the caring voice) and shifted to the taking-orders voice, which, while seeming to morally protect her at the time, clearly troubled her years later.[62] In her deposition, she retreated to this voice when asked if she withheld the diagnosis from the men. "No," she told the lawyers, "nobody ever told me not to tell them. This was just a part of nursing ethics."[63] She described clearly the differences between primary, secondary, and latent syphilis when questioned. But then, under lawyer Fred Gray's prompting, she slipped back into saying that she only knew what the doctors told her.[64] Her shifting temporal sense suggests that her moral qualms might have grown concerning penicillin, but her views were so formed by the Study's rationale and the earlier thinking that she could not change her position.[65] To do so would have forced her to imagine she had done something terribly wrong. As was the case with the physicians, it might have taken her years to come to this conclusion, if she ever did.

When she spoke of the men, she often told stories of their questions, providing a multivoiced narrative. When she referenced the Oslo Study, she used her science authority voice as she explained the medical understandings of syphilis in black and white populations. She was adamant that she knew when to look for the rashes and chancres that differentiated the disease's stages, although in her deposition it becomes clear that attorney Fred Gray was trying to protect her from saying that she had any medical knowledge at all.[66]

Very little slipped by her. She recalled: "If some white doctor told me something that I wasn't too sure of, or if he just told me because . . . [ellipsis in original] I'd go tell Dibble. 'What is it now, Miss Rivers?' I said, 'Dr. Dibble, I've got a problem.' 'All right, nurse, sit down.' So I'd come back and tell Dr. Dibble. He said, 'Well, what did you say?' I said, 'I didn't say anything.' He said, well you do such and such a thing and such and such a thing and it will be all right."[67] Such a tale suggests that Rivers learned when to speak, when not to speak, and what to do. A nurse in the community, whose mother was a good friend to Rivers, recalled that Rivers "did not discuss what she did not want to and kept her privacy."[68]

Her nursing voice, inflected by her science voice, shaped what she knew about the disease and what was happening to the men. If she listened to what the PHS doctors or Tuskegee physicians Eugene Dibble and J. Jerome Peters told her or read the PHS reports, she possibly gained a complex and evolving understanding of syphilis's effects. In the early reports, it is clear that the men in the syphilitic arm were doing worse, and this appeared to be true again in the early 1960s but not in the late 1960s. But in the 1955 report (a decade after penicillin became available), the autopsies showed that the men in both arms of the Study were dying at around the same age and that those left untreated with syphilis "would have, roughly, a 50-50 chance of demonstrating syphilitic cardiovascular involvement at autopsy." The existence of other cardiac difficulties was assumed to be due to "hypertension and/or myocardial degeneration."[69]

Rivers then projected backward from these reports to state her belief that the Study had done little harm from the beginning. Indeed, in her deposition, she recalled: "The thing that was always interesting to me in the study, that whenever the doctors came down to examine the patients, they said that the syphilitics were in better physical condition than the negatives were. . . . We used to laugh about it all the time. They tell me, Nurse, if you get syphilis, it ain't going to kill you. And they would say and many of them made the remark that syphilis was not near as bad as some people would have it. That is certainly true among the people that we had."[70] Her statement could reflect her post-Study construction of what had happened, what she thought at the time, or both.

Inverting Gender/Race as Power

Rivers's rapport with the men allowed for her position of power. She spent hours driving them into Tuskegee over rutted and muddy roads. For the men, the time with her was also a break from their heavy everyday labor. In a short description of how the men kidded one another about "what they got" when they took their clothes off, she described a conversation in her car: "I said, 'Lord have Mercy.' So what we did, we would all be men today, tomorrow, maybe we'll all be ladies. . . . Well, you see, when you've got one group together you can say anything. Tell 'em about anything. But if you got women and men, well you have to [be] careful about what you say, see . . . You see. So when they want to talk and get in the ditch, they'd tell me, 'Nurse Rivers, we're all men today!' . . . Oh we had a good time. We had a good time. Really and truly. When we were working with those people, and when we first, and when we got started early that was the joy of my life."[71]

Her position as a professional woman, representing the "super-moral" black woman, would not normally have allowed such a shift in class behavior.[72] Although her place in the community and her representation was as a professional woman, in her car, while she was at the wheel, in a state of transition from rural country to the more urban Tuskegee, her gender, class, and sexualized hearing (if not her actually voicing) could invert in order for her to bond with the men. In her car, she created a sense of self and connection, almost invisible and able to transcend moral judgment.

Her description of her power reflected the delicate balance needed by a public health nurse and her efforts to control male authority. Her story of entering nursing acknowledged her father's advice but portrayed it as her decision.[73] She believed she controlled the white doctors' behaviors toward the men. In her statements about the doctors and their relationships to the patients, the themes of caring, power, and treatment come together. As she explained in one of her oral histories, she told the physicians: "'Don't mistreat my patients. You don't mistreat them.' I said, 'Now cause they don't have to come. And if you mistreat I will *not* let them up here to be mistreated.'"[74] She knew that both the men and the doctors needed her. She appears to have acted, as other nurses in Tuskegee did, by "distinguish[ing] [between] those traditional expected acts of deference vis à vis physicians from unquestioning obedience to doctors' orders."[75] She had little authority as a nurse, but she believed in her power to make the Study's longevity possible.

Rivers told her Tuskegee students to maintain their dignity and their distance from the doctors. A public health nurse she trained recalled that Rivers reminded her students: "Never work with a physician who wants to use you. Don't let them pat you on the head because they'll think you want to drop your drawers. That way you can always stand up for what you believe."[76]

This nurse's memories suggest that Rivers knew there were ways to maintain one's dignity and limit the doctors' sexualizing of them, by setting careful limits. Rivers told them: "People may not like you for what you do, but if you are right they will respect you for what you do."[77] In dealing with the white doctors, she became not only hypervisible but also hypermoral, redefining black womanhood out of a sexual realm.[78] She demonstrated, when she had to, what historian Evelyn Brooks Higginbotham has called the "perceived centrality of female morality and female respectability to racial advancement."[79]

Rivers as a "Race Woman"

Just as Dibble thought of himself as a "race man," Rivers thought of herself as a "race woman," concerned about advancing the rights of African Americans. Because of her assumption that the Oslo study was also comparative, she did not see the Study as "a civil rights issue." She accepted the idea that there were racial differences in the disease's progression. She said directly in 1977, "I don't think it was a racist experiment."[80] And it may also be that part of her story as a race woman and nurse is her coded silence.[81] The use of indirect speech, of negatives, of "suppressed discourse," show the ways she produced what she had to say.[82] Rivers's refusal to speak out and provide testimony may be because she had a different understanding of what had happened *and* because she also felt she had to keep silent.

This is suggested in her struggle to explain her differences with one of the physicians about whether she let some of the men get treatment. It is here that her testifying voice most clearly comes through. In his testimony before the federal investigating committee, Reginald James, who worked with Rivers on venereal disease control out of the Macon County Health Department, claimed she would tell him not to treat his patients who were in the Study.[83] James's view is corroborated by the repeated testimony of some of the surviving men from the Study, who also recalled that she actively kept them from getting treatment.[84] To her friends in Tuskegee who interviewed her, Rivers declared:

> And Dr. James told folks up there in Washington I would not let him see the patients that I would not let them get treatment. And when they told me that I said I can't I hate to dispute it. I said we're supposed to respect the medical profession but Dr. James is lying, saying I . . . the only thing I would do I would tell Dr. James this is one of the patients. Now it was up to him if he wanted to treat him. . . . So this is ah ah I don't know but nobody knows what I went through here you'd have thought I was a doctor mistreating the patients. [H*er voice gets quieter.*] And I cause a lot of them I don't know I think that there was a lot of the jealousy and the medical profession and me, [*her voice gets stronger*] see because they felt that I was not letting the patients get the treatment. I never told anybody that you couldn't get treatment. I told them. "So who's your doctor. If you want to go to the doctor go and get your treatment." So they didn't tell you you couldn't be treated. . . . That they [the physicians] had to fall back on something, have an excuse, and maybe the medical profession was all men so they put it on me that I wouldn't let the patients get treatment.[85]

As in her other interviews, when she grew concerned about the Study's moral morass, she retreated to another of her voices, that of "the nurse who just took orders and did not prescribe."[86] As in her deposition, she was very clear that she may have identified the patients as being in the "study group" but that she never told the doctor directly not to treat.[87] Or perhaps there is another explanation.

There is a possibility that her hedging was not merely defensive. Irene Beavers, a nurse who had been Rivers's student at Tuskegee and then became her supervisor when Beavers became director of nursing at the institute's hospital, described Rivers as a dignified "Harriet Tubman" of nursing, an "underground railroad person who advised these people, not to be used." She recalled Rivers telling her students during a lecture in her Tuskegee course on venereal disease control in the late 1940s (before the Study was exposed):

> And there were several of them that . . . got treatment because she
> told the family to pick them up and bring them back. And take them
> to Birmingham. . . . And they were treated for syphilis. . . . And she
> had to do it this way or she would have lost her job. . . . And the thing
> she was trying to get us to understand [was] that as nurses you had
> a responsibility to yourself and to your counterparts and to your
> patients. . . . You had certain rights and there were some things you
> knew not to do. And you could make diagnosis too, although the
> physician felt he was the only person who could.[88]

Other public health officials in Tuskegee said it would have been possible for her to have given the men penicillin from the local health department supplies, or to have gotten other public health nurses to care for the men, although this may have been true only in the 1960s after supplies of penicillin became more affordable and available. Beavers also recalled a quick conversation that occurred after 1972 when she said to Rivers, "You were involved with the bad blood?" And Rivers replied, "I don't know why they call it bad blood. That's a bad name to put to anything. You remember what I told you all a long time ago. Well they can't write everything."[89] A woman of her generation, Beavers knew that "there are techniques you use in fighting [racism]. And this is what most folks are missing[:] the point that there is a way to get anything."

One interview is not enough historical evidence to prove that Rivers found ways of treating the men. But another clue comes from one of the members of the federal investigating committee, who, after interviewing her in 1972, wrote about her in a private letter to the committee's chairman, stating that he was "convinced . . . that she made treatment arrangements for any person in the untreated group upon his request."[90] But he did not make clear whether he was talking only about the controls, and this also assumes that the men would know to ask.

The next piece of possible evidence comes in a report from a PHS physician, Joseph Caldwell, who worked on the Study toward its end. Writing to his superiors in 1970, he stated about Rivers: "Once more, however, I began to doubt Nurse Laurie's conflicting loyalty to the project. Several times I have wondered whether she wears two hats—one of a Public Health Nurse, locally coordinating the Study[,] and one of a local negro lady identifying with those local citizens—all of her race—who have been 'exploited' for research purposes."

Caldwell cited a patient who had been lost to follow-up since 1944 but who somehow turned up in 1970 while Nurse Rivers was elsewhere. The man lived "four blocks from the old Macon County health department where all of [the] survey examinations were generally held." The man told Caldwell that he and his wife were good friends to Rivers and her husband. Then the man told the PHS doctor: "He got penicillin shots, a full series, at the Macon County Health Department as soon as possible after 1944, when he first learned he had 'bad blood.' Perhaps I am being supersensitive," Caldwell concluded, "but this all seems to be a bit more than mere coincidence."[91]

Nearly twenty years earlier, in 1952, another PHS official had expressed a similar concern about Rivers. Writing to critique Rivers's inability as a "colored person" to provide "100% effort" without "constant supervision," the CDC's Eleanor N. Walker complained: "I have never felt that Nurse Rivers was an adequate 'policeman' for these people. . . . In a community of this type where everyone knows everybody's business I can't see how we could have lost from contact so many of the group if Nurse Rivers had been even moderately interested in perpetuating this Study."[92] When historian James Jones interviewed Rivers in 1977, he asked her about treatment. As they discussed the heavy metal treatments, she again emphasized her understanding of the nursing role, but she did so, interestingly, by answering him in the negative. "Nurses have so much responsibility today," she said. "But no, and I never told somebody *not* to take any medication." When Jones asked her the penicillin question by saying, "So how did you all go about keeping them from getting penicillin." Rivers replied, "I don't know that we did." Jones then asked, "Did you try?" And Rivers answered: "No I did not try . . . to keep them, because I was never really told not to let them get penicillin. And we just had to trust that to those private physicians."[93]

Her stories waffled about treatment. Although Jones is sure she had no moral uncertainty during the Study years, he recalled that she told him to shut off the audiotape he was using. She then turned to him and said: "We should have told those men they had syphilis. And God knows we should have treated them."[94] She also recalled the treatment that became possible, but not her role in it. She told her friends in 1975: "As I go through the records, I see where various ones had gone to Birmingham for rapid treatment in Montgomery and [were] *still* in the study. . . . Some of our patients in the study did go to rapid treatment centers. One of them even now, why he's doing very fine. I know one, but there may be others."[95]

All of these various sources suggest that although there was a "Miss Rivers' Lodge," to which the men paid with their lives and illnesses to gain a decent burial, there may also have been a "Miss Rivers' List," which may have made it possible for some of the men to receive medical treatment.[96] Was Rivers part of the process, or just wishing that she had been? The evidence supports both: that she regretted after 1972 that all the men were not treated and that she aided several to get to treatment before the Study ended.

Moral Triage

It is possible to explain Eunice Rivers's willingness to serve as the link between the PHS and the men by assuming that she knew very little or, if she knew anything, that she was powerless to act. Reading backward into the violence that underlies racial power and the gender deference that girded nurse-doctor relationships, it is not difficult to see her as a victim too. Doing so protects the racial and gender binaries and allows for a tragic recounting of a familiar drama. It allows us to wonder: if only she had had more power, if only she had known more, if only she had not gone along in order to keep her job. Would it have made any difference if she had yelled out loud, "Stop"?

The other side of this assessment plays out a female version of what critic Linda Williams calls the "Tom/anti-Tom dialectic" in America's "racial melodramas," in which "moral outrage" at her becomes a substitute for "social change."[97] The tensions can then cause Rivers to be seen as either the evil mulatto allowing the men to die at the hands of the white doctors or the tragic mulatto who never really understands that her choosing the white doctors over the black men dooms her moral self.

If we accept that she cared deeply about the men and the community, we are then reminded that caring can be blinding to complexity and context.[98] Her sense that her beneficence mattered may have allowed her to ignore everything else. Yet Rivers did not just care. She did on some level believe she was contributing to science in the face of medical uncertainty. She was a science woman as well as a caregiving race woman. She seems to have accepted that the Study would show the meaning of, or lack of, biological racial difference. The award from the federal government for her role in the

Study gave her immense pride. Her testifying voice, the one that speaks of the difficulties in the community and of hard choices, becomes the one that seems to be her most honest one. The moral triage she performed is central to her nursing.

If she did help some of the men get to treatment, her innocence and powerlessness are undermined. We would have to accept her complexities and even her sources of power. We have to allow for the possibilities that her views changed over time and that she picked some men to save but not others.

Those who were with Rivers when the story broke in July 1972 said that she went into a back room of the Macon County Health Department and wept.[99] The fragmentary evidence suggests that she tried after this time to reconsider her participation, to help the men as much as possible, and to rethink the meaning of treatment. At least one reporter, on interviewing Charlie Pollard and his wife, wrote, "After the study was disclosed publicly, she was nice enough to drive him to the lawyer's office."[100] Once the legal proceedings and investigations began, she retreated, speaking only selectively. When the world descended upon her, she could do little more than defend what she had done and perhaps only hint at what else could have happened.

Rivers kept in contact with many of the men after the Study ended and told the lawyers during her deposition, "They call me quite frequently and want to know what has happened to the doctor and nurse. . . . You come to see about us. And I go to see them. I haven't visited them much lately, but I go to see them and check on them when they call me."[101] Charlie and Luiza Pollard stayed friendly with her, going to dinner, and as he recalled, "We never talked about the study. I never accused her of doing anything wrong."[102]

Historian James Jones tells a sad story about the two of them driving around the back roads of Macon County several years after the lawsuit had been settled. She spotted a former subject of the Study out in a field. Jones stopped the car and Rivers walked out between the cotton rows to greet the aging man whom she had cared for those many years. They embraced in the field and the man asked: "How come you don't come see us no more." And Rivers answered, "You don't get the money and Nurse Rivers too."[103]

In "testifying" on the tapes about her position, she gave "verbal witness to the efficacy, truth and power of some experience in which [the group has] shared."[104] In the context of a Tuskegee Institute culture that allowed for both racial accommodation and hidden resistance, perhaps Rivers really was finding the only shifting positions she thought possible and then testifying to them. Her choice to wear the Hobby award medal for her public photograph in 1984 argues that she went to her grave with pride, not shame, in her work.

She passed away on August 28, 1986, and was buried in the Greenwood Cemetery in Tuskegee, not far from some of the men. On her flat gravestone, her husband had her name carved as "Eunice Verdell Laurie." But as the story of the Study traveled into American culture, "Rivers" became code for explaining moral and scientific failure, racial and gender caste systems, and misuse of power.

Another group of photographs captures this coding. In one picture taken by the PHS of Rivers at work, probably in 1953, she stands next to a medical scale, her hands up to pull the lever down on a man's head to measure his height. As in most published medical photographs from the time, the subject's face is blocked so that he cannot be identified. At the desk on the man's other side sits a white physician, his blood pressure machine visible and his back to us and his eyes still shaded by the glasses worn to take a fluoroscope.

California photographer Tony Hooker used this picture in 1999 for part of his montage exhibit on the Study called "The Greater Good." He superimposed it upon a photograph he took of John A. Andrew Memorial Hospital's crumbling walls, *after* it had been closed for more than a decade. The resulting composition, with the subject's entire face now covered in black and the ceiling light fixture almost attached to his head, takes on a different meaning. Rivers, as she raises her arm to get to the scale lever, looks as if she is performing a lynching that is watched by a masked white man as the walls are falling down.[105] As the story of the Study took on cultural meaning in the next decades, both images of Rivers—of her doing her work and of her work literally using death to control black men—would become iconic.

PART III

Traveling

10

Bioethics, History, and the Study as Gospel

Physician Eugene Dibble thought that the Study would be remembered forever, but attorney Fred Gray worried that without the lawsuit somehow it and the men would be forgotten. They were both right. "Tuskegee" entered the American lexicon after 1972. The story had too many elements—a morally and physically loathsome disease, the powerful state, the sexualized black male body, white betrayal of black trust, seeming co-optation of the black middle class against "the folk," experimentation, "mad" scientists, a "betraying" woman, ghoulish autopsies—for it to be erased forever from collective memory.[1] The Study, in all its intricate facticity, has not been remembered correctly or evenly throughout the decades, nor could we expect it to be. Whether in academic lecture, oral story, Internet assertion, news broadcast, or fiery sermon, the facts have dropped in and out of the telling in service of differing political goals.

In the public's imaginary about race, the Study's sustained salience as a term to be invoked to express anguish and fear over medical care, research, and indifference lived on because it never stayed just as a memory. It would provide explanation for the fears generated by a physician's actions when a patient or family member experienced poor medical care or the failure to acknowledge the cultural power of collective history.[2] In the health professionals' imaginary, it would be taught and remembered with anxiety and as a cautionary tale about hubris and paternalism in research. It would become an explanation by researchers for why African Americans seemingly did not volunteer for clinical trials. Naming "Tuskegee" could be an easy way to imagine a health care provider's cultural sensitivity while ignoring structural barriers.

Neither the public nor the health care communities thought about the Study as just history or just memory. "Tuskegee" paralleled historian Ira Berlin's comments on history and memory of slavery: "If the history of slavery speaks to the world transformed, the memory of slavery addresses what was done to my people, to my family, to me."[3] In the Study's case, however, memory brings the research community and the public *together*, as narratives of ethics and memories of oppression become interlocked. The Study did not become just a conflict between memory (an oral tradition within parts of the black community) and history (as translated into ethics texts, institutional review board training, and history lectures). It is the very histories in their truncated forms that become the memories. The memory is what was done to "my people" in the lay black communities and a "what could I possibly do to subjects" in the public health, nursing, and medical research communities.[4] They do not, of course, have the same valence or effects.

The Study's entry into American lore fueled the growth of the "bioethics enterprise."[5] Once there, the story would become one of the failures of researchers to consider informed consent and of the callous disregard of the vulnerable, often devoid of any analysis of race and with barely a nod toward justice. Concerned health care providers and researchers, who would attempt to reach out to what became labeled as *the* black community, would invoke the Study's name frequently or use pictures of it ironically. Two historians would tackle the story, each in his own nuanced way, and differing elements of these histories would be picked up. Over the decades, the cherry-picked or ignored evidence would come to structure the narratives, which would be told by conspiracy theorists to national broadcasters who bungled the facts.

In a widely performed play and then television movie, in poems and jazz pieces, in the publicity surrounding the failed nomination of a surgeon general, and in the organizing of a federal apology from the White House, "Tuskegee" would be told over and over, with varying degrees of historical accuracy. Often, "Tuskegee" became a simple word whose meaning need not even be discussed, as when some research project was referred to as "just like Tuskegee."[6] The Study haunted the American cultural landscape as a supple symbol and object lesson, available to whomever wanted to use it to tell a particular tale of woe or warning.

The Study and the Beginning of Bioethics
Anxieties, expressed as whispers, fears, fiction, and facts, over what physicians might do to their patients and researchers might do to their subjects lurk throughout the history of medicine. Syphilis in particular was the ob-

ject of several nineteenth- and early twentieth-century studies that raised alarms about the misuse of subjects.[7] What counted as research and what as medical practice was not always clear to either physicians or their patient/subjects.[8] "To do no harm," the Hippocratic Oath that underlies Western medical ethics declares, although it has nothing to say about research.[9] Oaths and codes were supposed to be enough to protect the innocent and imbue physicians with a sense of moral standards and norms toward their patients and research subjects.[10]

With the Nuremberg Trials of the Nazi doctors at the end of World War II, efforts began to differentiate between therapeutic research (that might help a patient) and nontherapeutic research (that might help populations but harm individuals). The Nuremberg Code, a list of ten principles written to protect human subjects from nontherapeutic experiments without their consent, is often seen as the beginning of modern discussions of ethics.[11]

Yet, to most American physicians, the Nuremberg Code was seen as irrelevant. The horrors of the experiments under the Nazis became thought of as Nazi science, not science.[12] American medical researchers, flush with the excitement of the expanding funding and medical breakthroughs of the postwar period, did not think they needed such outside authority or that names of those doing problematic research could be given out because of the possibility of criminal prosecution. Even with the Nuremberg Code and in 1964 with the more research-friendly code that came from the World Medical Association's Declaration of Helsinki, the concept that such codes were relevant to American researchers remained illusive.

Codes are guidelines to research ethics, not enforceable regulations. Throughout the period before the late 1960s, the question of whether formal governmental regulations or merely better moral education for medical researchers could best protect the public and advance scientific knowledge was debated among researchers.[13] With all the support for research and all the media coverage over what it meant to do it, most "subjects" were seen as volunteers, providing what sociologist Sydney Halpern argues was labeled "service to the community."[14] Even with the worry about drug trials raised by the dangers of thalidomide (the German sedative that had horrible effects on fetuses), it was still assumed that American research was being done correctly.

Within the federal government in the late 1960s there was discussion on the need for informed consent during research. Most of this discussion focused on "risk rather than consent," especially if the "risk . . . was deemed insignificant." It was assumed that investigators could determine risk, even though, as scholars of this period have noted, the researchers themselves were "hardly impartial judges of risk."[15]

The "bioethicists' tales" that are their own "begat" stories credit the Study and other horrific reports with making the need for outside regulations seem credible. As one scholar succinctly wrote, "Bioethics was born in scandal and raised in protectionism." And "Tuskegee," another bioethicist argued, "changes it all."[16] When the Study surfaced in the media, it completed the bioethics "holy trinity" of American horror stories of research—joining the stories of injection of cancer cells into aging patients at the Jewish Chronic Disease Hospital in Brooklyn in 1964–65 and of the oral intake of live hepatitis virus given to children with retardation at the state-run Willowbrook Hospital on Staten Island in New York in 1963–66, which both became major scandals in the same decade as the Study.[17]

Knowledge about ethical lapses in research took time to develop. Henry Knowles Beecher, a well-known Harvard anesthesiologist, shocked his colleagues with an article, "Ethics and Clinical Research," in the June 1966 issue of the *New England Journal of Medicine*, which listed "unethical or questionably ethical studies." Beecher provided actual problematic studies, which he hoped would be discussed in order to induce "compassion" in his colleagues. For his cases, he pulled examples from major medical journals in a rather unsystematic manner to show how normative the moral errors had become. To make sure his points would be taken seriously (and prosecution avoided), he hid the actual names of the studies and their researchers.[18] The widespread media coverage of Beecher's claims opened up more national discussion of what counted as "ethical" and of what steps should be taken. The Jewish Chronic Disease Hospital and Willowbrook cases were two of his then masked twenty-two examples. "Tuskegee" was not.[19]

In 1972, just one month after the AP's Jean Heller broke the story of the Study, Beecher's student Jay Katz and Katz's students Alexander Morgan Capron and Eleanor Swift Glass published their 1,159-page compendium, *Experimentation with Human Beings*. The Jewish Chronic Disease Hospital and Willowbrook cases were included. Much to Katz's great regret later, he and his colleagues had completely missed "Tuskegee" as a problem.[20]

Beecher's exclusive and unsystematic use of the more easily available major journals may account for his failure to "see" it. In the case of Katz and his students, the omission may have been because they did not survey the specialty journals in this era before Internet and electronic data bases. Although the Study articles in the 1950s and 1960s appeared in *Journal of Chronic Diseases*, AMA *Archives of Dermatology*, and *Archives of Internal*

Medicine, along with *Public Health Reports* and *Journal of Venereal Disease Information*, neither Beecher nor Katz found them.

Communications theorist Martha Solomon Watson argued that the "rhetoric of dehumanization" in the published articles about the Study makes the men the "scene" and the "agency" through which medical science does its work. Although rhetorically the Study reports normalize the use of "male Negro syphilitics" as subjects and make the object of the Study the advance of medical knowledge, this does not explain why Beecher and Katz never found the reports. It does suggest why other medical professionals reading the articles might not have thought anything was wrong.[21] Further, since the later articles on the Study often used the term "volunteers," it would have been impossible for Katz and Beecher to know that they were not, even if they had found the reports. However, historian Susan Lederer has argued that "researchers sometimes used *volunteer* as a synonym for *research subject*, with no special meaning intended regarding the decision of the participants to join in an experiment."[22] Thus, although the Study was "visible" in the medical and public health literature, it remained primarily "invisible" to the broader research communities until the story became public.

Even though the Study did not gain visibility from these two major critiques of American research, it came to be the "scandal" with the longest life in bioethics and public memory.[23] Unlike for the children at Willowbrook or the aging patients at the cancer hospital, the Study had a large and vocal constituency in the African American population, which would remember it as it resonated through other experiences. It affected southern black men, went on for forty years, and built on novelist Richard Wright's insight that "the Negro is America's metaphor."[24] "Tuskegee" became in bioethics the word for the nonconsenting research subject victim. As a key bioethicist made clear: "When somebody wants to point at a project and say, 'This is the worst thing I can imagine,' they say, 'That reminds me of Tuskegee.'"[25]

With all the publicity, the Kennedy hearings, and the federal investigating panel's report in 1973, the Study had perhaps its greatest policy impact on the growth of bioethics through the passage by Congress of the 1974 National Research Act, which mandated the establishment of local institutional review boards for all federally funded research. It meant that checking with "the best men" in the field on a research project, as the PHS had done with the Study, was not adequate. The act also created the National Commission for the Protection of Human Subjects of Biomedical and Behavior Research. Five years later, this commission issued what came to be known as the Belmont Report, with emphasis on the three key principles for research — respect for persons, beneficence, and justice—the founding beliefs for modern American bio-ethics.[26]

When asked about their memories of the work on the Belmont Commission, its members make the Study figure large. For some, the details of all the studies become mixed together. Paul Rogers, a former congressman, managed to recall that it was a study where they "just gave syphilis to people," and Texas internist Donald Seldin thought that "the injection of prisoners—or subjects—with an infected organism without their knowledge, without any kind of informed consent was terrible." Others clearly understood that both Congress and the public were deeply angered by what Georgetown University ethicist LeRoy Walters called "a gross violation of the rights of those men." At the highest reaches of the federal rethinking of research ethics, "Tuskegee" meant that a response was needed.

The Study as "America's Nuremberg"

Bioethicist and Belmont commissioner Albert Jonsen summed it up: "Tuskegee was a constant echo that informed the way in which we viewed research ethics."[27] After "Tuskegee," it was impossible to expect that researchers alone could make "appropriately paternalistic decisions for the public good" in the name of science.[28] Nor could the arguments that certain expendable individuals owed the state and the broader communities the right to their bodies, with or without consent, continue to hold.[29] In addition, the story of the Study became public at a time when broader social currents were focused on racism and the questioning of authority. The bioethics "moral entrepreneurs" would, in sociologist Sydney Halpern's words, use this historical moment to shift "moral boundaries" in order to gain "influence over arenas of public discourse."[30]

On a rhetorical level, "Tuskegee" became "America's Nuremberg" and seemingly brought the issues raised by the Nazi experiments "home" for the first time.[31] Yale bioethicist and Belmont Report commissioner Robert Levine recalled that by the 1990s "Tuskegee" replaced "Nuremberg" (as code in bioethics for Nazi medical horrors) in the American context as the "number one metaphor for evil in research."[32]

This linkage to the Nazis brought attention to the Study and also created a problem. When the litany went directly from Nazis to Tuskegee, the details of the Study entered a historical fog. Alabama became a prison, the men were concentration camp victims, and the PHS physicians morphed into Nazis. The underlying focus on race that suffused the Study, and its location deep within the Alabama Black Belt, often became a way to distance researchers from the PHS physicians.

Although no one told a historian that "they were racists"—as the PHS's John R. Heller commented to James Jones when asked about the Nuremberg Code ("they were Nazis")—"Tuskegee's" southern racialized location provided a mechanism for distancing health care professionals from the Study. And its beginnings were frequently taken as meaning the entire time of the Study, making it closer to the Nazi period and obscuring all that happened during the civil rights era and the ability of the men to leave their farms or use Medicaid or Medicare to get care by the end of the 1960s. It made it easier to see the PHS physicians only as "barbarians" and not "like us."

"Tuskegee" became what psychologists label a "flashbulb" memory, a highly significant event (as opposed to a long series of events) that gets remembered because it is constantly reinforced in discussions and in the media.[33] The Study's "use and abuse" came to be routinely applied to a myriad of other events as the details faded away and the vague metaphor remained.[34] Availability as a supple metaphor requires neither historical accuracy nor the "right use." The linkage between Nazis and "Tuskegee," which took place especially when it became part of the "begat" stories told in an opening lecture in a professional ethics course or in a listing of abuses in an institutional review board-training document, can obscure, rather than highlight, what had happened. Given "bioethicist tales" that emphasized the lack of ethical understandings in the "bad old days," the Study became an example of both how far ethics had traveled and why bioethicists were needed.

Bioethicists kept knowledge of the Study alive in research publications and teaching, but only in narrow ways. The field grew, debating whether principles based in metaethics—the definitions of what is right and good—or in what was labeled the "new casuistry"—reasoning based on specific cases used to draw out the key lessons—should guide its work.[35] For those who focused more on specific cases and on research, "Tuskegee" figured more prominently. A survey of the key bioethics encyclopedias in their multiple editions and the major edited collections and texts reveals that the Study came in and out of use, primarily named as an example of the lack of informed consent and the ability of researchers to take advantage of the vulnerable. It provided a way to say that race matters and then to never really interrogate in what ways.

Critics of the bioethics enterprise argue that its often narrow focus on the problems of autonomy builds on American liberal theory and its concern with individual choice and rights.[36] Concern for individuals tended to obscure both the rights of communities and the context of "choice." With so much emphasis on autonomy, this principle tended to, in Albert Jonsen's word, "swamp" the principles of beneficence and justice.[37] The arguments about the problems of informed consent and the development of the entire institutional review board infrastructure provided little focus on the links between race and science or the problems of equity.

Experimentation as a "practice," not just an ethical dilemma, requires an analysis of "the relationship among medical researchers, doctors and the state as well as between the state and society."[38] This would prove more difficult to make real. The easier story of evil often swamped the parallels that the Study might provide for the problems of gaining consent from a community leader, the realities of agreeing to research in the face of few options, and the actual belief by the researchers that they were not doing anything wrong.

In these bioethics' tellings of the Study story, African Americans were seen as carrying an "undue burden" as the subjects of research. The justice principle could be seen as fulfilled when the seemingly defenseless were protected, often itself a problem. Racial minorities, along with children, the mentally retarded, and prisoners, came to be seen as vulnerable to coerced consent or no consent.[39] The Belmont Report translated concern with the Study into protectionism. Bioethicists did not raise the problem that racism might also leave a community *out* of clinical trials, until after it became a political issue during the beginning of the AIDS epidemic.[40]

Belmont Report commissioner and Georgetown law professor Patricia King articulated how limiting it was to link the Study to protectionism and informed consent alone.[41] She recalled that the commission did not spend much time on "Tuskegee," because the federal investigating committee had already reported and civil rights laws had provided for hospital desegregation just ten years before. For these reasons, King thought, "we didn't go beyond thinking about informed consent in Tuskegee to thinking about what informed consent really means in a situation in which the men in Tuskegee found themselves." With the dangers of the "undue burden" of inclusion so vividly in their minds, King and the other Belmont Commission members could not figure out how "to strike a good balance between inclusion and protection, and it was easier to protect."[42]

"Tuskegee," she argued, was seen as a problem of lack of consent rather than within a broader context of justice tied to the everyday experiences of African Americans with medical care.[43] And, for King, justice required considering not just a more equal distribution of resources and protection. An examination of the everyday practices and institutional arrangements that made individuals from minority groups vulnerable needed to be explored. As the "Tuskegee" story was told, the men's vulnerability was accepted as a given rather than as something that had to be explained.[44]

Thus the Study's other lessons were obscured, despite the existence of much more information on what had happened. Those trying to understand the Study did not have to rely only on the newspaper stories or even on the federal report. Not only bioethicists had a tale to tell.

History and the Study

The story of the Study captured the historical imaginations of two scholars, Allan M. Brandt and James H. Jones, providing the Study with its major "official" storytellers and in turn the basic testimony for those who took the trouble to understand what happened and why.[45] Once these histories were written, they were selectively—and frequently incorrectly—mined for "the facts" to serve other rhetorical ends, with the subtlety of their arguments often ignored.[46] However used, Brandt's often-reprinted article, "Racism and Research," and Jones's book, *Bad Blood*, still in print after more than twenty-five years, were part of the reason why "Tuskegee" stayed in the public consciousness.[47]

Each historian would be captive to passions the Study aroused in the politics of the 1970s and the evidence then available. In the late 1960s, James H. Jones was searching in the archives for material for his dissertation on Kinsey and sex research around the same time as Peter Buxtun was trying to bring attention to the Study, although they did not yet know one another.[48] Jones stumbled upon some of the 1930s Study correspondence within the PHS records that were scattered throughout hundreds of boxes in the National Archives. With only the letters of the early years, and before the public exposure, there was no way for him to know that the Study was still ongoing or that Buxtun was raising questions. He filed a note card about the Study on his lampshade, an idea to be returned to some other time.

After finishing his thesis, Jones took a postdoctoral position in a new bioethics program at Harvard. Expected to write on Kinsey when he got there, he read the news about the Study as he was driving across the country in the summer of 1972. By the time he arrived in Cambridge, "Tuskegee" beckoned as a much more lively book project.

A white liberal southerner with roots in a segregated mining community in Arkansas and in an integrated working-class community in California and raised within the Welsh-American storytelling traditions, Jones understood immediately the critical importance of the Study to a history of racism, medicine, and the emerging field of bioethics. Having struggled with his own family on questions of race, Jones knew that this book could be critical to an ongoing historical engagement with America's racial politics.[49]

After the Harvard position ended, Jones took a full-time job at the National Endowment for the Humanities and put his book on the Study on the "backburner." But after he made contact with attorney Fred Gray over the lawsuit, a deal was struck: if Jones would supply the 1930s PHS correspondence for Gray's lawsuit, then in turn Gray's legal work would provide Jones with what had been culled from the CDC files, the men of the Study to interview, an eyewitness seat on the depositions, a chance to help shape the questions that Gray was to ask, and a framework.[50]

This bargain had a problem. Gray, in arguing the case, had to make the story black and white — to portray the men only as racial victims, to illustrate the gravity of the injury to them and to their families, indeed to all African Americans by extension.[51] But Jones could not do this. He had to step back from some of the sources of his information. Too skilled a historian and committed to telling the story as he saw it, he had to find a way to layer the racism, the professional hierarchy, the bureaucratic inertia, the context of medical research, and the efforts of public health in the South and try to make the "why" clear. As with Henry Beecher's condemnation of the pervasiveness of unethical research, Jones struggled to find the right "tone," as he put it, so that the story would be believable and compelling and not merely something perpetrated in a backwater by a group of racist monsters.

As Jones was working on his book, the *Hastings Center Report*, one of the new major bioethics journals, published in 1978 what would become the first scholarly assessment of the Study by another historian. Allan M. Brandt, completing his dissertation on the history of venereal disease, had also found the materials on the Study in the archives. Aware of the fact that the federal investigating committee had complained about the lack of any materials on the Study's beginnings, Brandt had found what Jones had seen years before. His article, "Racism and Research," became the first scholarly effort to explain "*how* the study was undertaken . . . and *why* it continued."[52] Using a survey of the racist views of physicians toward African Americans, Brandt would place the PHS researchers squarely within the practice of racial medicine at the height of the Jim Crow era. Acknowledging in a footnote that black professionals were involved, Brandt did not cover their roles extensively. He wrote that without access to the racial context and information from the beginnings of the Study, the federal investigating committee had focused on penicillin and informed consent and had missed key points. He made it clear that there was no way to see the men as "volunteers" once the history was uncovered. Racism, he stated strongly, suffused the entire process, and "the degree of deception and damages . . . [was] seriously underestimated."

Brandt made a forceful and definitive argument that would continue to resonate. His evidence came from reading the early correspondence in the National Archives in Washington and the materials and testimony given to the federal investigating committee, including the articles published by the PHS researchers. But materials that were then at the CDC, including the medical records that were not yet available, had eluded him, which might have changed some of his claims.[53]

His contact was with ethicist Jay Katz and reflected what had worried Katz in his dissent from the investigating committee's majority report. Brandt's article clearly summarized the Study, placed it directly in the middle of America's racial past, and argued that researchers could not be left to monitor themselves. Published in a major bioethics journal, it would then be picked up in bioethics, sociology, and history of medicine collections as the summary of the Study. It would continue to be widely reprinted and would be used repeatedly to demonstrate the Study's racism and the PHS's power and deceptions.[54] Brandt, possessing an engaged and deeply moral lecture style and the imprimatur of Harvard, where he taught, would continue to speak on the Study.

Bad Blood, which Jones published three years later, would come to be considered the definitive book, and its reviews in the early 1980s brought the Study back to public attention. As *Boston Globe* science commentator Chet Raymo wrote: "Like many Americans, I missed the story in 1972. I became aware . . . nine years later when I read a review in the *New York Times* of . . . *Bad Blood.* . . . I have never read a more profoundly distressing account of racism in American science."[55] Sold by Black Muslims on the streets of Harlem and in medical school and university bookstores, Jones's book was also widely taught and praised. Medical historians might pick at the nature of the argument and whether or not his claims about racism were not made strongly enough or made too strongly as the key motivator of the PHS doctors, but the reviews were primarily glowing.[56] The book won prizes and landed Jones on major television and radio talk shows and on the lecture circuit. In his jeans and cowboy boots and without notes, in his southern drawl and dramatic raconteur style, Jones told the Study's story in compelling fashion.[57] Ethicist Arthur Caplan summed up the key connection between *Bad*

Blood and the birth of bioethics: "Tuskegee gave birth to modern bioethics and James H. Jones was the midwife."[58]

Bad Blood and the "Racism and Research" article shaped what could be learned about the Study for decades after the newspaper stories faded.[59] Whether what these historians wrote and said, however, then informed what people *knew* about the Study was an entirely different story.

Gospel as Rumor: The Push for Inclusion

After the initial rush of stories, accounts of the Study appeared in major newspapers primarily when there was news of the search for the heirs of the men for the payout from the lawsuit or when *Bad Blood* was published.[60] The Study continued to be taught in college courses and bioethics training sessions and discussed in whispered and head-shaking stories passed as warnings from family member to family member.[61] It became, as a newspaper columnist described it, "the mother lode of all rumors spiraling in and out of black America."[62]

Even with the book and article available, the focus became more on deception and the need for informed consent. The issue of trust did not emerge until the 1980s. In 1985 a high-level federal study probed the links between race and health status, which began much of the contemporary national discussion on "health disparities," as the older term "health inequalities" faded. The Study was not mentioned.[63] Then came the HIV/AIDS epidemic and a growing realization of its major effect on African Americans. This fueled the increasing debate over the reasons for health disparities and why African Americans were disproportionately now missing in medical research clinical and drug trials. To answer these questions, the Study came back into the public story as a form of explanation.[64]

These debates gathered steam among members of a coalition of health reformers and politicians. The "inclusion-and-difference" paradigm, as sociologist Steven Epstein labeled it, shifted concerns from overprotecting African Americans from too much inclusion in research in the post-"Tuskegee" era to the problem of exclusion.[65] The new paradigm accepted that racial groups and women might have different experiences with drugs and disease and needed to be studied separately. Epstein argues that there was a "sharp irony" in this new story: difference was now a way to improve medical care for women and minorities. This reversed the history in which differences were viewed as oppressive. As two bioethicists would argue, there was a "swinging of the pendulum from justice-as-protection to justice-as-inclusion."[66]

AIDS activism led to demands for entries into, not out of, clinical trials. Groups such as ACT UP loudly and publicly raised the question of why minorities did not get tested for AIDS or participate in research. Feminist and other health activists, the Congressional Caucus for Women's Issues, and the Black Caucus took up this question of the missing minorities and women (white and of color) in research and clinical trials for new drugs and devices. With the passage of the National Institutes of Health Revitalization Act in 1993, which required recruitment of women and minorities for federally funded research, the question of why minorities did not willingly participate took on more urgency.[67]

"Tuskegee" was then assumed to be part of the answer, more of a "placeholder," as Steven Epstein labeled it, "in discussion of resistance to participation in clinical research."[68] It was to be, however, not a simple connection. The Study entered the AIDS discourse when it became an available part of the language to explain neglect, indifference, and racism in health care for African Americans. It became linked to a larger sense of a genocidal conspiracy, along with concerns of sterilization abuse, birth control testing, biological warfare, and the origins of AIDS. The Study as fact and "Tuskegee" as fiction made a more public appearance in the 1990s, as health educators and researchers sought to find out what African Americans actually thought about AIDS and medical care and what blocked the usage of health care services.

The Study as tragedy and genocide began to circulate again. At the first CDC conference on AIDS and minorities in 1987, members of a black coalition caucus argued that the "black clergy and church" needed to assure African Americans that "AIDS testing and counseling initiatives are not just another Tuskegee tragedy being perpetrated on the black race."[69] In the late 1980s, "Tuskegee" began to run through both public testimony and newspaper stories as *the* explanation for black fears.[70] The rhetoric shifted as the AIDS epidemic grew, and the story moved again from one of tragedy to genocide. "Tuskegee" would become, in one of the most virulent claims, a form of "germ warfare" and as practice for the unleashing of AIDS through vaccinations from Fort Detrick's biological warfare research laboratory in Maryland.[71] These connections between "Tuskegee" and contemporary health problems would continue and break out periodically.[72]

In 1990, health educators Stephen Thomas and Sandra Crouse Quinn gave a paper, based on what was a "convenience sample" of black church members, that linked the Study to fears over AIDS. In their widely quoted published article, they argued that "public health professionals must recognize that Blacks' beliefs in AIDS as a form of genocide is a legitimate attitudi-

Bioethics, History, and the Study as Gospel {199}

nal barrier rooted in the history of the Tuskegee Syphilis Study." Concerned that the Study had actually been forgotten in public health circles, they used Jones's book to retell the story. Their emphasis on "Tuskegee" would be repeated in their other articles and with citations to their studies and in public health circles, press accounts, and doctor commentaries.[73]

In many of these new surveys, the Study took the weight of other events in black history, as historian Vanessa Northington Gamble has argued, without an understanding, as she put it, that there was more "under the shadow."[74] A sophisticated phone survey done in the late 1990s suggested that the issue was not so much knowledge of the Study but whether or not that knowledge affected a "reduction in the level of trust." In fact, these researchers found that increased knowledge of the Study could actually *increase* willingness to participate in research if the concern with trust did not decline. Other more nuanced studies, following this, questioned whether or not the Study really was so critical to the mistrust among African Americans, which actually was caused by "broader historical and personal experiences."[75]

"Tuskegee" became for some a verbal cue, linked to genocide through AIDS on the one hand and to the Nazis on the other. It explained terrible fears and indicated a sense of historical understanding, whether or not anyone really remembered it, knew what happened, or understood the ways racism structured the health care system. It was, however, sure to raise "moral outrage," which was used to demand both more research and more focus on black health needs.[76]

Nor would "Tuskegee" stay linked only to health care and research. The flooding of New Orleans after Katrina led to widespread beliefs that the government had blown up the levees to intentionally flood the Lower Ninth Ward. When filmmaker Spike Lee argued with libertarian pundit and commentator Tucker Carlson on television over this possibility, they got into a shouting match over whether the history of the "Tuskegee Experiment" demonstrated what the government was capable of doing.[77]

Rumor as Gospel

The biggest rumor continued to be that the government had directly infected the men with syphilis. This belief is everywhere: the Internet, the national nightly news, academic papers, and in deeply held beliefs among health professionals and the public.[78] Stories circulated claiming that those injected included black women, prisoners, Tuskegee Institute students, and the Tuskegee Airmen of World War II fame, whose effort was called "The Tuskegee Experiment."[79]

One of the iconic photographs taken by the PHS in 1953 helped to per-petuate this belief. Widely reproduced from Jones's book and now available from the National Archives, it showed a white doctor inserting a needle into the vein of an unidentified black man. Although the photograph was clearly identified as blood withdrawal and rubber tubing is tightened around the man's arm to make his vein stand out, it could be misread as an injection.[80]

There is absolutely *no* evidence that injection of syphilis occurred in the Study. Inoculation of human beings with syphilis is possible, and there were other experiments in the nineteenth and twentieth centuries in which the syphilis spirochetes, obtained from either humans or rabbits in the more acute stages of the disease, were deliberately injected into the bodies of "sub-jects" through a wide variety of complicated techniques.[81] The spirochete of syphilis is an anaerobic parasite that must be kept moist. If outside of the body for more than two hours, the bacteria will die. Nor can the cells be grown to make an in vitro culture for more than a few generations.[82]

Syphilis's transfer through injection in an experiment also requires tech-niques that have to be done quickly. When this was done on prisoners at Sing Sing Penitentiary in New York in the mid-1950s, an infected rabbit was killed, its testes were ground up, and the bacteria were injected into the 62 subjects within two hours. This usually produced a nodule that became ulcerated at the point of the injection. The inoculum in the Sing Sing study had to be made at 2,000 times the normal infection level to make sure the prisoners got syphilis.[83]

Given the PHS's assumption that the disease was so widespread in Macon County, why would they have bothered? Given the ulcerated sores that would have appeared on the injection sites, why would the men have returned year after year with such a visible and direct initial sign of something wrong?

There are several cultural reasons why the assumption of infecting has outlived the Study and its men.[84] With the linking of the Study to the delib-erate infecting of children with hepatitis and the injecting of older patients with cancer cells, the idea that this third of the trio of bioethics horrors was also an infecting story becomes plausible and the confusion understandable. As the 1994 revelations of the federal government's role in the secretive 1950s LSD and human radiation experiments drew widespread publicity and a gov-ernment investigating committee, the idea of "infecting" by the government through nefarious means took on another mantle. These disclosures came at the same time as AIDS spread and as the twentieth anniversary of the public's knowledge of the Study drew more news analysis.[85]

To understand the symbolic power of "Tuskegee," it is necessary to understand why this fiction persists and what it teaches us about the making of historical meanings. "The wrong tales," Italian oral historian Alessandro Portelli writes, "allow us to recognize the interests of the tellers and the dreams and desires beneath them. . . . Errors, inventions, and myths lead us through and beyond facts to their meanings."[86] If the men being given syphilis are an "invention," what are the "dreams and desires," as Portelli would have it, beneath them? This "wrong tale" has a basis for belief. Health educators have called the assumption that the men were intentionally infected a "disaster myth," a way to explain the "pervasive sense of black mistrust of public health authorities."[87]

The belief that the men were deliberately infected thus fits both folk and historical knowledge. As folklorist Patricia Turner argues, there is "the pervasiveness of metaphors linking the fate of the black race to the fates of black bodies, metaphors in use since the very first contact between whites and blacks."[88] If difference is ultimately presumed to be in the body, then injecting syphilis into the blood, in this case making it "bad," becomes one of the ultimate forms of control to define the nature of that difference. The belief that the men were given a disease that fit racist assumptions about black male sexuality slips without question into the pantheon of horrific modes of control over black bodies.

It is a story used to cope with some of the experiences of racism and the literal and continual danger to bodily integrity that overshadows the experiences of many African Americans. It is not true, but it is certainly plausible. If you assume that the men were not infected but *were* allowed to continue to expose their families, then the government is responsible. The line from a man with syphilis to his wife/sexual partner and then his children becomes the PHS's route of infecting.

In a strange way, the horrific notion of deliberate infection makes it easier to understand the Study and yet to isolate it. To imagine the infecting makes the Study abnormal and a failure of ethics on a grand scale. In this way, the men in Alabama become victims of a different kind of Holocaust. To make this analogy "fixes" both the men in the Study and the PHS physicians as "others."[89]

To understand that the men were not deliberately infected but also were not told that they were in a research study integrates the Study into the logic of American medical science and connects it to the zeal of public health. Then indeed the racism, and its role in the evolution of medical science, becomes much more of a normative experience. This way of making decisions about care—giving it to some, denying it to others—is also an increasingly familiar experience, even a necessity, some would argue. To avoid this kind of understanding, it is easier to deny the Study's reality by making the PHS doctors into monsters and the men into total victims. In this way, the Study becomes a problem only of a specific group, time, and place.

Historians and bioethicists who write about the Study, as well as the media commentators and bloggers who read about it and respond, have tried to correct this assumption about "infecting." This correcting has gone on now for decades. The facts do matter in understanding what happened and, more important, can happen; the story created, however, reflects what Americans need to know and tell themselves. As historian Jill Lepore has written, "The difference between history and poetry, Aristotle argued, is that 'the one tells what has happened, the other the kind of things that can happen.'"[90] The Study's entrance into American lore needed not just the facts. It also needed the fictions.

The Court of Imagination

"Tuskegee," throughout the 1990s and into the new century, evolved into a noun that reverberated through the evening news, films, music, prime-time dramas, and Internet rumors. Uttered by characters on *House, Law and Order, CSI,* and *Saturday Night Live* and by sonorous news anchors, it became *the* word for racism, experimentation, and government deceit.[1]

Questions of trust and experimentation demanded a cultural explanation.[2] In this process, the linkage of race and medical science played out within the paradigm of a racial melodrama that called upon the suffering black male body as a claim for rights.[3] In the "court of the imagination where blacks seek to punish whites for their misdeeds and whites seek to punish blacks for theirs," as scholar/critic Henry Louis Gates Jr. argued about another event, "Tuskegee"-imagined became a crucial site for this kind of reckoning.[4] "Tuskegee" became part of the definition of American blackness, a piece in the "temporal map" of identity that could be formed in the vortex of a cultural "racial passion play."[5] It was these representations that became central to justice for this cultural trauma, which could be neither acknowledged nor healed without them.

A New Sound Track

Don Byron, famed New York–born jazz clarinetist and *Downbeat* magazine's jazz artist of the year in 1992, copyrighted his music under "not tuskegee-like" and titled his highly acclaimed first 1991 album *Tuskegee Experiments.*[6] Byron is a student of history with an extraordinary talent for rehabilitating music forms in a jazz idiom, and the Study attracted his musical genius.[7] The plural name of his album title plays on both the Study and the formal name "the Tuskegee Experiment" that was used for the Tuskegee Airmen.

On the title track, Byron enlists the poetry and voice of Sadiq Bey, a performance poet who often links historical imagery to contemporary problems.[8] The resulting composition is powerful and rhythmic and fits Byron's concern that the jazz of the early 1990s had become too "apolitical," as rap music began to take over the airwaves as the voice of black oppression.[9] The track starts slowly with a wailing clarinet, which gets louder and louder. The percussion picks up the sound and reverberates the painful clarinet's almost human howling as the poet's voice gets more insistent and powerful.[10] The music and the poetry are attacks on the white doctors and the assumed collaboration of the black professionals.[11]

In the poet's rhythmic beat, the stanzas become: "A Dr. Clark conviction, a Dr. Wenger conversion, a Dr. Vonderlehr conception, a Dr. Peters spinal puncture, a Dr. Dibble hanging from his ankles in the town square, the Surgeon General's *schwarzegeist* rising, while Tuskegee falls asleep." Using lines from Jones's interview with Rivers in *Bad Blood*, Sadiq Bey wrote: "Nurse Rivers, who even had a car to shuffle her syphilitic children across Macon County, her 'bad blood' cotton pickers, the 'joy' of her life, was clearly chosen. An appointment befitting this darkest century. . . . They didn't receive treatment for syphilis, but they got so much else. Medicine is as much art as it is science." This was "not a crime, but a rite of sacrifice." He concluded with a mantra of "no treatment! no treatment! no treatment! no treatment," as the screeching clarinet in the background grates on the ears, now more angry than plaintive.

The Study became, in Byron's skilled hands, both familiar and what Freud labeled *unheimlich*, the uncanny that lies between dream and reality, the dread that comes from a border of unreality but yet seems real.[12] Subtleties of why the Study happened and why choices were made drop out in the wailing of Byron's clarinet and in the insistence of Sadiq's voice. The listener is not allowed to forget that something terribly wrong happened to those who, although nameless, ought to be recognized.

Byron's music ultimately provided an updated sound track for the Study, not allowing it to live only in the early twentieth-century blues or gospel of the southern farmlands. With *Tuskegee Experiments*, the Study moved into more urban and modern jazz, reflective of the musical roots of much more contemporary concerns.[13]

History as Television

As Byron was completing his album, news magazine producers at ABC's *Primetime*, documentary filmmakers at *Nova*, PBS television's science program, a BBC film crew, and the National League for Nursing were all getting ready to produce television and video versions of the Study.[14] These documentaries reached millions of viewers—more than did the books and articles, the bioethics courses, or Byron's music. For the first time in nearly twenty years, both the Study's survivors and the PHS doctors emerged from historical fog to become named and visible.

Primetime Live's February 6, 1992, fifteen-minute segment on the Study demonstrated the difficulties of this medium and the construction of a binary of innocence and evil. As the ABC correspondent Jay Schadler would say later, "Television can make anybody into a monster." This certainly happened with physician Sidney Olansky, described as the Study's last director.[15] The doctor, with his grin, white face, and bowtie, provided melodramatic contrast to three of the soft-spoken men of the Study. Schadler's words portrayed the men as peasants. Charlie Pollard was described as a sharecropper, when in fact his family had owned land for several generations. Price Johnson was asked if the $25 for his twenty-five years in the Study was "a lot of money back then," making it sound as if it had been given during the Depression rather than in 1957, when it would have been equal to about three days work at minimum wage.

Olansky clearly had not yet understood what they had done and clung to a doing-the-best-science position. Medical complexity, as an excuse rather than an explanation, was emphasized.[16] Indeed, when Schadler asked Olansky about penicillin, his honest reply, "It would have ruined the study," made it impossible to understand why penicillin might or might not have helped anyone, which in later comments Olansky made clear.[17] The segment created a deep sense of betrayal and wrong.

If the racial differences between the Study's men and its doctors was a subplot to the monster-doctor theme of *Primetime*, it became a much more important part of the longer story told in PBS's *Nova* version. In 1992, as the Study's twentieth anniversary was coming up, veteran ABC medical reporter George A. Strait Jr. took his idea for an hour-long documentary to colleagues at *Nova*. Strait had not covered the story in 1972, but he knew that the men were aging and dying off. As a former scientist, he was concerned with issues of ethics in research and trust. It took more than a year of research and multiple trips to Macon County before the film emerged.[18]

In "The Deadly Deception," *Nova*'s 1993 version of the Study, writer-producer-director Denise DiIanni relied upon historians Allan M. Brandt and Vanessa Northington Gamble (with James Jones in a more minor role) as the "talking heads" and on their writings and interpretations as the film's analytic spine.[19] Strait served as the film's credible key reporter, leading viewers down Alabama roads and into the homes of survivors and to the grave sites of others. The opening lines promise with great drama that he would "find out the truth of the deadly deception." Although the historians make it clear that the Study was not a hidden conspiracy, the film indicts it as deceptive both to its subjects and to the public. Throughout the film, a blues guitar is the musical reminder that you are in the generic black South of long ago.

The film attempts to make clear the ways in which institutional culture at the PHS perpetuated the Study. Interspersed with early 1930s documentaries made of the PHS/Rosenwald Fund syphilis control work in Georgia (the hanging moss on the trees makes it clear that this is not Macon County, Alabama, even if the viewer may not know this), the film made the PHS's intention not to treat and the consequences for the men and their families powerfully clear.[20]

Several of the physicians agreed to be on camera, including John C. Cutler, Sidney Olansky, and David Sencer. Cutler's coldness and "smirk," George Strait remembered, made it difficult to do the interview, and Denise DiIanni characterized him as "beyond defensive to dismissive." Olansky and Sencer, in contrast, Strait thought, were the voices of "institutional bureaucrats who had lost their way."[21]

Since the film was made before the *Primetime Live* segment aired, likely consequences of the doctors' appearances was not yet apparent. As in the ABC segment, the callousness of the PHS is made visual through editing, contrasting the doctor and the unknowing subject. If the physicians had hoped that this film would finally give them a chance to explain their position, they were wrong. No narrative of science or the complexities of syphilis emerged. Instead, at least for Cutler and Olansky, their failures to see the paternalism and racism in their views and their efforts to separate out the "morals" from their "methods" were patent. As Cutler later told a reporter, "These men in Tuskegee helped us learn how to treat syphilis among blacks. They were serving their race."[22]

To make the film more dramatic and to give Rivers a voice, three men from the Study—Charlie Pollard, Herman Shaw, and Carter Howard—are shown going to see *Miss Evers' Boys*, a fictional play about the Study, which, by serendipity, the Alabama Shakespeare Company was staging in nearby Montgomery during the filming of the PBS show. The fictional and factual are laced together to give the viewer a chance to see the men of the Study responding to seeing themselves portrayed on stage. When Mr. Shaw tells again the story of being kept from treatment, the next film cut is back to the play and to the Miss Evers character, who is now stopping him in Birmingham, even though Mr. Shaw has made clear to others that she never did this. In using the play version of Rivers, the fiction imagined by the playwright becomes her words in this documentary.

The views of the health professionals are edited in next to those of the men and next to Strait's narration. Mr. Pollard speaks of being promised free medicine and having his "bad blood" cured. He is the only one who says, "I couldn't have done that to them," as the veneer of southern black politeness slips off for a moment. For the first time, the film gives voice to Bill Jenkins, the epidemiologist at the CDC whose group had tried unsuccessfully to stop the Study in 1969 and who was not in Jones's book. Gene Stollerman, the only physician on the 1969 committee who thought the Study should have ended, again says he was "afraid they were in real big trouble" giving medicine, his, apparently, at least one voice of reason. John Cutler continued to argue that the men were not "merely guinea pigs" and had done the right thing "for their race." Peter Buxtun, the Study whistle-blower, dramatically tells a story of Cutler lambasting him for his interference: "I couldn't understand how they could do something like this," although the CDC's David Sencer cannot imagine Cutler giving such a tongue-lashing.[23] There is a sense that it was lone men who stood up against the system. Any links to a powerful civil rights movement and a growing health rights movement that would have empowered them to speak are ignored.

The connection of Tuskegee Institute/University to the story is mainly visual. Strait speaks to the camera in front of the campus's famous statue of Booker T. Washington lifting the veil off a kneeling black farmer, and Rivers is identified as a Tuskegee Institute–trained nurse, but the Tuskegee Institute–PHS connections are never made clear. The images are much more black and white.

The sense of whether or not the men can speak for themselves is made ambiguous. Attorney Fred Gray argues: "Those men could not speak. I speak for them . . . and they would say my government should never have done it." In this view, the men become the silenced victims, given voice by their attorney, who can enter the courts on their behalf. Yet Mr. Shaw on his tractor and Mr. Pollard in his home both give powerful voice to their personalities and needs. The dignity of the men and their faith are emphasized in a final scene at mealtime as they pray, after which we are told that nearly two dozen of the men died because of the government's indifference.

In the end, the racism underlying the Study and the state's power to make it happen are clear. There is no real discussion of other options, of escape, of concern of medical science at the time, of why this was so normative. The PHS/CDC lost the chance to be seen as saying, "I'm sorry," or "we learned from it." Even if their view of the science could be understood, their failure to see how "Tuskegee" carried into the public realm left them seeming indifferent and immoral. If ever the art of medicine needed to trump its science, it was here.

The politics of these documentaries make a plea for identity and justice for the survivors because of the men's dignity and pathos and due to the price of their pain in the face of what seems certain death. The men become framed as racial innocents because of the PHS's deception. In this portrayal, the usual ways syphilis as a sexually transmitted disease normally leads to stigma are erased, in one of the few cases where venereal disease is not judged. Justice-denied because there was no punishment for the unrepentant doctors becomes the beginning of justice-provided in the documentary imaginary.[24]

"The Grey Zone" of Miss Evers' Boys

The PBS documentary made the rounds of college classrooms and bioethics training programs. But five years later, the story of the Study became a fictional drama and the most common visual way it circulated. Begun as a widely staged play in the 1980s and early 1990s, physician and playwright David Feldshuh's Miss Evers' Boys became the 1997 HBO film starring well-known actors Laurence Fishburne and Alfre Woodard.[25]

Feldshuh had read a review of Bad Blood and then the book while he was in medical school and was fascinated by Jones's view that Nurse Eunice Rivers was the "one who . . . had ethical qualms" and who could provide a sense of "moral ambiguity." The doctors, Feldshuh thought, seemed to have a more straightforward explanation for what they had done.[26] Searching for a way to tell the Study's story that dealt with both current and past time, Feldshuh centered his play on the liminal position of a fictional Rivers, renamed Eunice Evers.

To allow for the dramatization of her moral musings, Feldshuh moved the narrative back and forth between "real" time in Macon County and the august hearing rooms of the U.S. Senate. This allowed him to *imagine* his nurse's "journey of awareness" to moral reasoning and to give speech to her "inner dialogues." In fact, Rivers herself was never called before the Senate and never gave testimony.[27] This fiction allowed a dramatic public self-reflection on her part, as the nurse character says, "I loved those men. . . . [They] were susceptible to kindness." This kindness phrase is so chilling that Feldshuh later used it for the play's accompanying educational video.[28] Rivers, however, never spoke these words. They were actually the thoughts of one of the doctors in the Rosenwald Demonstration, which preceded the Study and in which treatment was given.[29]

"Nurse Evers'" deep connection to the men is portrayed when Feldshuh transformed the "Miss Rivers' Lodge," which served as a burial fund, into "Miss Evers' Boys," the name the men give themselves as a "jilly" dance troupe. Aware that both dancing and boys were black stereotypes, Feldshuh nevertheless needed to dramatize syphilis's progression, without making the play "a lecture on disease." As the fictional Study subject's knees buckle, so does his hope that dancing would be "that desperate ladder out that has hunger about it."[30]

Feldshuh sought to depict the nurse's power and her dilemmas vividly. The play becomes a classic jury trial drama in which the legality and morality of the Study are played out in front of the "court" of senators, with the nurse as both the accused and one of the victims.[31] What Feldshuh called her "moral truths" become most visually told, because, he said, "There is something about pain that comes in spite of love that I found . . . fascinating."[32]

She takes on the moral burden of the Study as both innocent temptress and failed savior. Caught between her sense of nursing duty and love, the fictional nurse ultimately remains a virginal caregiver, always on the edge of lost innocence. She is given a romantic interest in Caleb Humphries, the Study subject who manages to find out more about the disease, to join the army, and to get penicillin.

It would be hard to imagine the talented and attractive stars Laurence Fishburne and Alfre Woodard without sexual sparks. In the film, Evers's dilemmas deepen into tragedy as she rejects her suitor's sexual advances, his entreaties to marry ("I can't be with you and have a lie in my heart," she tells him), and her chance to leave Alabama. She stays single (unlike the real Rivers, who married) and devoted, the film leads us to believe, until the end of her life, caring for the Study subjects who survive. Duty, not a fear of syphilis, has shaped her decision.

In the HBO film version of the play, rewritten by 1950s blacklisted screenwriter Walter Bernstein, sexuality as a theme is even more obvious.[33] The Evers character is given a scene in which she dances seductively in her party clothes (not her blue serge nursing uniform), with her braids down, in a rural juke joint with one of the subjects. The joint's patrons surround her, bang on the tables, and demand that the tempo of the music be made more provocative, while her love interest cheers her on. Centering the film around the romance, Bernstein declared, makes her relation to the men more powerful and "works better." Bernstein was well aware himself of the government's power to turn people against one another, and his version of the story provides romance to lure the viewer in and to express the subtlety and personal costs of the government's power.[34]

Evers becomes the tragic nurse caught between identities: caregiver and race woman, scientific assistant and patient advocate, sexual virgin and race traitor. Although she is the one who speaks, in many ways the play and film silence her ability to speak out. It is her silence and acceptance that condemn her and deepen our sense of tragedy.

The play/film attempts to capture the internal racial politics that enforced immoral decisions during the Study years. African American doctor Sam Brotus, a possible fictional Dr. Dibble, explains the problems of race and science carefully to Miss Evers. When she expresses outrage that the men are not to be treated and that she may leave because of this, he demands that she stay to care for and love them. "Stay with them," he orders, "and carry our burden yourself. Don't ask those men to carry it." Evers replies, "I'm a nurse. I'm not a scientist." But the physician reminds her: "There is no difference. Not here. Not now. Not for us." Although she still protests, she stays, even stopping the men from going to the rapid treatment centers. "You serve the race in your way. I serve it in mine," he reminds her. "I can't rock the boat while I'm trying to keep a people from drowning. There are trade-offs you can't even imagine. Don't you see that?"[35] With the grave-looking actor Joe Morton playing the doctor in the film, Brotus's difficulties become believable.

Class lines in black communities are erased in the film version. The fictional Dr. Brotus is seen as traveling to Washington for the first time, although the real Dr. Dibble was a world traveler. The fictional Nurse Evers is made to be a Tuskegee native and given a father to live with in the community. The class lines that would have separated the educated Rivers from the men in the rural areas are blurred. When the money for the Study dries up for a time, Evers is seen doing domestic work for a group of haughty white women rather than performing other nursing duties, as the actual Rivers did. But then, as an HBO vice president argued about another historical drama, "when we look at historical accuracy, we look at history as it plays in the service of a narrative."[36]

With the focus on the tragedy of the nurse, it is not possible to fully understand the doctors' "why and wherefore." Feldshuh understood that this could be a major difficulty and made clear he differentiated between the "big blames" and the "little blames."[37] He made an effort to explain how racism impinges on scientific thinking, as when Evers tells the senators at the end of the film, "We proved there is no difference between how whites and blacks respond to syphilis." Yet, for most of the play/film, the content of scientific thinking, so hard to dramatize, is left uninterrogated. The dramatization only discusses the overt power of a white establishment. The fictional senator, clearly modeled after Ted Kennedy, asks, "If they were white would they have been treated as anyone?" Here is where Evers shows a touch of anger: "You wouldn't have dared. You wouldn't have voted for it for forty years, if they were white. Somebody would have said something about this before now. Everybody knew what was going on. It wasn't no secret. But because they were black nobody cared."

Before the federal apology in 1997, the play/film appears to have functioned both to put the Study into wider cultural circulation and to provide a form of healing. Actor Obba Babatune, who played one of the subjects in the film, "chased this project. . . . I wanted to be one of the people to tell the story, and in a sense, pay homage to the men who sacrificed their lives."[38] One reviewer of the play's Atlanta production concluded: "The play is partial redemption, not for the unredeemable study but for its victims. The play saves them from pointlessness in their suffering and death. . . . [It] *must* succeed. It is the victims' last chance. And bless it, 'Miss Evers' Boys' does succeed."[39]

Without quite so much hyperbole, Tuskegee's mayor, Johnny Ford, recalled, having performed as the black physician when he brought a version of the play to the city, that it helped to absolve a sense of shame. It made the men into survivors of a tragedy that meant they had served their country. The "embarrassment and shock" that had rocked the city when the story of the Study was made public in 1972 was given a "ritual purge." Ford made sure that some of the survivors came to see the production, and they were given keys to the city and a standing ovation by their fellow citizens. They were for him the story's "unsung heroes." Ford, who remembered the lines he had spoken and many other key ones, took Feldshuh's words into his own memory of what had happened.[40]

Feldshuh's focus on the nurse pushes viewers into what Holocaust survivor/essayist Primo Levi calls the "grey zone." With a focus on those caught in the middle, "grey zones" provide seemingly more dramatic tensions. It allowed for, as in the film made of Levi's essay, a chance for "the viewer to reflect on the larger question of moral culpability and engage in an exercise of historical empathy."[41] Levi was writing, of course, after a generation of complex Holocaust histories and fictions had appeared. Feldshuh was telling the one fictionalized version of the Study that would make it to the screen and that had to represent the untold stories and approaches that would never appear.[42]

Fictional Problems

The film and the play were not without their controversies and difficulties. An actress in one of the early productions of the play accused Feldshuh of lying because he did not show that the PHS had given the men syphilis. Kenny Leon, who directed the play at the Alliance Theater in Atlanta in 1992, argued that it was a chance to open up the possibility of white folks saying, "We did this and we're sorry," and for black folks to reply, "We hear you." But who, he asked, was going to be blamed, "especially when blacks don't want to be the bad guys?"[43] Scott Glasser, who directed the play in Madison, Wisconsin, had to deal with the tensions between himself and his black actors, who were angered that this history was being told at all.[44]

The limits of the film's truths came into focus in Tuskegee as well. Two months after *Miss Evers' Boys* aired on television, lawyer Fred Gray called a press conference to discuss, in part, problems with the film as homage to the men and as an apology for the Study. From the pulpit of the Shiloh Missionary Baptist Church in Notasulga, where dozens of the men were recruited to the Study and then buried in its graveyard, Gray and several of the Study survivors criticized the film's historical veracity. Speaking on behalf of the men, Gray declared: "Miss Rivers was always professional and courteous to them. She did not accompany them to nightclubs. They did not dance, play music and entertain people. . . . The entire depiction of them as dancers and 'shuffling sams' is a great misrepresentation, and does not accurately represent them, nor the other persons who were participants in this study." Herman Shaw declared, "I'm a living witness . . . [and] what they said about Miss Rivers was absolutely wrong." Although the play and movie made it clear that they were "based on" historical events and that Feldshuh had sought to dramatize the Study's moral lessons, to Gray and some of his clients the difference between their realities and those portrayed in the movie were too great. They expected the film to be authentic to their experience and to support legal and political views of them as innocent and dignified survivors of a racial tragedy.[45]

When David Feldshuh and Fred Gray publicly discussed these differences in Tuskegee at a bioethics conference in 1999, the conversation got heated.[46] For Gray, born in 1930 and raised in segregated Alabama and who had seen racism's terrible—literally killing—power in intimate and personal ways, it was the PHS and the state government who had to carry all the blame for the outrage of the Study, not Nurse Rivers or any of the black physicians. Angry at the portrayal of the survivors, whom he knew and respected, as hard-drinking dancing "boys," Gray saw all of it as historically wrong and reprehensible. Feldshuh's attempt to defend his efforts, to explain the racial "vise" he thought his characters were in and the irony of the title he had created, failed to convince Gray.[47]

Feldshuh had his own stories: a bomb threat against the play one night in Los Angeles and a white woman who grabbed him and demanded, "How dare you portray white doctors like that?" Yet such tales carried little moral weight when put up against Gray's life experiences. Even when Cynthia Wilson, the Tuskegee University archivist, attempted to insert more of the "facts" and "evidence" of the Study into the discussion, it was clear that Feldshuh's effort would continue to be denounced by Gray as ahistorical.

Memory, experience, and the need to see one's own story reflected accurately in film trumped an effort to dig out the historical "facts." The usual tensions in film about what is "authentic" in black experiences were played out in the arguments between Gray and Feldshuh. Gray, and the survivors who spoke, wanted any sense of playfulness or drinking out of the film. They did not want the movie to add to any sense that the Study had undermined their dignity and control.

Instead, the dramatic need to show the impact of syphilis led to a "cinematic mimesis" that repeated the old view of black men as hard-living, easily manipulated, and sexualized "boys," except for the one character who gets away.[48] For the Study's survivors who had overcome the stigma of a sexually transmitted disease to become pure racial icons of victimization, this stereotype in a film that they had expected to be ethnographic was anathema. In searching for a representation that focused on the limits of white stereotyping of blacks, the film in many ways recapitulated the very stereotype it was attempting to critique.[49]

The play/film's focus on a fictional Nurse Rivers provided a rich sense of moral complexity. In many ways, *Miss Evers' Boys* was an attempt to show how the power of racism could corrupt a good and caring person. It allows us to consider: Which Nurse Rivers is more fictional? The racial and gender nurse victim of memory or the more deeply morally troubled fictional character? We cannot expect that one film or one telling, even from the memories of those who were there, can answer these questions.

The play/film became a "radical injustice" in which the PHS doctors avoided judgment and scrutiny.[50] The biological assumptions about race, the complicated public health questions surrounding syphilis, and its treatment over time were all ignored as well, because this story could not so easily be dramatized. It left viewers to imagine that somehow we already know this story about doctors doing the wrong thing in experimentation and we do not need for it to be told.

Miss Evers' Boys went on to a continued life, often shown during black history month in February on HBO and easily available as a DVD for teachers to use in class. Don Byron's linkage of the Tuskegee Airmen to the Study as "the Tuskegee Experiments" would also gain its visual parallel with another HBO film. Starring Laurence Fishburne again, this film, *The Tuskegee Airmen*, became a drama about one of the proudest exemplars of African American manhood.[51] With the terminology of "Tuskegee" and "experiment" so similar and with actor Laurence Fishburne starring in both films, the two stories began to merge in the public imagination.[52] Thus, newly reracialized and resexualized, the Study added a visual memory to its cultural repertoire and fueled the factual confusions.

The separation of fact and fiction in the Study becomes even more difficult when visual images burn a particular telling into our minds. Yet those pictures, of a dancing man slowed to a standstill by syphilis, of the courtly comments of Herman Shaw on his own farm, and of the obtuseness and lack of repentance of the PHS doctors, all kept the Study alive. The film, play, and documentaries told the story as tragedy, but at least they created visual memory, while Byron's music created the sounds of urgency, not mourning.

During his run for the presidency in 2008, Barack Obama reminded the nation that Americans prefer our race stories as "tragedy" or as "spectacle." The visuals provided this tragedy and left the responsibilities more ambiguous, but it would be in the halls of Congress and at the White House that the spectacle of responsibility would be named directly.

12

The Political Spectacle
of Blame and Apology

The Study seared its place into American culture through its appearance in the political realm, adding different kinds of visual events to the saga. With the election of liberal white southerner Bill Clinton to the presidency in 1992 and his efforts to speak about racial divides, it would be no surprise that the Study could gain political prominence. The debate over Clinton's choice for surgeon general and then his willingness to extend a federal apology brought new media attention and scrutiny. The Study returned to its origins in the federal government, but in ways that provide insight into how differing understandings could become potent political fodder. At first glance, the apology would seem finally to provide some closure, giving us what novelist William Dean Howells once described as the American desire for "a tragedy with a happy ending."[1] But redemption is never this simple.

Moral outrage as a response, however momentarily satisfying, can be manipulated into very different meanings to serve multiple political ends. The very acknowledgment of what happened can be the beginning of a meaningful societal conversation, but it did not and could not guarantee that the talking would continue.

Henry W. Foster Jr.: Going after the Wrong Surgeon General

Just as *Miss Evers' Boys* had focused on the black nurse in the Study, confirmation hearings in 1995 for a new surgeon general spotlighted the black doctors.[2] An open airing of what the government and medicine could do to overcome the legacy of mistrust turned instead into the rejection of a black doctor who had worked at John A. Andrew Memorial Hospital at Tuskegee

Institute during the last years of the Study. Once again, apparent black complicity became the focus of concern.

In 1994, President Bill Clinton, under intense political pressure, forced the resignation of Jocelyn Elders, the nation's first black surgeon general. She had dared to speak out in favor of health reforms and suggested that masturbation could be an alternative to risky sexual practices in the face of the AIDS epidemic. Clinton turned to Henry W. Foster Jr. as the next physician to nominate for this medical bully pulpit. An obstetrician-gynecologist at Vanderbilt University in Nashville, Foster's "I Have a Future" organization to prevent pregnancy in urban young women had been cited several years earlier as one of President George H. W. Bush's "thousand points of light" programs for volunteerism. Foster seemed a safe candidate after Elders, given this Republican award, his support for sexual abstinence, and his long years of work in black communities.

Foster's nomination came in December, just after the 1994 midterm elections in which the Democrats lost control of the House for the first time in forty years to the Republican "Contract with America" juggernaut. Foster's confirmation process began in the press, even before his hearings in the Senate. Because of his specialty, the issue of abortion and sterilizations came up almost immediately. Foster made several public fumbles on the number of procedures he had performed and why. The press waved the hot button issue of abortion before Foster's formal confirmation even began.[3]

It was at this point that the Study became part of Foster's undoing. Searching for ways to discredit Foster's nomination further, Gary Bauer, a former Reagan administration domestic policy adviser and head of the conservative Family Research Council, followed Foster's career back to his eight years as the only obstetrician at John A. Andrew Memorial Hospital.[4] Releasing excerpts from Jones's *Bad Blood* to the press, Bauer's organization noted that Foster had been vice president of the Macon County Medical Society in 1969. This was at the time that two CDC officials had come to Tuskegee to discuss the Study with the by then almost entirely black medical group. Foster's link to the Study was made, even though in his book Jones mentioned only Jones's vice presidency status, not his being at the meeting where the CDC presumed that support for the Study was obtained.[5]

For the next several months, until Foster's confirmation hearings in early May, his nomination continued to be damaged in the public mind. Most of the focus was on the abortion and sterilization questions, but his "possible" role in approving the Study in 1969 served as the emotional coup de grace.[6]

Through the White House, Foster immediately issued a statement that he had only learned about the Study in July 1972. "Had I learned the facts of the study any earlier," he declared, "I would have been equally outraged then, and I would have insisted on appropriate treatment, as I did in 1972."[7]

Reporters and congressional staffers immediately began searching the National Archives to find the names of other physicians who had been there and asking scholars of the Study what they knew. Dr. Luther McRae, a physician whom Foster had crossed swords with before in Tuskegee when McRae attempted to get funding for a local hospital that only served whites, told reporters he was certain Foster had been at the meeting, named the restaurant, and remembered where Foster sat. Howard Settler, a Tuskegee ophthalmologist who was also at the meeting, was much less sure. He could not remember if Foster had been there and recalled the meeting as more of a "report" than a question of getting the doctors' approval.[8] Reporters and the scrambling Clinton administration staffers asked the same questions of the historians, lawyers, and ethicists who had written on the Study: what did he know, when did he know it, and did we have documents?[9]

Clearly, the Clinton administration staffers handling the nomination were becoming increasingly concerned that it would be difficult to explain how Foster, at such a small hospital in a small community, could *not* have known about the Study. None of the historians had ever seen minutes of the medical society meetings or a list of who had been there. All had seen the same CDC bureaucratic note the officials had produced in 1969.[10]

When Foster finally appeared on May 2 and 3, 1994, for his confirmation hearings, the senators continued to use the Study to question his credibility. A *Washington Post* editorial concluded: "It is crucial to pin down when Dr. Foster learned about the study. His fitness for the job hangs on it."[11] In this context, the focus on what the doctors knew and did was directed not at the federal government, but at Foster and the physicians of the Macon County Medical Society.

Foster explained carefully and forcefully that he had not known about the Study until 1972, when as president of the medical society he had worked to get the survivors to treatment. He testified that he had not been at the 1969 meeting and provided an affidavit from one of his patients to show that he had been doing a Cesarean section at the time of the meeting. There was no "cover-up," he contended, because the medical society doctors who did remember the meeting were sure they were not told that the men were not being treated. As he would write later in his memoirs, "No doctor in Tuskegee would have tolerated such a deplorable experiment; in fact, I am sure every doctor would have gone ballistic. I couldn't understand how anyone would have thought we would have turned our backs on the very community we had come to serve."[12] Under the circumstances of the attacks and the hearings, Foster was not in a position to discuss what Dr. Eugene Dibble and other black physicians in the community had done or not done. He did not know.

Republican senator Dan Coats of Indiana pressed Foster at the hearings. Citing the documents that appeared to show that the CDC came away from the 1969 meeting believing the Macon County Medical Society was on board, Coats came close to accusing Foster of lying and being a racial sellout. Yet a clearer reading of the documents that Coats put into the *Congressional Record* tells a more nuanced story.

In the deposition he gave in the Study lawsuit, CDC head David Sencer made it clear that his subordinates who went to the meeting had not left a written record but had told him the Macon County Medical Society evinced "a total lack of interest in getting involved." This is a far cry from the assumption that they were on board, the idea that somehow got translated into the CDC's thinking, Jones's narrative in *Bad Blood*, and then the charges against Foster.[13]

In his exchange with Coats over all of this, Foster finally lost his "cool," insisting that he had no knowledge of the Study before 1972. His strong response to Coats reflected his anger that, as he would write, "this was the first time my sense of morality had ever been impugned."[14]

The question of whether or not the local physicians did or did not approve the Study would never be answered. Because the focus was on the 1969 meeting, no one asked Dr. Foster if he had discussed the Study with Dr. Dibble, who had hired him, before Dibble's death in 1968. But there was, as many of the scholars of the Study explained to the members of the press who asked, no reason to assume that Dibble would have discussed the Study with an obstetrician-gynecologist. As Foster made clear, none of the men were his patients, although no one asked him if he had seen any of their younger wives or children. Foster knew Rivers from the hospital, but there is no reason to assume that she would have discussed the Study with him. In the process of looking back, the Study takes on enormous power as a major event in Tuskegee. But those caring for an underserved population would have been focused on many other more pressing concerns.

At the hearings, Dr. Foster told his own story—of a black man of his generation who had struggled against segregation and racism. Through the support of his family he had become a physician who cared deeply about the health care of black communities. In the end, his story and his assurances silenced the concerns about "Tuskegee," but for naught. His nomination made it through the committee, but there were enough questions about his willingness to do abortions and sterilizations, wrapped in doubts about his credibility, to threaten a filibuster. His nomination died, tabled and never voted upon.[15]

The public was left to wonder why black doctors had allowed the Study to continue but not to consider why the Study had happened in the first place. In the glare of the publicity and the lights of a Senate hearing, the complicated reasons behind the Study were never discussed. Foster's hearings deflected any real conversation about what had happened. The real Nurse Rivers never had to explain herself to the Senate, and it became ironic yet emblematic of racial spectacle that a real black doctor who had had nothing to do with the Study did. A potential surgeon general, not the ones who had approved the Study, took the blame and became the villain.

Anatomy of an Apology

The Study as political spectacle began almost immediately to take on a new form, which would overshadow the Foster debacle. On February 23, 1994, while Foster's nomination was being tossed about in the media on its way to the Senate, a small academic conference was being held at the University of Virginia. "Doing Bad in the Name of Good: The Tuskegee Syphilis Study and Its Legacy" sought to evaluate the Study's history and consequences.[16] The usual array of academics spoke, and it might have been just another conference. When a British documentary on the Study shown at the conference demonstrated yet again Sidney Olansky's lack of remorse or regret, University of Virginia bioethicist John C. Fletcher was "dismayed and appalled." An Alabama-born former Episcopal priest who had worked on bioethics in its earliest incarnations while at the National Institutes of Health, Fletcher dropped his assigned talk on the Nuremberg Trials and spoke on the history of informed consent and ethics within the United States. At the end, he declared in heartfelt tones, "It is never too late to apologize."[17] Fletcher's suggestion did not give rise to an immediate response.[18] The conference moved right on to the next speaker.

Fletcher's deeply felt statement might have stayed at the conference had he not had connections within the federal government and in "informal networks" where the idea could take root.[19] After the conference, Fletcher spoke to his contacts within the federal health hierarchy and to Don Demeter, vice president for Health Sciences at the University of Virginia. Demeter, a physician, a former officer in the PHS, and a clinical associate at the National Institutes of Health, then wrote to Dr. Phil Lee, an undersecretary for health in the Department of Health and Human Services in the Clinton administration, to begin an inquiry about the possibility of the apology. Others began to discuss it within the CDC. AIDS activist/organizer A. Cornelius Baker remembered that he heard a CDC physician talk about it at a CDC-sponsored "Syphilis in the South: New Ideas, New Partners" conference in Washington eleven months later, in January 1995.[20] Enough people thought it a good idea that by May 1995 a working group within the CDC had formed.

In the early 1990s, official apologies became much more common worldwide as truth and reconciliation commissions were organized, part of what one scholar calls an "age of apology" that "spring[s] from the interpretive fluidity of history."[21] The advantage of a call for an apology for the Study and at that time became clear. Unlike demands being made for reparations and apologies for slavery, an apology for the Study would focus attention on a particular set of acts by the federal government and on a particular set of victims, some of whom were still alive. The Study had been over for decades, and it had gone on during both Democratic and Republican administrations. Getting an apology from a government led by a southern-born president who appeared "to get" racism might be possible.

The idea swirled around for about a year within the CDC and within the health education and provider communities, which were becoming increasingly aware of how distrust and stigma might be related to memories of the Study.[22] The reauthorization bill for the National Institutes of Health in 1993 required more inclusion of minorities and women in medical research. But researchers claimed they were running into mistrust and refusals.[23] Yet there was anxiety within the CDC that if it apologized it would affect its work. The idea appeared to be at a dead end and "going no where," in the words of Rueben C. Warren, then associate director of Minority Health at the CDC.[24]

"Outside agitation" came by late 1995 from the collaboration between Ralph V. Katz, an academic dentist and epidemiologist at the dental school at the University of Connecticut, and Warren, a longtime colleague of Katz who is also a dentist and has a public health perspective.[25] Katz, who had come to the University of Virginia for the conference on the Study, was then the director of the National Institutes of Health–funded Northeastern Minority Oral Health Research Center. Katz and Warren conceived a plan, cobbled together some funds from the CDC, and funneled the monies through the Minority Health Professions Foundation.

Their idea was to bring together historians, CDC officials, Tuskegee University, and state and local health administrators for a workshop in Tuskegee to discuss, as the invitational letter read, "the impact of the USPHS-Tuskegee Syphilis Study on minority PARTICIPATION in Federally-sponsored health research." The carefully worded invitation made it clear that its purpose was both "to develop a strategy for issuing an apology to the African-American community from the U.S. government for the research abuses" of the Study and to consider ways to increase "minority trust." The call for the workshop explained that part of the agenda was to advance the "biomedical research agenda, which now mandates inclusion of minorities and women as research subjects."[26]

On January 18 and 19, 1996, a group of twenty-six met at the Tuskegee University Kellogg Conference Center. Attorney Fred Gray was not invited to the conference because of the 1973 lawsuit and CDC funding, nor were any of the survivors or their families. Whistle-blower Peter Buxtun told his story, general discussion occurred over trust, and the Study's major historian, James H. Jones, spoke of "Tuskegee" as a symbol and metaphor. John C. Fletcher reiterated his call from the Virginia conference. "It needs to be done because it has never been done," he declared. Historian/physician Vanessa Northington Gamble pointed out that the apology for the government's radiation studies was done at the presidential level and that the group ought to, as her grandmother had taught her, "go to the top."

The urgency of the request was underlined when, on the night between the two days of meetings, the highly popular cop/crime television show *New York Undercover* screened an episode called "Bad Blood."[27] The plot involved a murder and an older black physician who had been in Tuskegee and who was now injecting unknowing patients in Harlem. "What could we do," Fletcher asked directly the next morning after the episode was discussed, "to pierce the belief that science equals genocide?" The answer came in the wording put forth by Jones and seconded by Gamble: "The apology should be from the President of the U.S., as soon as possible, issued at Tuskegee, with directives (Executive orders) from the President to the appropriate governmental services and agencies."[28]

The group passed the motion to ask for the apology and then discussed what else needed to be done. Everyone seemed to sense that such an apology would be momentous but only an empty gesture if it lacked a way to provide other concrete mechanisms to back it up. The ideas ranged widely: bioethics conferences, educational modules on the Study, a museum, scholarships on bioethics for minority students, and a bioethics center at Tuskegee University.

As a result of the meeting, a subgroup formed as the Legacy Committee, with Fletcher and Gamble as the cochairs.[29] Over the next months, Fletcher tried his hand at a draft, which was reworked by others on the committee and sent to Gamble. With Fletcher's draft, the comments, and the assistance of her graduate student Judith A. Houck, Gamble edited what would become the final call for the apology. There was concern over the tone of the call and the question of to whom the president would apologize.[30] Would it be to the survivors and their families, or to the "larger black community"? Those helping to write the call also struggled with how much of the complex history to put into such a short document.[31]

By the end of May, a final report had been hammered out and sent to the CDC. It linked the call for a presidential apology to the litany of the Study's ability "to symbolize racism in medicine, ethical misconduct in human research, paternalism by physicians, and government abuse of vulnerable people." The report's request was for a formal apology from President Clinton to the "living survivors, their families, and the Tuskegee community," made "to redress the damages caused by the Study and to transform its damaging legacy." The history was briefly laid out and the possibility that the men had been contagious and passed the disease on to their wives and children was noted. The statement went on to point out the way in which Tuskegee University's name had been tarnished by its connection to the Study, even though "primary direction" had come from the "government under the auspices of the USPHS." Apologizing was seen as a first step toward regaining trust within the entire African American population. To "transform the legacy," the committee called for a center at Tuskegee University that would be both museum and educational institution.[32]

Apologies, of course, do not occur just because a group of concerned citizens writes a request to the president. The organizing had to happen in earnest once the letter had been sent. By May 1996, the committee agreed that the push for the apology had to wait until after the 1996 presidential elections, because, as Gamble wrote, "it would trivialize an apology if it were viewed as election year maneuvering."[33] Inside the CDC, Rueben Warren and then Dixie Snider, the CDC's Chief of Science, continued to stay in touch with Gamble, Tuskegee's president Benjamin Payton, and Representative Louis Stokes, whom the CDC's Rueben Warren called the "godfather of the apology."[34]

As the proposal went through what Snider called "umpteen iterations," the importance of the past and its contemporary legacy became the focus.[35] Within the CDC, not everyone was certain that making so public a statement about such a seemingly colossal failure was the right thing to do, and some feared its negative impact on their work. At critical moments in the internal discussions, those pushing for the apology joined with the Congressional Black Caucus and other political organizations.[36] AIDS activist A. Cornelius Baker began getting his contacts to weigh in.[37] The caucus, which had been working its connections to the White House, issued a formal letter. As the caucus's two cochairs, Maxine Waters and Louis Stokes, argued to the president, "There can be no justice and no faith can be regained in this nation's public health system until those Black men, who were subjected to the Tuskegee experiment, have had their humanity recognized, validated, and restored. Now is the time to bring this sad chapter in our nation's history to an end by issuing a formal apology." Fred Gray, who knew about the Legacy Committee and who still represented some of the Study survivors, also leaned on his Washington connections.[38]

The lobbying and timing worked. National attention was refocused on the Study as HBO's film was aired that February. Staffers and those with contacts in the government continued to press the request. During February and March, the details were worked out, as Clinton agreed to do it. On April 7, the press was alerted that it would happen in May. The location was set as the White House, not Tuskegee, as originally requested, because of Clinton's schedule and the fact that the press corps was more likely to cover a major racial story in Washington.

The apology was thus staged, on May 16, 1997, with all the pageantry that an event in the East Room of the White House makes possible. Crammed into this formal room, along with the president and vice president, were Study survivors, Clinton cabinet members, federal officials, high-ranking black political leaders both in and outside of government, the Legacy Committee, Dr. Henry Foster, attorney Fred Gray and his son, representatives from Tuskegee University, and family members of the Study's men. A satellite downlink brought the event into the conference center at Tuskegee University for hundreds more and was available on C-SPAN. Sticking to his principles, John Fletcher refused to attend because the event was not in Tuskegee.[39]

The event was worthy of a tableau in a southern novel. Five of the Study's six living survivors, with carnation boutonnieres in their suit lapels and accompanied by family members and friends, came in after everyone was seated as both applause and awe filled the room. Called to speak, 95-year-old Herman Shaw walked slowly to the podium, exuding his usual great strength and dignity. As the spokesman, he reminded the world that the

African American men in the Study were not "dancing boys," as portrayed in the HBO film, nor should they have been the government's "human guinea pigs." As he said clearly and directly, "We are hardworking men, not boys, and citizens." Linking manhood to citizenry in a united America, Shaw declared that trust and caring had to span "black, red and white together" so that "the kind of tragedy which happened to us in the Tuskegee Study [would never] occur again." Then, with his characteristic charm, awareness of what he labeled his "great pleasure," and no small sense of irony, he introduced "the Honorable William Clinton, President of the United States."[40]

Clinton's speech of apology was a masterpiece of political rhetoric and expression of heartfelt sadness for the bitter legacy of the Study. He welcomed each of the survivors or those representing survivors by name. "Without remembering the past," he declared, "we cannot make amends and we cannot go forward." He acknowledged the betrayal and the denial of the rights of citizenship. With great depth of feeling he reminded his audience: "What was done cannot be undone. But we can end the silence. We can stop turning our heads away. We can look you in the eye and finally say on behalf of the American people, what the United States government did was shameful, and I am sorry." Stunned silence and then applause filled the room.

Clinton declared that there would be assistance for a "lasting memorial at Tuskegee," as he reclaimed the honor of the institute/university of Booker T. Washington and George Washington Carver. He authorized a planning grant for a "center for bioethics in research and health care" and a "museum of the study and [to] support efforts to address its legacy and strengthen bioethics training." He asked for a report on how to best involve minority communities in "research and health care," for "training materials for medical researchers" on "ethical principles," and for "postgraduate fellowships" for minority students in bioethics.[41]

The president's rhetoric, as communications scholars noted a few years later, put racial injustice, not "medical ethics and abuse of power," at the center of the problem. Clinton's language made it clear that the apology was not just from the PHS or the government. It was from the American people. The institute's role in the Study was made to be peripheral and the desire for racial reconciliation was made simpler. Science became value-free, as only racial politics, not something inherent in the way scientific ideas are constructed, became the cause of the Study and at the center of what went wrong.[42] The apology thus became an apology for racism and not really about the role of medicine and science in the creation of beliefs about race.

Perhaps it could not have been more. Clinton could not turn the event into a lecture on racial stereotypes, medical racial beliefs, and the passion of science. A formal setting in the White House did not allow for a discussion of the complexity of syphilis and the idea, even for a moment, that the PHS doctors were not merely racist monsters. The possibility that there had ever been any escape for the men and their families was not to be mentioned. The federal government needed to acknowledge its role in deliberately causing illness and death and then repent. This Clinton, with all his southern political skills, could do with soaring rhetoric and deep emotion.

Indeed, the coverage centered on the emotionalism. Both at the White House and in Alabama, many commented on the high and varying feelings at the event, the closure it provided for some, the simple but powerful effect of a president saying that this was racist and that "we are sorry." Much of the coverage milked the event for its passions. On CNN *Live*, survivor family members were asked over and over, "How did you feel?" The word "emotional" became the mantra repeated by the reporters.[43] It was as if only in the context of emotionality could the pain of racial injustice become real or discussed. The Study apparently could only be communicated to a television audience in the familiar daytime format of confession and repentance.

A front-page *New York Times* photograph captured the poignancy of the event. Herman Shaw was in full view embracing the president, with only the side of Clinton's head (not his face) visible, as Vice President Al Gore and CDC director David Satcher fade into the background. For that moment, in that photograph, the trust and humility seemed to be captured. Yet Albert Julkes, whose father and uncles had been in the Study, told a reporter, "Can you close out slavery? There never will be a closure. But this offers a salve on a festering sore."[44]

Damaged trust would become a more difficult and deeper wound to heal. Apologies, historian Johanna Schoen has argued, can be just "rituals without coming to terms with history."[45] Anger that the doctors never suffered, either in their careers or by going to jail, for what many saw as murders fueled some of the responses. The apology for the Study mattered because it acknowledged the pain and renewed the necessity for a discussion of the history. The meaning made of that history, however, would never be uniform, and the Study's availability to be imagined continued.[46]

Epilogue

The Difficulties of Treating Racism with "Tuskegee"

By the early twenty-first century, "Tuskegee" had become deeply embedded in the cultural life of the United States, and it had traveled across borders to be used in battles over drug studies. With the growing number of clinical trials in the Global South, medical racism and neocolonialism renewed the need for regulation. This time, in a trial for anti-HIV drugs in Uganda, "Tuskegee" came to be part of a new worldwide contestation. In this version, however, the CDC, the National Institutes of Health, and the African physicians who had agreed to these studies replied immediately, arguing something eerily similar to what Dr. Eugene H. Dibble might possibly have said if asked in 1932: you do not understand what bargains need to be made in a community with few medical resources and what kind of studies are needed.

These experiences in Uganda caused "Tuskegee" to be used to raise new questions. Under such politicized and powerful circumstances, new "counternarratives" about the Study appeared.[1] With racism in research now seen as a moral error of international consequence, the "methods" of the Study and its "facts" came under increasing scrutiny. "Tuskegee's" power as symbol was refueled.

With this focus on racism, the concepts of race that had begun the Study in the first place dropped out. When the apology and lawsuit proved to be not enough justice and with consciousness of the disparities in health outcomes growing, the idea of a drug treatment just for African Americans emerged as a new form of reparations for the Study's racism. Without a critique that included both what had happened and how the concept of race and the social reality of racism are linked, the Study's life as symbol was still available. Meanwhile, in Macon County, an effort to provide a new history and future for its citizens would also make use of the "Tuskegee" story.

"Tuskegee" Goes International

Less than a month before the apology, a clinical trial for an antiretroviral drug for HIV treatment in Uganda and other developing countries brought the Study to international attention. In April 1997, physicians Peter Lurie and Sidney Wolfe, from the Health Research Group of Ralph Nader's Public Citizen organization, fired an opening salvo in what is still a major debate over a failure to treat in international drug studies in developing countries. The National Institutes of Health and the CDC were both funding drug trials to stop vertical transmission (mother to child) in women with HIV, especially in Uganda.

Several of these studies were designed to test whether a short course of one of the newly available antiretroviral drugs, AZT, rather than the expensive long courses then being used in the developed world, would stop newborns from developing HIV. But instead of matching short courses with long courses of the drugs in the study, some of the trials matched the short course with placebos, which meant no treatment for some of the women, who had approximately a 26 percent chance of passing the disease on to their newborns. It was not clear that the women understood that they could be in a placebo arm or if it was ethical not to give this arm of the study the standard of care (long courses) available in the Western world.

After learning about the studies, which were funded with U.S. government money, Lurie and Wolfe wrote to Donna Shalala, secretary of the Department of Health and Human Services, to denounce these trials and to call for their suspension. Aware that the apology for the Study was about to take place, they argued that another "atrocity" was occurring, that the government was "perpetrating a new African-Asian-Caribbean Tuskegee in which many more people will die." As Sidney Wolfe put it bluntly, "It is Tuskegee, part two."[2]

When the letter did not receive much attention, Lurie and Wolfe appealed to President Clinton and then to the medical community in the highly visible and well-circulated *New England Journal of Medicine* the following September. Accompanying the doctors' letter was journal editor Marcia Angell's denunciation of the studies, and the parallel to "Tuskegee" became her central trope. It was the medical world's way of arguing, as it had in 1972, that "genocide" was occurring without using the actual term. The word "Tuskegee" would do.

The directors of the CDC and the National Institutes of Health rejected the "Tuskegee" analogy in their response article a month later. They defended the ethics of the placebo trials in developing nations as the quickest way to find drugs that were "safe and effective" and that took into account both the nature of illness in the areas and available resources. The standard for determining ethical research could not be the same as in the developed world since the risks and benefits were not equal, they argued.[3]

The debate remained a primarily medical one until media coverage spurred by the *New England Journal* controversies were picked up. Then journal editor Angell brought the criticism even more into the public eye with an op-ed piece in the *Wall Street Journal*. This time the analogy was clear: the editorial was titled "Tuskegee Revisited." Here she made the parallels to the Study even more explicit, from the false promise of medical care to a critique of the defense that treatment was not otherwise available to the Ugandan subjects.[4] The debate spilled over into other media outlets and into congressional hearings, as physicians and ethicists around the world took up their positions. Defenders of the studies pointed out the efficiency of placebo studies in providing proofs and expressed the belief that HIV's course was varied in different populations. Critics argued for the need for universal protections that brought the research standards of the United States and Europe to the rest of the world. "Tuskegee" was a constant refrain.

Part of the justification for the Study in Alabama had been, of course, the assumption that the men would not have gotten to treatment even if there had been no study. In the international context in 1997 this justification raised the "standard of care" argument: whether the drug trials' standard of treatment would be "defined in universal or local terms."[5] Some supporters of the new studies charged the critics with "ethical imperialism." Local supporters of these protocols believed they better understood conditions and needs in their own countries than the foreign ethicists did. Indeed, one philanthropic official who worked on disease in the developing world declared that "ethicists had become a significant threat to global health."[6] In Kenya, an official from the Ministry of Health who supported the studies believed that "the issue of ethics is compounded by the fact that African women simply cannot afford AZT."[7] But the critics of the trials denounced the dangers of "ethical relativism" and lack of justice.[8]

The debate continued well after the uproar over the AZT trials had died down and after each side had claimed that the placebo was needed or was not needed. After these debates, the World Medical Association, in a revised Declaration of Helsinki, tried to come up with a compromise that would allow for placebo trials "in studies where no proven prophylactic, diagnostic or therapeutic method exists." But as soon as this policy was declared, it was being honored in the breach. Even now, more than ten years later, there is still no worldwide consensus on an acceptable standard of care in research trials in poorer areas, or even about who should make that decision.[9] Bowing to a variety of pressures, however, in May 2008 the U.S. Food and Drug Administration (FDA) agreed that despite the Declaration of Helsinki it would accept "new drug applications even if the trials only compare new products to placebos instead of the best available treatments," in both U.S.- and foreign-based trials.[10]

The lack of consensus reflects the difficulty of what hardly are "choices" in many developing countries. In these studies, as in Alabama, it has been local physicians who have had to triage care by accepting research in the hope that it would lead to other assistance. Most of these physicians believed that they were doing the best for those under their care.[11] This is not meant to justify the research then or now, but rather to refocus our attention on how hard the decisions are—and were. This issue of the under-resourced local doctors' tough decisions never made it into Angell's denunciation of the 1997 studies nor into her argument about their similarities to the Study. When the "Tuskegee" analogy was used as a cudgel against the new studies, Dibble's dilemmas and his willingness to agree to the Study were not mentioned. Once again the Study was being used to paint a black-and-white portrait.

Above all, the debate over the AZT trials showed that when Americans commented on international research issues that involved the Global South, the "Tuskegee" of the American South could be invoked.[12] As with much transnational ethical discussion, the terminology from the West—and in particular from the United States—flowed at first in only one direction. Ethics considerations can also flow back, however, which allows a reconsideration of what "really" happened in the Study.[13]

Rise of the Counter-Narratives

"Tuskegee" is too powerful to be ignored, and another generation of historians has revisited its facts. The differences between what physician-historian Thomas Benedek in 1978 had called the Study's "morals and methodology" came back again in the late 1990s in what anthropologist Richard Shweder labels the "counter-narratives."[14] Questions of racial assumptions and racism became part of the morals, and the medical facts separated into the methodologies and the limitations of medical science.

These "counter-narratives" refocused attention on the medical uncertainties among syphilologists and on the questions over heavy metals therapies and penicillin for late latent syphilis. Were the medical scientific decisions so dreadful, those writing the counter-narratives asked. Was the "discourse of horror," as Shweder labeled the narrative of the Study, used to justify modern "research regulation," unfair, once more of the "facts" were known? Should there even have been an apology, Dr. Robert White asked.[15]

Rejecting the liberal rhetoric that had underlain historians' work nearly twenty years earlier, the new critics revisited the debates in the medical literature about the type and duration of efficacious treatment, how common "nontreatment" was, and whether the provision of penicillin would have made a difference. Using these analyses, they then argued for a different kind of historical judgment. Their conclusions supported an earlier review of studies on cardiovascular syphilis treatment, which concluded that "the therapeutic efficacy of penicillin in the treatment of cardiovascular syphilis is not established" because of the lack of control trials, even though a wide range of dosages of the drug were being used.[16] These new narratives took the uncertainty and subthemes of earlier histories and brought them front and center to the analysis.[17]

The counter-narratives hoped to make the same key point: the symbolic "Tuskegee" is wrong because the *real* Study was not so horrific or out of character for the times for both whites and blacks. The oft-quoted belief that 60 to 70 percent of those with late latent syphilis did not die from it was used to counter the sense of the public narrative that hundreds of the men died because of the PHS's malfeasance. Racism is labeled a "presentist" worry, while the medical science gets elevated and shorn of its racial assumptions. The "efficacy" of the drugs—both the heavy metals and the penicillin—became a central concern rather than attempts to withhold treatment.[18]

Nontreatment studies at other institutions, even though none went on as long as the Study or were run by the government, were cited as examples of the normality at the time of such research efforts. The medical belief that latent syphilis would not kill everyone and acceptance of the claims of the PHS that the contagious were treated serves the arguments that the Study was not so terrible. These counter-narratives argued that most of the men either died early, before the availability of penicillin, or might not have been helped by it, and that the danger to their lives was not born out by the epidemiological evidence.

Rather than simply dismissing these counter-narratives as confused, as racist, or as efforts to protect scientific research, the arguments need to be analyzed, especially since they have also been picked up by conservative blogs to suggest there is "mere" black paranoia.[19] This has to be done by appeals to what we *can know* about what happened rather than the "truths" that have prevailed, however useful they are to current political considerations.[20] We will probably never know, because of the incomplete men's records and reports, whether the PHS's assertion that the failure to treat made the men sicker and that the syphilitics died earlier until the antibiotic era is really true for everyone in the Study. The conflicting evidence in the autopsies, the lack of records for those who dropped out, the ways in which controls were switched to the syphilitic group, and the evidence that some of those in the syphilitic group probably never had the disease in the first place and should have been in the controls—all muddy the data. It is impossible to know if penicillin would have changed the health outcomes of those still alive in the antibiotic era and whether those who were decades out from their initial infections would have been helped. But even a syphilis study that used white patients at Stanford in 1948 and withheld treatment concluded: "Should penicillin prove effective, all arguments against the routine treatment of latent syphilis should vanish."[21] By the mid-1950s, penicillin became routine in medical practice, even for those in latency.

The symbolic power of "Tuskegee" works because of the revulsion over the idea that the PHS deceived the men and their families, waited for years as they died, whether from syphilis or not, and then carved up their bodies at autopsies. These are the images that float through cultural consciousness. It cannot be forgotten that the men were treated as a public health problem to be watched. Even if only one man was harmed at the time (and we know it was more), or only one man passed the disease on to his wife and children, it would matter, just as the death of one man—Jessie Gelsinger—mattered in the critique of gene therapy trials in 1999.[22] In the Study, what is crucial is the way racial difference was assumed when it was needed to explain why the Study after Oslo was necessary, and then forgotten so that its results could justify the need for syphilis treatment in the country for everyone. The men were treated as a population, rather than as individuals, and without their knowing, and the deception that went on for so long will haunt "Tuskegee" forever.

The assumptions of racial difference shaped the Study's science from its beginning. The reigning medical belief before penicillin was that "if the patient has had syphilis for 25 years without clinical disease, he is to be congratulated not treated." But even a leading syphilologist who defended the Study in the 1970s would write: "I followed the advice, with exceptions, of course."[23] The historical fact is that the men were not given a choice and they were intentionally lied to, because the PHS doctors thought they were doing little harm to people who expected to get little attention and whose other ills they diagnosed. If the men became "exceptions," it was not because the PHS wanted it this way. If we see the men as individuals and understand that the situation in Alabama changed over the forty years, we can then see how some managed to get to treatment. Our focus becomes the men and their families, not just the intentions of the PHS.

The counter-narratives bring up what their authors claim are the "medical facts" of this deeply flawed study, as if the science can be separated from its political context, as if the history does not form a kind of testifying, and as if the facts are easy to know. In this way, those writing these new narratives are doing what sociologists call "boundary-work," that is, pursuing an "ideological style found in scientists' attempts to create a public image for science by contrasting it favorably to non-scientific intellectual or technical activities."[24] Whether it is morals or methods, racism or medical science, these counter-narratives are a way to separate out concerns about the ways science can create race and perpetuate racism, whether it is done overtly or in more subtle ways.

The facts about syphilis do matter, of course, and no one should back away from trying to learn them, even with—or especially with—"Tuskegee." These "medical facts," as they were defined in the Study, were suffused with racial assumptions and rested on beliefs about racial difference. Above all, in the Study, race mattered and it made the science. Even if "Tuskegee" is now based on what Shweder somewhat scornfully labels "identity politics [rather] than on critical reason," so, in fact, was the science itself.[25]

We cannot look at the Study as if the symbolic "Tuskegee" does not exist. The symbolism informs how we understand the facts, what questions we ask, what explanations we offer. In turn, as with any historical event that becomes mythic, examination of the "facts" often does little to undermine a powerful and useful story. There is a truth to what actually happened, and trying to understand it does matter. In this sense, the counter-narratives should be read, their facts should be measured, and the arguments should be considered, if for no other reason than to understand why they are being made.

The symbolic "Tuskegee" and the historical Study, however, feed on one another, as they did from the beginning. It is not possible to understand one without the other, to read the "facts" without knowing the myths and tropes that shape them; nor is it possible to create the myths without ignoring some of the facts. Depending on where we stand politically, the facts can serve political needs of all kinds. At best, we can find the new facts and be aware of the paradigms we use to understand them.[26]

Bidil, "Special Treatment," and the Logic of Race Redux

If counter-narratives tried to reanalyze the "facts" of the Study to deny the racism and explain the medical thinking, the demand that a drug be given only to African Americans was raised to counter that racism. "Tuskegee" as a foundational story of racial injustice central to righting past racial medical wrongs reached its apogee in 2005 in the case of a drug, BiDil, manufactured by the NitroMed company. Approved by the FDA, BiDil was the first, and still the only, drug for one racial or ethnic group: "self-identified" African Americans with heart failure who were not treated successfully with the standard drug regimens. The approval process sparked controversy, not only over the evidence but also over what it meant for the FDA to certify a drug for what would then be assumed to be a biological category called "race."[27]

At the FDA advisory committee hearing in June 2005 at which the drug passed into the approval process, "Tuskegee" as a historical reality was both ubiquitous and invisible, exerting its power even though no one spoke its name, and BiDil's governmental stamp of approval became an unstated reparation for past evils. Only after the committee had met did the FDA advisory committee's chairman, Cleveland Clinic cardiology chief Steven Nissen, acknowledge, "We were putting [Tuskegee] . . . to rest."[28]

Once the drug was approved, NitroMed encouraged doctors to use it for anyone they thought needed it. But it was expensive, and BiDil had a difficult time being sold and accepted. Despite heated arguments at subsequent conferences about the criticism, in the end the cost of the drug was its undoing. Less than three years after FDA approval, BiDil was selling so poorly that the company was itself sold as its stock dropped precipitously. But the government had once again approved the use of racial difference as biological.

BiDil is of course not "Tuskegee." The Study happened, in part, because racism left a population under-educated, ill, and in need of any help it could get, while at the same time doctors and researchers could use clinical certainty about race—both behavioral and physiological—to explain these conditions, even when contradictory data on purported racial differences and alternative explanations to prevalence rates existed. Statistical manipulations and questionable research in the Study, even in an era when clinical trials were badly organized, protected racialized assumptions about disease. In the face of clinical and autopsy evidence that might have undermined that certainty, race and some unknown biological process in the "bad blood" shored up clinical experiences of racial difference, except when race was allowed to disappear to make a larger medical and public health need apparent.

In the case of BiDil, clinical "certainty" about race-based population differences and the desire and demand to do "something" combined. BiDil's supporters argued their position by pointing to the history of racism that had led to the denial of care, deceit, and questionable ethics in "Tuskegee," but they dismissed the ideas about race that made the Study happen in the first place and continue for so many years. "Biological plausibility," focused on genetic expressions yet to be determined, allowed race to become the real surrogate endpoint in a clinical study, and this metalanguage, once again, overwhelmed other variables.

The harm of BiDil's approval is certainly less apparent now than the harm done by the Study as fact and metaphor. Governmental support, however, for the substitution of race as a population concept for the needs of individuals may have its own deadly effects in the future, as it gives approval to a form of racial reification. Ironically, the acceptance of BiDil makes the racial logic that underlay the Study seem less outrageous. If we accept now in some simple way that there are genetic and inherited biological reasons for disease differences for a category labeled "African American," then what does it say about the assumptions of the PHS doctors in the Study? The complicated story of the BiDil experience demonstrates that using "Tuskegee" to make a simple moral argument can have its own serious limitations.

Facts, Humor, and Cultural Memory
In the aftermath of the AZT trials, the counter-narratives, and the BiDil debate, the role of the Study's history requires rethinking. In a 2004 story in the *New York Sun* tabloid, which picked up on the historical debate, health educator Stephen Thomas argued that the "facts" now are "moot" because "Tuskegee" has become "a metaphor."[29] Thomas is right in one way: it is a metaphor. However, the facts of the Study matter as much as their symbolic life, and their intertwining needed explaining. The Study's metaphorical status came about not just through memory but also through the written histories, the bioethics textbooks that pick up some of the facts, the films and plays that are part imagination, and the rumors that got spread.

Perhaps we are left with the need to see, as Marx reminded us more than a century ago, that "history repeats itself, first as tragedy, second as farce." On NBC's late-night comedy show *Saturday Night Live*, in October 2006, "Tuskegee" made an appearance. In a skit labeled "Trust Your Doctor," starring black comedian Kenan Thompson and white actor Hugh Laurie (television's fictional Dr. House), a black patient lies in a hospital bed in pain with a broken leg, although he keeps up his joshing with his wife (played by Laurie in drag), as a black nurse and a white doctor come in. The assumption in the skit seemingly is that the doctor is doing good for a patient who does not really understand medicine. The patient's name is Dallas Rivers (Dallas as a symbol for a government led by Texan George Bush and Rivers as Nurse Rivers). After the couple laughs to one another about why it is called a medical practice (because "they practice on you," we are told), the doctor offers medications. "We know what this is," the patient and his wife tell one another, and then begins the mantra "Tuskegee, Tuskegee, Tuskegee."[30]

The humor depends, of course, on the historical and cultural literacy the viewer brings to the skit, and it works on multiple levels. Are we to laugh because the patient is too untrusting in some minstrel sense to know that they are going to help him? Or are we just to find it hilarious when an actor who plays a gruff television doctor who eventually helps his patients is now a hairy-legged wife in a blond fright wig, aiding and abetting medical distrust and demonstrating the patient's stupidity? Or might we consider that the "Tuskegee" mantra is a form of signifying on the doctors, a way to remind us that the patient is not paranoid to be mistrustful and that he is telling us this in a black vernacular? "Tuskegee" as a metaphor cannot be changed, however, if we do not reconsider what we know and, more important, what conceptual framework we place it in and why we tell the stories that we do.[31]

The stories are not the same, however, for every individual. As critic/lawyer Karla F. C. Holloway has argued about the dangers of "the romance and appeal of community," it is imperative that there be no simple assumption that every individual African American will remember the Study or see it as having relevance for him or her.[32] There will always be a tension between the individual and collective memory, between the needs for autonomy and the construction of "community" as some racial "other." To know "Tuskegee" does not mean to know whether it has relevance to an individual or how it will be used.

Does History Matter: What Now and Where?

In January 2007, I had an experience that illustrates the continuing complexity of "Tuskegee" and the ways we retell the stories of the Study. I was invited to speak informally about my work to a group of CDC professionals in Atlanta who were planning the country's response to a possible flu pandemic and also to give a Sunday afternoon sermon on the Study two days later from the pulpit of the Shiloh Missionary Baptist Church in Notasulga, just outside of Tuskegee. David Sencer, the CDC's former director and the doctor who oversaw the 1969 meeting that allowed the Study to continue and then negotiated its close, issued my invitation to his old workplace. Liz Sims, a relative of several Study subjects and head of the Shiloh Community Restoration Foundation, organized my visit to her church.

The contrast between those two worlds was still evident—even as both have ties to the Study. At the CDC, David Sencer guided me through the sprawling campus of buildings and then through a metal detector to a windowless room. My talk on the Study's story of complexity was met with interest and the usual detailed questions. More important, even as I spoke on "the Study," the symbolic "Tuskegee" became the real cipher through which black and white professionals within the CDC spoke to one another. Concerns about who could represent black communities, how the planning for the pandemic ignored the realities of black life, and what could be done were in the end much more crucial than anything I could say. "Tuskegee" once again provided a vocabulary that acknowledged its racial pain yet had different individual meanings. It allowed a discussion about why misunderstandings exist and what might be done. At least in this somewhat safe space, where history provided cover, a painful conversation took place.

Then I drove the 127 miles from Atlanta to Tuskegee. I always get off the interstate highway for the last twenty miles onto a two-lane back road and meander through the rolling hills of Macon County. It prepares me for where I am. I pass mobile homes and older wooden ones with wraparound porches that signal families and friends, a juke joint with a falling-down sign, the kitchen gardens and barking dogs. I drive over Osceola Creek. This name calls up the power of government doctors— Osceola was a Seminole Indian leader, born in Macon County, who died in captivity in 1838. Before his burial, his head was taken and kept by a military doctor and then given to a medical school. Just before I enter the city of Tuskegee, there are the trees of the Tuskegee National Forest, signs for the VA Hospital, and the new Tuskegee Airmen National Historic Site, all of which remind me of the federal government's power in the county. I know that it is no longer the Depression in Macon County, or even the 1970s, and that all of the men from the Study and almost all of the physicians who oversaw it are gone.

Yet this portion of the Alabama Black Belt, which is 84.6 percent African American, continues to have economic and social difficulties and health needs. The median household income in 2005 was $24,781, "61.2 percent lower than the median income in the State of Alabama" and "98.3 percent lower than the median household income level in the US."[33] Johnny Ford, the first black mayor of the city, who was elected in 1972 on the heels of the Study's disclosure, was in his seventh and last term as mayor. He was trying to deal with the problem of abandoned buildings in Tuskegee, and the Confederate statue in the town square looks out on a beautiful courthouse, legal offices, and a deathly quiet business district. Wal-Mart, which thrives in bustling Auburn twenty miles away, closed here after a few years. The fast-food restaurants, along with a conference center at Tuskegee University, provide the major public eating options.

Health care in the county still is difficult. The John A. Andrew Memorial Hospital is gone, closed for lack of use in 1987 and its space rebuilt as the National Bioethics Center and classrooms. The Tuskegee VA Hospital merged with another institution and is now called the Central Alabama Veterans Health Care System. It does not provide urgent care. The Macon County Health Care Authority built a multimillion-dollar ambulatory care center in 2005 and then ended up in a fractious fight with its doctor and with the local newspaper and politicians over competence. The building stood empty for more than a year and now houses a local private medical practice. Emergencies mean trips to hospitals miles away, in Montgomery, Auburn, and Opelika.[34] Of the county residents, 85 percent have health insurance, but a feasibility study concluded that the county cannot support and does not need a "full-service hospital."[35]

The Study lives on—in the memories of family members, in the work of the Tuskegee University National Bioethics Center, in the memorial/museum to the Study's men and Macon County's multicultural history that attorney Fred Gray and his family have built in an old bank building off the main square, and in the efforts to preserve the Shiloh site. The Bioethics Center is attempting to "transform the legacy" of the Study. It provides courses on ethics on the campus and is reaching out to do research on racial health disparities.[36] Each year around the time of the anniversary of the apology it provides a major lecture and workshop and honors the remaining family members. Gray's Tuskegee Human and Civil Rights Multicultural Center has the men's names printed onto its floor, surrounded by panels and videos that cover the county's history of African Americans, whites, and Native Americans. Gray continues to struggle to fund this small museum and hopes it will become the visitors' center for the county.

For the families, the Study is etched in their memories and identities. I learned this once again as I came to the Shiloh church. It was in its school and yard that Nurse Rivers recruited dozens of the men, and it is in the church's graveyard up the road that they are buried. It is where Lucious Pollard, a man in the Study who died of syphilis, has his picture and the words "gone but not forgotten" carved on his headstone. In the church, Charlie Wesley Pollard, Lucious's son and Liz Sims's cousin, always sat in the second pew and remembered to dispense quarters to children on their birthdays.[37]

The occasion was a chance for the men to be honored again and for me, as the outsider and historian, to speak. Sims has worked tirelessly to get the church, the adjacent small school, which was funded by the Rosenwald Fund, and the graveyard on the Alabama Historical Register, and she is toiling to get them on the National Register of Historic Places as well. She hopes that the school can be cleaned up through the organizing she and others have done and made into a community center, with computers and other resources for the area's children to use.

The crowded church was filled with nearly one hundred people, more than a quarter of them family members of the Study's men. Sims had organized the Sunday afternoon so that the Tuskegee University Gospel Choir could inspire us, the preacher would have his powerful say, and others would sing and read poetry. I spoke on the history of the Study, showed the CDC pictures of the men, and then fielded questions, which ranged from "why us" to "what now" to "why are you telling it this way" for nearly an hour.

Realizing I would be standing in the pulpit of a Baptist church, I reached for a biblical metaphor. I told them that the men had wandered in a medical desert for forty years, sometimes finding manna, other times not. I promised I would do what Jews are supposed to do at Passover—remember the travails and exodus from Egypt by retelling the story of this wandering and the escape from slavery to their children. As with modern versions of the ancient slavery story that Jewish feminists and reformers reconsider every year, by adding an orange to the traditional items on the Seder plate or by linking good fortune to responsibility for good works elsewhere in the world, I hope that this book has told a new version of the Study and of "Tuskegee." I, and all of us, owe that congregation in Notasulga at least that much.

We also owe ourselves. Nations are built on the myths and stories they tell themselves. "Tuskegee" is one of the foundational stories of American racism in the twentieth century, and it anchors our beliefs about race, medicine, and science. This retelling—with its emphasis on contingencies, possibility for escape, racial assumptions, and the whys of the doctors thinking that they did nothing wrong—will probably not change the myths, or the ways "Tuskegee" tends to travel, or the political work it makes possible. I do hope, however, that in places as disparate as an open church sanctuary and a windowless medical room we start having these long overdue conversations that will lead to change, or at least to more understanding.

The continued existence of "Tuskegee" ultimately depends more on what happens every day in medical encounters than on what occurred during those forty years.[38] I have then what is perhaps a strange hope for a historian: may the Study be remembered but may "Tuskegee" be forgotten—because we no longer need it to interpret injustice.

Chronology

1891–1910, 1925–1927	Caesar Boeck hospitalizes approximately 2,000 white patients with primary and secondary syphilis until lesions heal, without treatment, in Oslo, Norway. His deputy, E. Bruusgaard, attempts follow-up, beginning in 1925. The results become known as the Oslo Study.
November 1929	The Rosenwald Fund votes to spend up to $50,000 from January through December of 1930 for syphilis control and treatment demonstration programs. The PHS recommends six locations for the program: Macon County, Alabama; Scott County, Mississippi; Tipton County, Tennessee; Glynn County, Georgia; Pitt County, North Carolina; Albemarle County, Virginia.
February 1930–September 1931	The Rosenwald Fund Demonstration Project in progress in Macon County, Alabama. 39.8 percent are presumed to test positive for syphilis. 1,400 men, women, and children are treated; 3,684 are tested.
May 1930	Dr. H. L. Harris Jr. makes a site visit for the Rosenwald Fund to Macon County.
Fall 1930	Harris visits the Macon County site again, questions the procedures, and recommends that a comprehensive health plan be implemented. It is not because the Rosenwald Fund cannot afford to continue the project or expand it beyond September 1931.
1931–1932	Black Sharecroppers' Union is organized and has shootouts with sheriffs in Talladega and Tallapoosa counties, near Tuskegee.

| 1931–1937 | Nine young black men are falsely accused of raping two white women and are arrested, tried, and jailed near Scottsboro, Alabama. |

September 1932 — The PHS proposes to study untreated late latent syphilis in Macon County. Tuskegee Institute officials and the local and state health departments agree to the Study. Nurse Eunice Rivers is appointed to the Study as a liaison to the men.

October 1932 — The PHS study of untreated late latent syphilis begins in Macon County. The projected length of the study is 6 to 8 months and is supposed to include black men at least 25 years old who have positive blood tests, have had syphilis for at least 5 years (determined by onset of chancres), and who have not been treated. Not all the Study subjects meet this criterion. Subjects are then administered less than the recommended amount of therapy. Both men and women are being treated, although men's names are selected for the Study.

May 1933 — The Study's men are subjected to spinal taps to diagnose neurological complications of syphilis.

June 1933 — Dr. Taliaferro Clark retires from the PHS; Dr. Raymond A. Vonderlehr succeeds him as head of the Venereal Disease Division and continues the Study. Autopsies are added to the Study. Men are now given aspirin, vitamins, protiodide, and iron tonics.

August 1933 — 28 percent of those tested are found to be positive for syphilis.

September 1933–March 1934 — PHS begins selecting a group of men as controls for the Study.

May 1934 — The Milbank Memorial Fund gives $50 burial stipends to families of subjects and controls consenting to autopsies.

1936 — The first report of the Study is published: R. A. Vonderlehr et al., "Untreated Syphilis in the Male Negro: A Comparative Study of Treated and Untreated Cases."

1937 — "Bad Blood Wagon" bus, funded by the Rosenwald Fund and staffed by the PHS, returns to Macon County to begin treatment program. Men from the Study are supposed to be kept from treatment.

1941	Draft for World War II threatens to undermine the Study since draftees (ages 18–45) are tested and treated if necessary for syphilis. Macon County draft board is asked and agrees to not draft men in the Study.
	The Tuskegee Airmen program to train the first black military fighter pilots begins in Tuskegee at Moton Field. These men are not in the Study, although the program is called the "Tuskegee Experiment."
1943	The PHS's John Mahoney and his colleagues report that penicillin is highly effective in killing the spirochetes in those with early syphilis.
1946	The second and third reports of the Study are published: John R. Heller et al., "Untreated Syphilis in the Male Negro: Mortality during 12 Years of Observation"; and Austin V. Deibert et al., "Untreated Syphilis in the Male Negro: III. Evidence of Cardiovascular Abnormalities and Other Forms of Morbidity."
1948	The Nuremberg Code promulgates the principle that "the voluntary consent of the human subject is absolutely essential in medical research."
1950	The fourth report on the Study is published: Pasquale J. Pesare et al., "Untreated Syphilis in the Male Negro: Observation of Abnormalities over Sixteen Years."
1951	The PHS reviews the Study procedures and recommends changes.
1952	The Study's files are reorganized, autopsy reports are transferred to punch cards, and a single set of diagnostic standards for syphilis and syphilitic heart disease are adopted.
1953	The fifth report on the Study is published: Eunice Rivers et al., "Twenty Years of Follow-Up Experience in a Long-Range Medical Study."
1954	The sixth and seventh reports on the Study are published: James K. Shafer et al., "Untreated Syphilis in the Male Negro: A Prospective Study of the Effect on Life Expectancy"; and Sidney Olansky et al., "Environmental Factors in the Tuskegee Study of Untreated Syphilis." This is the first time "Tuskegee Study" is used in the article titles.
	In *Brown v. Board of Education*, the Supreme Court bans segregation in public schools.

Appendix A {243}

1955	The eighth and ninth reports on the Study are published: Jesse Jerome Peters et al., "Untreated Syphilis in the Male Negro: Pathologic Findings in Syphilitic and Nonsyphilitic Patients"; and Stanley H. Schuman et al., "Untreated Syphilis in the Male Negro: Background and Current Status of Patients in the Tuskegee Study."
	Bus boycott in Montgomery, 40 miles from Tuskegee, after Rosa Parks, a Tuskegee-born activist, is arrested for refusing to give up her seat on the bus to a white person.
	Trygve Gjestland publishes last follow-up on the Oslo Study, *The Oslo Study of Untreated Syphilis*.
	Count Gibson writes to Sidney Olansky to question the ethics of the Study.
1956	The tenth and eleventh reports on the Study are published: Sidney Olansky et al., "Untreated Syphilis in the Male Negro: X. Twenty Years of Clinical Observation of Untreated Syphilitic and Presumably Nonsyphilitic Groups"; and Sidney Olansky et al., "Untreated Syphilis in the Male Negro: Twenty-two Years of Serological Observation in a Selected Syphilis Study Group."
1957	The PHS distributes certificates of appreciation and cash payments of $25 to the subjects and controls for their "service."
1958	Eunice Rivers Laurie wins the Third Annual Oveta Culp Hobby Award, the highest commendation that HEW can bestow on an employee.
Early 1960s	PHS begins a regular distribution of small cash payments of $1 to $2 per subject to induce cooperation.
1960	In *Gomillion v. Lightfoot*, the Supreme Court bans gerrymandering to change borders as a means to disenfranchise citizens. The Tuskegee Civic Association brings the case to court.
1961	The twelfth report on the Study is published: Donald H. Rockwell et al., "The Tuskegee Study of Untreated Syphilis: The 30th Year of Observation."
1962	Food and Drug Act amendments order doctors to inform patients when they are being given drugs experimentally.

August 1963	March on Washington draws thousands to denounce segregation and racism.
1964	World Health Organization issues Declaration of Helsinki, which contains stringent provisions regarding informed consent in research.
January 1964	Twenty-fourth Amendment abolishes poll taxes.
July 1964	President Johnson signs the Civil Rights Act, which prohibits discrimination based on race, color, national origin, and religion.
1965	Malcolm X is murdered. Congress passes Voting Rights Act of 1965, making voting restrictions illegal, after March in Selma, Alabama, and the killing of two civil rights workers. Meeting held on the Study at CDC concludes: "Racial issue was mentioned briefly. Will not affect the study." Irwin Schatz writes to Donald H. Rockwell to question the Study's ethics. Peter Buxtun begins to make inquiries about the Study.
1966	Surgeon general issues Policy and Procedure Order No. 129 establishing guidelines for, among other things, peer review for publicly funded research (revised in 1969 and 1971). Henry Beecher publishes an article in *New England Journal of Medicine* exposing various unethical medical studies and experiments. Sammy Younge Jr., a black civil rights worker and Tuskegee student, is shot and killed in Tuskegee for refusing to use a toilet for blacks in the bus station.
1968	Martin Luther King Jr. is murdered. Rioting breaks out across the country. President Johnson signs the Civil Right Act of 1968, outlawing discrimination in housing sales and financing.
1969	The CDC convenes a panel of physicians to reconsider the Study. The panel recommends continuation. One panelist objects to the decision. The CDC tries to gain more support for the Study by visiting the Alabama State Board of Health and the Macon County Medical Society. Elizabeth Kennebrew is added to the Study as the new nurse to assist the aging Rivers.

	Bill Jenkins and others at DRUM raise objections to the Study.
1970	The assistant chief of the Venereal Disease Division of the PHS says the Study is incongruous with the goals of PHS and is bad science, but he opposes ending it.
1972	Peter Buxtun tells an AP reporter about the Study.
July 25, 1972	The AP sends the story about the Study to major newspapers.
August 1972	After a public outcry, HEW appoints an Ad Hoc Panel to review the Study.
1973	The thirteenth and last report on the Study is published: Joseph G. Caldwell et al., "Aortic Regurgitation in the Tuskegee Study of Untreated Syphilis."
February–March 1973	Kennedy holds hearings in the Senate on human experimentation. New HEW guidelines are established regarding research projects involving human subjects.
March 1973	HEW halts the Study by authorizing lifetime medical treatment to Study survivors after members of the federal investigating panel and Senator Ted Kennedy object that the Study is still ongoing.
April 1973	The CDC offers to find the subjects and controls, treat them, and pay for their medical care but does not have the authorization to offer the Study's participants compensation.
July 23, 1973	Civil rights attorney Fred D. Gray files a $1.8 billion class action lawsuit against the United States, HEW, the PHS, the CDC, the State of Alabama, the State Board of Health of Alabama, the Milbank Memorial Fund, and individual physicians connected with the Study.
December 1974	A settlement is reached and the government agrees to pay approximately $10 million. Each living syphilis subject receives $37,500, the heirs of each deceased subject with syphilis are awarded $15,000, each living control is granted $16,000, and each deceased control is awarded $5,000: 6,000 people will receive some compensation.
1974	Congress passes the National Research Act and sets up the National Commission for the Protection of Human Subjects of Biomedical and Behavioral Research, charg-

ing it with creating regulations for human research subjects.

1975   The government extends medical benefits program to the men's wives, widows, and children who have contracted syphilis.

1978   Allan Brandt's article, "Racism and Research: The Case of the Tuskegee Syphilis Experiment," is published.

1979   The National Commission releases the Belmont Report. The report creates guidelines for the ethical treatment of research subjects and sets out principles of respect for persons, beneficence, and justice.

1981   James H. Jones's book on the Study, *Bad Blood*, is published.
        First cases of what will become the HIV/AIDS epidemic are identified.

1992   David Feldshuh writes the play *Miss Evers' Boys*, a fictionalized account of the Study that has a fictionalized nurse as its central character.
        ABC's *Primetime* special on the Study airs.

1993   PBS's *Nova* film on the Study, "Deadly Deception," airs.

1994–1995   Henry W. Foster Jr. is nominated to the position of surgeon general. Questions about the Study affect the confirmation process, and it is permanently tabled in the Senate.

1995   Federal benefits program expands for survivors, wives, and children to health, not just medical, benefits.

1996   The last payments from lawsuit are made to subjects, controls, and their heirs. Interest payments from the settlement are still provided.
        Legacy Committee is organized by academics and health professionals to urge a formal federal apology. Others groups become part of this process.

1997   *Miss Evers' Boys* is adapted into a film and aired by HBO in February.
        President Clinton and Vice President Gore offer a formal federal apology for the Study in a White House ceremony, and 5 of the 6 remaining Study survivors attend on May 16.

1997–1998	Controversy arises over the clinical testing in developing countries of AZT, a drug to prevent the transmission of HIV from mother to child. The Study is invoked as a parallel because placebos are given in one arm of these studies.
1999	The Tuskegee University National Center for Bioethics is founded with funding from CDC. Fred Gray organizes the Tuskegee Human and Civil Rights Multicultural Center.
2004	Ernest Hendon, the last survivor of the Study, dies.
2005	FDA approves BiDil, a heart medication, only for "self-identified African Americans."
2006	Shiloh Community Restoration Foundation is incorporated in Notasulga, to place the Shiloh Missionary Baptist Church, its Rosenwald Fund school, and its graveyard on the Alabama Trust for Historic Preservation and the National Trust for Historic Preservation. Restoration of the Rosenwald school begins.
2009	Last widow receiving health benefits dies.

SOURCE: Susan E. Bell, Susan M. Reverby, and Elian Rosenfeld, revision of Susan E. Bell, "Events in the Tuskegee Syphilis Study: A Timeline," in *Tuskegee's Truths: Rethinking the Tuskegee Syphilis Study*, edited by Susan M. Reverby (Chapel Hill: University of North Carolina Press, 2000), 34–38.

Key Participants' Names

ALABAMA HEALTH OFFICIALS
James N. Baker   Murray Smith
Ruth Berrey   W. H. Y. Smith
D. G. Gill

FEDERAL INVESTIGATING COMMITTEE, AD HOC PANEL
Ronald H. Brown, general counsel, National Urban League
Broadus Butler, president of Dillard University and one of the Tuskegee Airmen
Vernal Cave, M.D., director of VD Control, New York City Health Department
Jean L. Harris, M.D., executive director of the National Medical
    Association Foundation
Seward Hiltner, professor of theology at Princeton
Jay Katz, M.D., professor of law and psychiatry at Yale
Jeanne C. Sinkford, D.D.S., associate dean, College of Dentistry, Howard University
Fred Speaker, former attorney general of Pennsylvania and prominent Republican
Barney Weeks, president of the Alabama Labor Council

KNOWN WHISTLE-BLOWERS AND JOURNALISTS
Peter Buxtun   Bill Jenkins
Count Gibson   Edith Lederer
Jean Heller   Irwin Schatz

LAWSUIT ATTORNEYS   MEDICAL CONSULTANTS
Harold J. Edgar   Joseph Earle Moore
Fred D. Gray   J. Lawton Smith
                            Eugene Stollerman

PHS DOCTORS
Joseph Caldwell, 1960s–70   Austin V. Deibert, 1936–40
Taliaferro Clark, 1932–33   John R. Heller, 1930s and 1972
John C. Cutler, 1950s–60s   Sidney Olansky, 1950s

Arnold Schroeter, 1960s

Stanley Schuman, 1950s

Raymond Vonderlehr, 1932–1940s

O. C. Wenger, 1932–1950s

PHS, CDC, NATIONAL INSTITUTES OF HEALTH,
AND OTHER HEALTH PROFESSIONALS

David Albritton

Thomas J. Bauer

William Brown

Martha Bruyere

P. T. Bruyere

Walter Edmondson

Geraldine A. Gleeson

Alfonso Holguin

J. Donald Millar

Pasquale J. Pesare

Eleanor V. Price

Donald Printz

Donald Rockwell

David J. Sencer

James K. Shafer

Lloyd Simpson

Lida Usilton

Eleanor Walker

Anne R. Yobs

ROSENWALD FUND
VENEREAL DISEASE CONTROL
PROJECT MEMBERS

H. L. Harris

Reginald James

William B. Perry

TUSKEGEE-BASED NURSES
AND DOCTORS

Eugene H. Dibble Jr.

Elizabeth Kennebrew

Eunice Verdell Rivers Laurie

Jesse Jerome Peters

Joshua Williams

U.S. SURGEONS GENERAL

Hugh S. Cumming, 1920–36

Thomas Parran Jr., 1936–48

Leonard A. Scheele, 1948–56

Leroy E. Burney, 1956–61

Luther L. Terry, 1961–65

William H. Stewart, 1965–69

Jesse L. Steinfeld, 1969–73

VENEREAL DISEASE DIVISION
CHIEFS, PHS

Thomas Parran Jr., 1926–30

Taliaferro Clark, 1930–33

John McMullen, 1934

Raymond A. Vonderlehr, 1935–43

John R. Heller Jr., 1943–48

Theodore J. Bauer, 1948–52

James K. Shafer, 1953–54

Clarence A. Smith, 1954–57

William J. Brown, 1957–71

J. Donald Millar, 1972

Men's Names

Green Adair
Courtney Adams
James Adams
Louis Adams
Prince Albert
Ben Alexander
Joe Alexander
Marion Alexander
Jefferson Allen
Sam Allen
Seldon Allen
George Anderson
George T. Anderson
Will Anthony
Seaborn Askew
Alfred Austin
Dean Austin
George Austin
Hyth Austin
Nelson Austin
Wiley Austin
George Baker
Early Banks
Jack Banks
David Barrow
Seth Barrow
Enoch Battle Sr.
Lee Battle
Nathaniel Beasley
Robert Beasley
John Berry

Lornie Berry
Edward Bessick
Ernest Bessick
Ishman Black
Jim Black
Wiley Black
Will Blackburn
Primus Blackman
Tommie Lee Blackman
Pustell Bledsoe
Muncie Borum
Grant Boyd
Jimmie Boyd
Richard Bernard Boyd
Tobe Boyd
Eli Brooks
Bailey Brown Jr.
Doll Brown
John C. Brown
K. L. Brown
Logan Brown
Riley Brown
Vance Brown
J. R. Bryant
Willie Bryant
Winfield Bryant
Ben Buchanan
Charlie Buchanan
Columbus Buchanan
Gene Buchanan
John Buchanan

Sol Buchanan
Wash Buchanan
James Buford
William E. Burton
Bishop Buscom
Eli Butler
Sam Byrd
William Caldwell
Forney Calhoun
Alfred Campbell
Charlie Campbell
Ishmael Campbell
Jack Campbell
Judge Campbell
Will Campbell
Robert Carlisle
Gus Carmichael
Jim Carr
Eugene Caston
Henry Chambliss
Jerry Chambliss
Pollard Chambliss
William Chambliss
Hilliard Chappel
Seaborn Chappel
Rufus Charleston
George Chatman
John Cheeks
Ben Chisholm
Ed Chisholm
James Clabon

Joshua Clark
Moses Clark
Ludie Clements
Allen Cole
Samuel Coleman
Isaac Collier
Algie Collins
Jim Collins
John Collins
Julius Collins
Relice Collins
Willie Collins
Dan Collis
Sylvester Collis
Ben Comer
Amos Cooper
Frank Cooper
Gentry Cooper
Fletcher Cox
Jeff Cox
Redonia Cox
Tom Cox
George Crawford
Jimmie Lee Crawford
John Crawford
Logan Crawford
Wash Crawford
James Crawley
Ernest Crayton
Lonzie C. Crayton
Zettie Daggett
Albert Daniel
Clark Daniel
John Wesley Daniel
Mac Daniel
Floyd Darkey
Anthony Davis
Bonnie Davis
Elbert Davis
Henry Davis
Mariman Davis
Martin Davis
Frank M. Day
Benjamin Demps
Nat Dennis

Frank Dixon
Zettie Doggett
Kelly Donar
Mose Donar
Sam Donar
Wilbert Doner
Wiley Doner
Aleck Dorsey
Jim Dorsey
Will Dorsey
Crawford Dowdell
Willie Downer
Bill Dozier
Harvey Driscoll
N. D. Dubose
D. C. Echols
John Echols
Pressley Echols
Wade Echols
Wiley Echols
Willie Echols
John A. Ellington
Samuel Ellington
Henry Epps
Ben Evans
Henry Mark Evans
Lemuel Evans
Cleve Felton
Tom Felton
Green Fitzpatrick
Ned Fitzpatrick
Thomas Fitzpatrick
Willie Fitzpatrick
Bill Foote
Joe Foote
Abbie Ford
Arthur Ford
Percy Ford
Calvin Fort
E. Gary Fort
Jasper Fort
Nathan Fort
Sandy Fort
Archie Foster
Ben Eddie Foster

Bonnie Foster
David Foster
Lee Foster
Pomp Foster
Reuben Foster
William Foster
Jim Foy
Louis Foy
Ulysses Franklin
Percy Gaines
Ben Galgher
Bob Gamble
Elijah Gamble
Alfred W. Garner
Will Gaston
Nick Gauchett
Albert Germany
Fred Germany
Ben Gholston
Fred Giles
Quince Gilmer
Doc Gilmore
Sam Glenn
John Goode
Grover Goodson
Virgil Gordon
Desibe Gray
Clayborn Greathouse
Clifton Greathouse
John E. Greathouse
Mose Green
Walter Green
Will Green
George Greer
Colonel Griffin
Dave Griffin
Miles Griffin
Samuel Griffin
Willie Griffin
Charlie Griggs
Emmett Grimes
James Grimes
Harvey Griscoll
Frank Grove
G. B. Hagins

Andrew Hagood
Cary Hall
Columbus Hamilton
Sherman Haney
Freeman Hann
Albert Hardy
Clifton Harper
Robert Harper
Adolphus Harris
Alonzo Harris
Elisha Harris
George Harris
Jake Harris
James Harris
Lewis Harris
Theodore Harris
Will Harris
Will Smuch Harris
William Harris
Edward Harrison
Willie Harrison Sr.
Frank Hart
John Hart
L. Z. Hart
Charlie Harvey
Walter Harvey
Ludie Hatten
Sandy Hatten
Square Hatton
Henry Hawkins
Absalom Henderson
Dick Henderson
Hillard Henderson
James Henderson
Ernest Hendon
Louie Hendon
Johnnie Henry
Philip Hicks
William Hicks
Phillip Hill
Clayborn Hoffman
Joseph H. Holliday
Zan Holmes
Carter Howard
Tony Howard

John Hudson
Bennie Lee Huffman
Marcus Huffman
Arthur Hughly
Will Hurt
Zack Hutchinson
Minor Iszell
David Jackson
Fleming Jackson
Isiah Jackson
James Jackson
Jim Jackson
Martin Jackson
Randall Jackson
Roosevelt Jackson
Stephie Jackson
Tom Pony Jackson
Tommy J. Jackson
Clinton James
George James
Jesse James
John C. James
Jorden James
Wilbert James
Howard Jenkins
West Jenkins
William Jenkins Jr.
Willie Jenkins
Will Jernigan
Charles Johnson
Feagin Johnson
G. C. Johnson
Jimmie Johnson
Johnnie J. Johnson
Price Johnson
Simon Johnson
Spencer Johnson
Sylvester Johnson
Thomas Johnson
Thomas J. C. Johnson
Chancey Jones
Clifford Jones
Dan Jeff Jones
Hayes Jones
Henry Jones

Major Jones
Roosevelt Jones
Shepherd L. Jones
Willie Jones
Willie Moffett Jones
Jim Jonking
Albert Julkes
Ephrom Julkes
Warren Julkes
John K. Kelley
Ad Kelly
Mitchell Kelly
Usher Kennebrew
Charlie B. Key
George Key
Henry Key
Jesse Key
Nathan Key
Ned Key
R. T. Kindell
Edmond Kitt
Nathaniel Laine
John Edward Lane
Johnnie W. Lane
Wiley Lane
James Laster
Andrew Laury
William Levett
Peter Lewis
Sherman Lewis
Riley Ligon
George Lockett
W. P. Lockwood
Sim Long
Will Long
Milton Love
Ed Loveless
Ernest Loyd
V. M. Macon
Jesse Maddox
Dave Mahone
Fonzie Mahone
Charlie Young Manley
Governor Martin
Lewis Martin

Roosevelt Martin
Wesley Martin
Frazier Mason
Clabon Mays
Thomas McGrady
Essex McKee
Wash McMullen
Willie McNeill
Joe Menefee
John Menefee
William Miles
Richard Mims
Samuel Mindingall
Gary Mitchell
John Mitchell
Aaron Moore
Abner Moore
Alonzo Moore
Ezekiel Moore
Felix Moore
Frank Moore
Marshall Moore
Willie Bill Moore
Lenza Morgan
Hobbie Morrest
Frank Moss
Frederick Moss
Grant Moss
John J. Moss
Otis Moss
Peter Motley
Julius Mott
Dock Murphy
Albert Murray
Jim Mutry
I. S. Myrick
Rubin Neal
Rufus Neal
Ed Norwood
Willie Nunley
York Ogletree
Thaddeus O'Neal
Eddie Pace
Elmore Pace

Evans Pace
George Pace
Henry Pace
Lonzie Pace
Nelse Pace
Otis Pace
Steve Pace
Whitelaw Padgett
Eli Parker
Will Patrick
Cleve Patterson
Frank Paulk
Ludie Payne
Pender Pearsall
Ed D. Pearson
John Pendleton
Tom Philips
Charlie Phillips
Ed Phillips
John Williams Phillips
Ned Phillips
Prince Phillips
Roland Philpot
Charlie Pinkard
Charlie Lee Pinkard
Walter Plezes
Albert Polk
Charlie Wesley Pollard
Elbert Pollard
Lucious Pollard
Osburn Pollard
Vertis Pollard
Will Pollard
Woody Pollard
Bertha Porch
Jethro Potts
Taylor Pruitt
Armistead Pugh
Arthur Pugh
Joe Randolph
Johnnie Randolph
Major Randolph
Robert Randolph
George Ray

William Ray
Andrew Reed
Douglas Reed
Fletcher Reed
Charles Reynolds
Gus Reynolds
C. H. Rhone
Clinton Ries
Tom Robbins
Bob Lee Roberts
Lige Robertson
Albert Robinson
Butler Robinson
Ben Rockamore
Henry Rogers
Charlie Rowell
Edmond Rowell
Theodore Rowell
R. L. Ruff
Lieutenant Rush
Wash Rush
Clarence Russell
Jeff Russell
Willie Russell
Bill Samuel
George Samuel
Odell Samuel
Tom George Samuel
Emmet Sanford
Fletcher Sanford
Lester Scott
Nelson Scott
William Scott
John Seatts
Charlie Shaw
Herman Shaw
John Shelton
Purvis Shelton
Paul Shumpert
Fred Simmons
John Simmons
Bennie Simpson
Simmie Simpson
Anderson Sinclair

Oscar Sinclair
Henry Sistrunk
John Slaughter
Cain Smith
Dudley Smith
Eugene Smith
Hillard Smith
Jimmie Smith
Joe Smith
John Wesley Smith
Lieutenant Smith
Low Smith
Richard Smith
Robert Harvey Smith
Thomas Kelly Smith
Ed Sparks
Olin Speed
Jim Spivey
Mack Stewart
Millard Storey
Mark Swanson
Please Swanson Sr.
Tom Swanson
Tump Swanson
Will Bossy Swanson
Willie Swanson
Lawrence Swift
Son Swift
Andrew Swint
Oscar Talbert
Louis Talley
Eugene Tarver
Oscar Tarver
Edward Tate
Louis Tate
Robert Lee Tate
Mayso Tatum
Sylvester Tatum
Richard Taylor
Van Taylor
Warn Taylor
George Temple
Bob Theney
Jessie Thomas

Oran Thomas
Pat Thomas
Peter Thompson
Willis Thompson
Edison Tinsley
Walter Todd
George Washington
    Tolbert
Jim Tolbert
Ocie Tolbert
Willie Tramble
Percy Trammell
Alf Tredwell
Will Turk
Joe Turner
West Turner
Jim Turpin
Stephen Tyner
Freddie Lee Tyson Sr.
Milton Upshaw
Jim Veal
Coleman Veals
Mitchell Wade
John Waggoner
Andrew Walker
John Warren Walker
Joe Nathan Walls
Alex Ware
Atlee Warren
Ed Warren
Sonnie Warren
John Henry Watson
John L. Watson
Willie Watt
Alonzo Weathers
Sam Weatherspoon
William Webb
Dan Welch
Anthony West
Tobe Wheat
Jake Wheeler
Archie White
Leonard White
Sonny White

Ed Whitlow
Motelle Whitlow
Albert Williams
Andrew Williams
Bill Williams
Bill Henry Williams
Bill Jesse Williams
Coleman Williams
Eugene Williams
George Williams
Henry Williams
James Williams
Lewis Williams
Matthew Williams
Meshack Williams
Morris Williams
Reuben Williams
Steve J. Williams
Tom Williams
J. W. Willis
Wilbur Willis
Governor Wilson
Houston Wilson
Logan Wilson
Roy Wilson
James Wimbush
Charlie Wood Jr.
Charlie Wood Sr.
Grant Wood
Louis Wood
Nelson Woodall
R. D. Woodall
Jesse Woolfolk
Clarence Wright
Ernest Wright
Jim Wright
Ludie Wright
Rev. T. W. Wright
Will Wright
Tom Wyatt
Booker Yancey
Mark Yarbrough
Harrison York
Jack Young

SOURCE: "Tuskegee Patient Medical Files," Southeast Region, National Archives and Records Administration, <http://www.archives.gov/southeast/finding-aids/tuskegee .html>, accessed February 23, 2009. A slightly different list appears in Fred D. Gray, *The Tuskegee Syphilis Study: The Real Story and Beyond* (Montgomery, Ala.: New South Books, 1998), 6–10. I have used both sources to compile the list that appears here. It is very possible that there are names missing or incorrect spellings or that the same man is in the records twice under different names.

APPENDIX D

Tables and Charts

NOTE: *Unless otherwise indicated, data in all tables and charts is compiled from coding of the Tuskegee Medical Files,* CDC-GA.

THE PROBABLE OUTCOME OF UNTREATED LATENT SYPHILIS, 1943

Outcome	Approximate Percentage of Patients in Whom Specified Results May Be Expected to Develop
Spontaneous "cure" (blood tests and cerebrospinal fluid negative; no lesions)	25–35
Infection remains latent (blood tests positive; cerebrospinal fluid negative; no lesions)	25–35
Late syphilis (skin, mucosa, osseous)	10–15
Cardiovascular syphilis	10–15
Neurosyphilis	1–2
Visceral syphilis, other than cardiovascular	0.5–1

Source: Joseph Earle Moore, *Modern Treatment of Syphilis* (Springfield, Ill.: Charles C. Thomas, 1943), 2d ed., 256.

DATE OF RECRUITMENT TO THE STUDY

Year Recruited	Frequency	Percentage	Year Recruited	Frequency	Percentage
1932	84	13.46	1938	9	1.44
1933	362	58.01	1939	9	1.44
1934	81	12.98	1943	1	0.16
1935	2	0.32	1971	1	0.16
1937	1	0.16	Unknown	74	11.86
			Total	624	100.00

INFECTION STATUS BY CATEGORIES, NUMBERS, AND PERCENTAGES

Infection Status	Frequency	Percentage
Syphilitic	427	68.43
Control	185	29.65
Control to syphilitic	12	1.92

MEN'S AGES AT FIRST EXAM

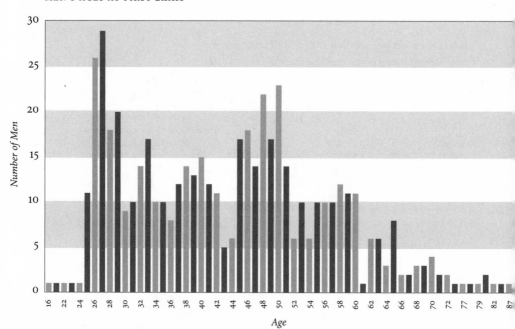

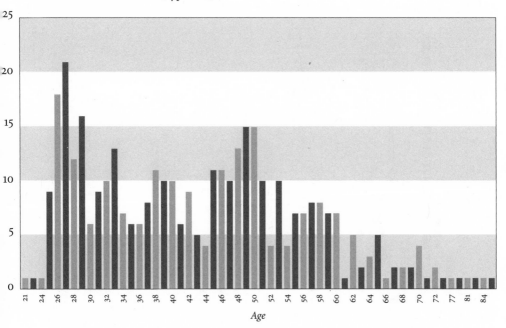

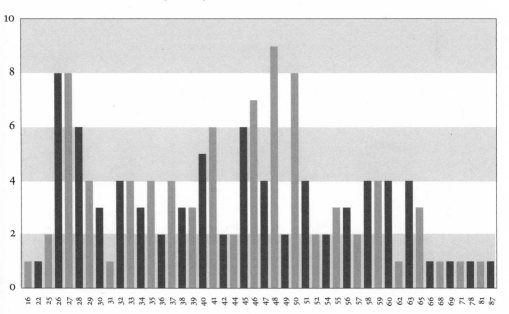

NUMBER OF YEARS BETWEEN FIRST LESION DATE
AND FIRST EXAM FOR SAMPLE OF 143 MEN

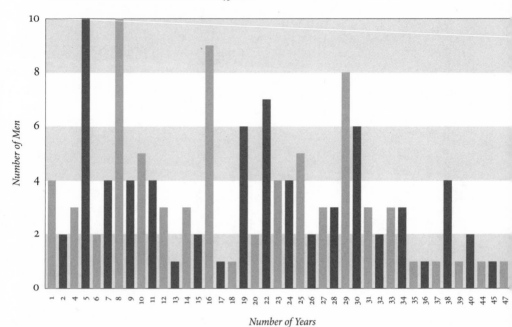

AUTOPSY BY CASE STATUS BEFORE 1973

Case Status	No Autopsy	Autopsy	Total
Syphilitic	94	162	256
Row %	36.7	63.3	100.0
Column %	75.2	71.1	72.5
Control	31	66	97
Row %	32.0	68.0	100.0
Column %	24.8	28.9	27.5
Total	125	228	353
Row %	35.4	64.6	100.0

Note: Autopsy information was available for 353 records: 256 syphilitics and 97 controls. The "risk" (rate) of autopsy was 162/256 = 63.3% for syphilitics and 66/97 = 68% for controls. Thus syphilitics were about 87% as likely to be autopsied as controls. This difference is not statistically significant (p~0.20). For the men who had died by 1973 (the end of the Study), the rate of autopsy was 64.1% for syphilitics versus 71.9% for controls (p-value = 0.09), a result significant at p<0.10.

COD	Control	Syphilitic	Total	COD	Control	Syphilitic	Total
Aortitis	2	3	5	Suicide	0	1	1
Row %	40.0	60.0	100.0	Row %	0.0	100.0	100.0
Column %	1.8	1.1	1.3	Column %	0.0	0.4	0.3
Aneurysm	1	4	5	Homicide	0	1	1
Row %	20.0	80.0	100.0	Row %	0.0	100.0	100.0
Column %	0.9	1.4	1.3	Column %	0.0	0.4	0.3
Heart, other	33	85	118	Diabetes	1	0	1
Row %	28.0	72.0	100.0	Row %	100.0	0.0	100.0
Column %	30.3	29.8	29.9	Column %	0.9	0.0	0.3
Cancer	13	31	44	Atherosclerosis	7	22	29
Row %	29.5	70.5	100.0	Row %	24.1	75.9	100.0
Column %	11.9	10.9	11.2	Column %	6.4	7.7	7.4
Cerebrovascular	13	25	38	Liver	0	4	4
Row %	34.2	65.8	100.0	Row %	0.0	100.0	100.0
Column %	11.9	8.8	9.6	Column %	0.0	1.4	1.0
Chronic lower respiratory	0	2	2	Alzheimer's	1	0	1
Row %	0.0	100.0	100.0	Row %	100.0	0.0	100.0
Column %	0.0	0.7	0.5	Column %	0.9	0.0	0.3
Tuberculosis	1	7	8	Nephritis	10	25	35
Row %	12.5	87.5	100.0	Row %	28.6	71.4	100.0
Column %	0.9	2.5	2.0	Column %	9.2	8.8	8.9
Lung, other	5	6	11	Syphilis	0	16	16
Row %	45.5	54.5	100.0	Row %	0.0	100.0	100.0
Column %	4.6	2.1	2.8	Column %	0.0	5.6	4.1
Unintentional injury	2	10	12	Other	6	14	20
Row %	16.7	83.3	100.0	Row %	30.0	70.0	100.0
Column %	1.8	3.5	3.0	Column %	5.5	4.9	5.1
Pneumonia and influenza	10	23	33	Unknown	4	6	10
Row %	30.3	69.7	100.0	Row %	40.0	60.0	100.0
Column %	9.2	8.1	8.4	Column %	3.7	2.1	2.5
				Total	109	285	394
				Row %	27.7	72.3	100.0
				Column %	100.0	100.0	100.0

Note: Controls to syphilitic conversions were grouped with the syphilitics. There are too many categories and small numbers to assess statistical significance by infection status.

Notes

ABBREVIATIONS

AP   Associated Press

CDC   Communicable Disease Center and, later,
Centers for Disease Control

CDC-GA   Centers for Disease Control Papers, Tuskegee Syphilis
Study Administrative Records, 1930–80, Record Group 442,
National Archives and Records Administration —
Southeast Region, Morrow, Ga.

Chesney Archives   Alan M. Chesney Archives, Johns Hopkins
Medical School, Baltimore, Md.

Cutler Papers   John C. Cutler Papers, Archives Service Center,
University of Pittsburgh, Pittsburgh, Pa.

Dibble Papers   Eugene H. Dibble Papers, Washingtonian Collection,
Frissell Library, Tuskegee University, Tuskegee, Ala.

HEW   U.S. Department of Health, Education, and Welfare

HEW-NLM   U.S. Department of Health, Education, and Welfare,
Ad Hoc Advisory Panel on the Tuskegee Syphilis
Study Papers, History of Medicine Collection,
National Library of Medicine, Bethesda, Md.

HHS   U.S. Department of Health and Human Services

Kahn Papers   Reuben Kahn Papers, Bentley Historical Library,
University of Michigan, Ann Arbor, Mich.

Laurie Papers   Eunice Rivers Laurie Papers, Washingtonian Collection,
Frissell Library, Tuskegee University, Tuskegee, Ala.

NIH   National Institutes of Health

PHS   U.S. Public Health Service

PHS-NA   U.S. Public Health Service, General Records of the
Venereal Disease Division, 1918–36, National Archives
and Records Administration, College Park, Md.

RF-Fisk   Rosenwald Fund Papers, Special Collections, John Hope and
Aurelia E. Franklin Library, Fisk University, Nashville, Tenn.

TMF   Tuskegee Syphilis Study Medical Files, Tuskegee Syphilis
Study Administrative Records, 1930–80, Record Group 442,
National Archives and Records Administration—Southeast
Region, Morrow, Ga.

TMF-Edgar   Tuskegee Medical Files, Harold Edgar, Rothman Office, Mailman
School of Public Health, Columbia University, New York, N.Y.

TUA   Frissell Library, Washingtonian Collection, Tuskegee University,
Tuskegee, Ala.

INTRODUCTION

1 This is the oft-used shortened version of Osler's longer quote: "Know syphilis in all its manifestations and relations, and all other things clinical will be added unto you." Osler, "Internal Medicine as a Vocation," 134. I am grateful to Jonathan Erlen and Lily Szczygiel for helping me track this down.

2 See Hammonds and Herzig, *Nature of Difference*.

3 See chapter 1 and Jones, *Bad Blood*.

4 The Veterans Hospital is now called Central Alabama Veterans Health Care System—East Campus.

5 For many, the possibility that the men could have passed this disease on to their wives and children is tantamount to the government's infecting them directly; see the story and comments on the blog, <http://blog.washingtonpost.com/fact-checker/2008/05/the_tuskegee_experiment_part_i.html>, accessed August 8, 2008. See also Reverby, "More Than Fact and Fiction," 2–8.

6 Benedek and Erlen, "Scientific Environment," 1–30.

7 Dowling, *Fighting Infection*, 82–104; Quetel, *History of Syphilis*; Parascandola, *Sex, Sin, and Science*.

8 Until the late 1920s, there was medical debate over whether syphilis was hereditary—that is, whether it could be passed on genetically through the sperm of an infected father or egg of an infected mother. By the time the Study began, it was understood to be congenital, passed by an infectious pregnant mother to her fetus or the infant during birth. If the father was not infectious when he had sex with the mother, even if he had the disease and she did not, it would be unlikely he would pass it on to her or the fetus. On the problem with wet nurses, see Reverby, "Syphilis of the Innocent," 11.

9 On the paradox of more syphilis but the assumption of fewer neurological complications in African Americans, see Crenner, "Tuskegee Syphilis Study."

10 Brandt, *No Magic Bullet*.

11 Parran, "Syphilis: A Public Health Problem," 149.

12 It alerts us to what historian David Blight argues: "How some selections [of historical memory formation] become or remain dominant, taking on mythic dimensions, and others do not, is the tale to be told"; Blight, *Race and Reunion*, 1. On the problem of stories, see Tilly, *Credit and Blame*.

13 King, "Race, Justice, and Research," 90.

14 The question of whether those who fear medical care and entry into clinical trials remember "Tuskegee" has been the subject of numerous studies since the 1990s; see chapter 10.

15 Holloway, "Accidental Communities," 7–17; quote on 11.

16 See Jones, *Bad Blood*; Gray, *Tuskegee Syphilis Study*; and Reverby, *Tuskegee's Truths*.

17 See Gamble, "Under the Shadow," 431–43. The Nazi doctor literature is extensive.

18 Burton, *Archive Stories*.

19 On the creation of memory in the South, see Brundage, *Southern Past*.

20 McAdams, *Stories We Live By*, 28; on the connections in the mind between memory and history, see also Schacter, *Searching for Memory*.

21 Hartman, *Scenes of Subjection*, 11.

22 I am grateful to Merlin Chowkwanyun for discussions on this overview.

23 Lee, "Racializing Drug Design," 2133.

24 Smitherman, *Talkin and Testifyin*, 58; Monroe, email to author, October 25, 2002.

25 See <http://www.examiningtuskegee.com.>

26 See further discussion in Parker and Alvarez, "Legacy," 37–38.

27 On the problem of a "post-fact" society, see Manjoo, *True Enough*.

28 For a thoughtful discussion of the difference between explaining and justifying horrific historical events, see Clendinnen, *Reading the Holocaust*; and Levi, *The Drowned and the Saved*.

29 "When versions of the past become embedded in current political debates, historians must continue to struggle to maintain their allegiance to a rigorous and independent scholarship while recognizing and accepting the political consequences and meaning of their work"; Curthoys, "History of Killing," 369.

30 Maier, "Doing History," 267.

31 Hayner, *Unspeakable Truths*.

32 I have heard this on numerous occasions when I have spoken to family members over the more than fifteen years that I have been traveling to Macon County. I have been asked this question about punishment over and over whenever I lecture on the Study. I thank sociologist Vivian Carter at Tuskegee University for discussions about the oral histories she has been doing in Macon County, which have also helped to shape my understandings.

CHAPTER 1

1 See William Warren Rogers et al., *Alabama*.

2 *Tuskegee News*, 100th Anniversary Edition, no. 3, n.p.; Atkins, "From Early Times," 58, 60, 72.

3 The word "Taskigi" (Tuskegee) meant "warrior" in the language spoken by the Muskogee people.

4 According to the 1860 census, there were 1,020 slaveholders in Macon County out of a white population of 8,624.

5 The term "Black Belt" has been given different meanings by a variety of authors. See Houston A. Baker Jr., *Blues, Ideology, and Afro-American Literature*, 94–95.

6 Norrell, *Reaping the Whirlwind*, 11.

7 Ibid., 4–5; Atkins, "From Early Times," 216–17.

8 Quoted in Myers, "The Freedman and the Law," 60.

9 Rogers and Ward, "From 1865 through 1920," 237.

10 Norrell, *Reaping the Whirlwind*, 9.

11 Ibid.

12 Butler, *Distinctive Black College*, 55.

13 See Bond, *Education of the Negro*; and Anderson, *Education of Blacks*.

14 Butler, *Distinctive Black College*, 56.

15 Andrews, *Up from Slavery*, 130.

16 Ibid., 65.

17 Bieze, *Booker T. Washington*, 20.

18 Mugleston, "Booker T. Washington," 124.

19 Cox, "Autobiography and Washington," 228–39; see also Norrell, *Reaping the Whirlwind*, 17.

20 Kowalski, "No Excuses," 181–96. I am also grateful to Kenneth M. Hamilton of Southern Methodist University for his long discussions with me about Washington. Washington remains one of the more complicated figures in American political life.

21 Campbell, *Movable School*.

22 Houston A. Baker Jr. makes a psychological/cultural argument about Washington, sexuality, and the "folk"; see *Turning South Again*, 56–58, 63.

23 Gates, "Trope of the New Negro," 129–55; and see the discussion in Kowalski, "No Excuses," 188.

24 See Harlan, "Secret Life of Booker T. Washington," 204–19, for examples of what Washington did in public and what he did behind the scenes.

25 Ibid., 165–78.

26 For insight into the politics of Tuskegee in the Washington years, see Alexander, *Homelands and Waterways*.

27 Quoted in Litwack, *Trouble in Mind*, 112.

28 The syphilis rumor persisted until 2006 when scholars at a University of Maryland medical conference, reviewing his medical records, determined that he died from "kidney failure brought on by high blood pressure," with no evidence of syphilis; see Alex Dominguez, "High Blood Pressure Claimed Booker T. Washington, Review Finds," *Seattle Times*, May 6, 2006.

29 Dibble, Rabb, and Ballard, "John A. Andrew Memorial Hospital," 103–18.

30 "John A. Andrew Clinic Boon to Medical Progress," undated clipping, box 12, Clippings Folder, Dibble Papers. See also Kenney, "Brief History," 65–68.

31 Kenney also organized a postgraduate course of four weeks' duration in 1921 that met several other times over the years. By 1950, Kenney's successor, Eugene H. Dibble Jr., was working to shift "the major emphasis at the annual meeting from a

treatment to a training clinic"; Eugene H. Dibble, "John A. Andrew Clinical Society Program, April 8–13, 1956," box 12, Folder 19, Dibble Papers.

32 On the links among freedom, health care, and citizenship, see Long, *Doctoring Freedom*.

33 Quoted in Susan L. Smith, *Sick and Tired*, 41. Smith provides an excellent history of National Negro Health Week, 33–57, and this section leans on her analysis. See also Tomes, *Gospel of Germs*.

34 My thanks to Louis "Mike" Rabb for discussing his memories of Moton with me; Louis Mike Rabb interview. On Moton's politics, see also Fairclough, "Civil Rights and the Lincoln Memorial," 408–16. Moton became principal of Tuskegee Institute following the death of Booker T. Washington, founder and first principal, in 1916. A full modern biography of Moton is needed.

35 Moton, *Finding a Way Out*, 240–41; Marable, *Black Leadership*, 81.

36 Quoted in Susan L. Smith, *Sick and Tired*, 46.

37 Gamble, *Making a Place for Ourselves*, 89.

38 Ibid., 102. On the guns, see also Helen Dibble and Lewis W. Jones, "Oral History of Annie Lou Miller," in Statewide Oral History Project, Alabama Center for Higher Education, January 17, 1973, TUA; and Daniel, "Black Power in the 1920s."

39 See Ralph Chester Williams, *United States Public Health Service*; and Kondratas, *Images*.

40 Kraut, *Silent Travelers*; Fairchild, *Science at the Borders*; JoAnne Brown, "Crime, Commerce and Contagionism," 52–81.

41 "U.S. Health Officer," 110; see also Lederer, "Hollywood and Human Experimentation," 282–306.

42 Ralph Chester Williams, *United States Public Health Service*, 247.

43 Ibid., 85. Debates continued throughout the PHS's history over how extensive its role should be and the nature of the federal/state/local relationship. The PHS reflected the debates that went on nationwide over the role of the government in public health and that of private physicians in providing care. Surgeon General Hugh Cumming, for example, opposed the use of federal funds provided in the Sheppard-Towner Act to states for maternal and child health programs; see Mullan, *Plagues and Politics*, 95.

44 "U.S. Health Officer," 104.

45 Mullan, *Plagues and Politics*, 61. The Hygienic Laboratory in its opening decades was kept busy primarily evaluating drugs; see Marks, *Progress of Experiment*, 48.

46 On the PHS officers as outsiders, see Rosenkrantz, "Non-Random Events," 244.

47 "Assailants," *Montgomery Advertiser*, May 21, 1922, clipping in Ku Klux Klan Clippings File, "Alabama 1922," TUA.

48 Ralph Chester Williams, *United States Public Health Service*, 545.

49 Altman, *Who Goes First*; Lederer, *Subjected to Science*, 126–38.

50 As Lederer has argued (*Subjected to Science*, 127), "Self-experimentation undermined accusations of research exploitation and demonstrated the nobility of investigators."

51 "At Georgia State Sanitarium in Milledgeville . . . Joseph Goldberger's mentally ill Negro women patients who ate the doctor's low-cost diet never knew what they

contributed to the eventual conquest of pellagra. . . . Some came down with pellagra, some did not"; Ralph Chester Williams, *United States Public Health Service*, 278.

52 Lederer, *Subjected to Science*, 137.

53 Marks, *Progress of Experiment*, 37.

54 Ibid., 38.

55 Rosenberg, *No Other Gods*.

56 See Dowling, *Fighting Infection*; Poirier, *Chicago's War on Syphilis*; Kraut, *Goldberger's War*; and Fee, "Sin versus Science," 141–64.

57 Marks, *Progress of Experiment*. Marks underlines the difficulties of making these kinds of connections because of the lack of research infrastructure and ways of adjudicating differences, but the PHS was often central to the efforts. See also Brandt and Gardner, "Antagonism and Accommodation," 707–15.

58 For an excellent example of the difficulties of this dance, see Kraut, *Goldberger's War*.

59 Joseph L. Graves Jr., *Emperor's New Clothes*, 122.

60 Marks, "Epidemiologists Explain Pellagra," 34–55.

61 See Hammonds and Herzig, *Nature of Difference*.

62 Folkes, "The Negro as a Health Problem."

63 See Lombardo and Dorr, "Eugenics."

64 For an introduction to the literature on eugenics, see "The Eugenics Archives," <http://www.eugenicsarchive.org/eugenics/>, accessed August 9, 2008.

65 Lombardo and Dorr (in "Eugenics") make a specific argument for the eugenics background of the leaders of the Study and in the PHS. For more on race and blood, see also Lederer, *Flesh and Blood*.

66 Limson, "Observations"; N. D. C. Lewis and Hubbard, "Epileptic Reactions"; Pearl, "Weight of the Negro Brain"; Heterington, "Kerato-Cricoid Muscle." On Pearl's complex history, see Hendricks, "Raymond Pearl's 'Mingled Mess.'"

67 Pernick, "Eugenics and Public Health," 1769. Pernick also notes, "Both eugenics and microbiology contributed to the assumptions about racial epidemiology that shaped the Public Health Service's decision to use African-American men for the Tuskegee Study of untreated syphilis" (1771).

68 The Curex Remedy Co. of Baltimore, for example, sold Curex Blood Purifier "with Stilligia and iodide of Potash," and 10 percent alcohol, as a cure for a range of symptoms from pimples and pustules to ulcers, scrofula, and syphilis (Curex Blood Purifier bottle, collection of the author).

69 Brandt, *No Magic Bullet*.

70 For an example of the debate, see Crenner, "Tuskegee Syphilis Study."

71 Ibsen's 1881 play *Ghosts*, which was, in part, about the horrors of congenital syphilis and its impact on a family, was considered so controversial when published that it could not be produced in Scandinavia, and thus it had its world premiere in Chicago a year later. The concern with the "innocent" is what drove the push for blood tests for syphilis before marriage in the United States, a requirement that now exists in only five states. See also Reverby, "Syphilis of the Innocent."

72 Solomon and Solomon, *Syphilis of the Innocent*, 1.

73 Ibid., 205; Parran and Vonderlehr, *Plain Words about Venereal Disease*, 213–14.

74 Parran, like many PHS officers, was a white southerner who began his PHS efforts doing rural sanitation work in the 1910s; see Brandt, *No Magic Bullet*, 122–60.

75 For Moore's importance, see chapter 7.

76 Brandt, *No Magic Bullet*, 131.

77 Marks, "Notes from the Underground"; Marks, *Progress of Experiment*, 53–60; Brandt, *No Magic Bullet*, 130–31.

78 The arguments on these points are made clearly by Brandt, *No Magic Bullet*, 122.

79 Parran was then the New York commissioner of health. See ibid.

80 Parascandola, "Syphilis at the Cinema."

81 Poirier, *Chicago's War on Syphilis*, 106.

82 Hazen, *Syphilis in the Negro*, 1–14.

83 Brandt, *No Magic Bullet*, 116. Miles and McBride argue further that the post–World War I rise in syphilis rates was directly related to where black soldiers had been stationed during the war, the failure to treat them, the lack of black doctors and nurses, and the "lure of the khaki" on young black women in the South where the soldiers were stationed. See Miles and McBride, "World War I Origins of the Syphilis Epidemic."

84 Carley and Wenger, "Prevalence of Syphilis," 1826.

85 Gjestland, *Oslo Study*, 12–13. The low percentage with neurological symptoms in an all-white population would later be ignored when it was assumed that African Americans suffered more from cardiovascular complications.

86 Ibid., 18; Stokes, *Modern Clinical Syphilology*, 18.

87 Vonderlehr, "Comparison," 1.

88 Quoted in JoAnne Brown, "Crime, Commerce and Contagionism," 70.

89 Ibid. On the issues of "Negro blood," see Wailoo, *Dying in the City of Blues*; Love, *One Blood*; and Lederer, *Flesh and Blood*.

90 Whenever a small "n" in Negro is used in the primary quotes, I have kept it, in keeping with historical practices. Marvin L. Graves, "Negro a Menace to the Health of the White Race." After discussions with Booker T. Washington, this doctor declared that public health education would be of use but that those who were vagrants could not be trusted and should be "emasculated."

91 Taliaferro Clark, *Control of Syphilis*, 27. Given contemporary debates over how to estimate the amount of HIV/AIDS in the United States, the problems of appropriate surveillance can be appreciated. I am grateful to my sister, Eve Mokotoff, for her decades of HIV/AIDS surveillance work and her willingness to talk to me about it.

92 Carley and Wenger, "Prevalence of Syphilis."

93 Ibid., 1828. In fact, the leading causes of death for African Americans in Mississippi at the time were tuberculosis and heart disease, not syphilis, unless every case of heart disease is assumed to have been caused by syphilis.

94 Ibid.

CHAPTER 2

1 The classic history of the Rosenwald Fund is Embree and Waxman, *Story of the Julius Rosenwald Fund*. Julius Rosenwald had been on the Tuskegee Institute board since 1911.

2 Taliaferro Clark, *Control of Syphilis*, 17. The demonstration ran for a year and half, between February 12, 1930, and September 1, 1931.

3 For more on the lives of those who were in the Study, see chapter 6.

4 Known as the Jessup wagon, the "movable school" had, by the 1920s, become a motorized bus. See Campbell, *Movable School*.

5 Taliaferro Clark, *Control of Syphilis*, 29.

6 Ibid., xviii.

7 On the role of violence and the use of root doctors and local healers, see Johnson, "Shadow of the Plantation: Survival." Root doctors, or those who practiced "hoodoo," used herbs and roots to provide cures.

8 Herman Shaw, one of the men in the Study (see chapter 6), described not being able to afford the tags and how they were shared.

9 It is not uncommon in rural areas for residents to make it into more "urban" centers only rarely. When I lived in rural West Virginia in 1973–74, my nearest neighbor, Okie Kerns, drove a thirty-year-old car; traded his furs and roots at the local store where he cashed his Social Security and miner's pension checks; grew, hunted for, or dug up most of what he ate; got his water from roof runoff and an outdoor pump; used an outhouse; and had not been to town (population about 5,000 and ten miles away) in over a decade. No one could have been a better guide to the cadences of rural life.

10 Ed Childray, box 526, Folder 6, RF-Fisk. Johnson's and his students' original interviews are in these papers.

11 The classic study of Macon County done for the Rosenwald Fund is Johnson, *Shadow of the Plantation*.

12 Dr. G. C. Branche, who worked at the Tuskegee VA Hospital, visited the men in jail. See Goodman, *Stories of Scottsboro*, 264.

13 See Rosengarten, *All God's Dangers*; Litwack, *Trouble in Mind*; and Kelley, *Hammer and Hoe*.

14 Reginald James, "The Mobile Clinic and Syphilis in the Rural Areas of Macon County, Alabama," TUA. Of 91 women who came to his clinic, James noted that 56 percent reported one miscarriage; 21 percent had two; 15 percent noted three or more; and 8 percent had experienced stillbirth (11). James does not make clear what percentage of his patients this accounted for, however. See "Number of Cases and Death Rates," ibid., 66.

15 Ibid., 28.

16 Hilliard Boyd, box 526, Folder 6, RF-Fisk. I have kept the quotes as recorded by Johnson's interviewers.

17 The Rosenwald Fund Demonstration Project concentrated in the southwestern third of the county. See Clyde D. Frost, "Report Concerning Medical Conditions," box 556, Folder 10, p. 1, RF-Fisk. The Rosenwald Fund paid for Johnson and his

students' work in Macon County as part of the Demonstration Project. The interviewers—all black—were clearly upset by the poverty, the attitudes toward sex, the jealousies, and the vagaries of daily life. Those interviewed were patients of the Demonstration Project (or their wives). The interviews were primarily the women, who were home during the day, and not the men, who were in the fields. The patients (men and women) in the Demonstration Project and the men in the Syphilis Study came from different parts of the county and with few exceptions were not the same men. I compared the names of the men in the Study to the names of those in the interviews on file in RF-Fisk.

18 For an example of the difficulties of medical communication, see Todd, *Intimate Adversaries*.

19 Box 526, Folders 5 and 6, RF-Fisk. "Scrofula" was a term used for what is now described as a form of tuberculosis in the neck that is due to infection in the lymph nodes.

20 Johnson, *Shadow of the Plantation*, 195. For example, he wrote, "Children die in great numbers and mothers accept their death with a dull and uninquiring fatalism" (192).

21 Box 526, Folder 5, RF-Fisk. Sheep nanny tea was a common rural concoction made by straining sheep dung through a cheesecloth. Yellow thrush was a fungal infection in the throat.

22 Frost, "Report Concerning Medical Conditions," 12.

23 Box 526, Folders 6 and 7, RF-Fisk.

24 Ibid., box 526, Folder 5. Dr. Lightfoot practiced in Shorter, Alabama, and his son was the mayor of Tuskegee during the famous civil rights gerrymandering case, *Gomillion v. Lightfoot*.

25 Box 526, Folder 6, RF-Fisk.

26 Will McQueen, Folder 6, and Will and Cora Gosha, Folder 7, RF-Fisk.

27 Pelly Anderson, box 526, Folder 7, RF-Fisk.

28 Box 526, Folder 7, RF-Fisk.

29 Jones, *Bad Blood*, 74.

30 Frost, "Report Concerning Medical Conditions," 8.

31 On white illness, see Gosha, box 526, Folder 8, RF-Fisk. On blacks and whites living together, see Lewis, ibid., Folder 6.

32 Jones, *Bad Blood*; Taliaferro Clark, *Control of Syphilis*.

33 Dr. Clyde Frost reported that the Rosenwald Fund Demonstration Project taught the local doctors more about what was needed. The PHS worked out an arrangement that provided drugs to local doctors at a lower cost and encouraged them to provide more treatments; Frost, "Report Concerning Medical Conditions," 9–10.

34 Ibid., 3.

35 Ibid., 5. I was surprised to find the expression "susceptible to kindness" in this physician's report on the Rosenwald Fund Demonstration Project. These words were given to Nurse Evers by David Feldshuh in his play about the Study, *Miss Evers' Boys* (see chapter 11). There is no evidence that the real Rivers ever uttered them. The video and discussion pamphlet prepared by Cornell University in conjunction with the play are also titled "Susceptible to Kindness."

36 Taliaferro Clark, *Control of Syphilis*, 24–26, 36.

37 Stokes, *Modern Clinical Syphilology*, 266.

38 Ibid., 67.

39 Frost, "Report Concerning Medical Conditions," 5.

40 Box 526, Folder 5, RF-Fisk.

41 Alabama state laws from 1919, 1923, and 1927 required "persons infected with vene-
    real disease to report for treatment to a reputable physician and continue treatment
    until such disease, in the judgment of the attending physician, is no longer commu-
    nicable or a source of danger to public health." Alabama, State of, *General Laws of
    the Legislature of Alabama*, 716. I am grateful to Bob Aller of Lompoc, California,
    for sending copies of these laws to me.

42 "Memo for Dr. Miller," May 23, 1930, box 526, Folder 2, RF-Fisk; Parran, *Shadow on
    the Land*, 62.

43 Box 526, Folder 5, RF-Fisk.

44 Taliaferro Clark, *Control of Syphilis*, 35.

45 Ibid., 29.

46 Brandt, *No Magic Bullet*, 152. See Roy, "Julius Rosenwald Fund Syphilis Seropreva-
    lence Studies," 319, for more on the limitations of the blood tests used and the many
    possible reasons for the high numbers.

47 Taliaferro Clark, *Control of Syphilis*, 53; Jones, *Bad Blood*, 76.

48 Taliaferro Clark, *Control of Syphilis*, 29.

49 Ibid., 36–41. Four doses was the county average, but 55.4 percent of the patients
    (663) actually received more than 15 doses of neoarsphenamine and more than 90
    mercury rubs. Neoarsphenamine was less toxic than the original arsphenamine and
    easier to administer.

50 Ibid., 38.

51 Ibid., 67.

52 Johnson, "Shadow of the Plantation: Survival," 58.

53 Jones, *Bad Blood*, 79. Jones covers the Rosenwald Fund Demonstration Project in
    detail on 78–90.

54 Quoted in ibid., 82.

55 Ibid. In response to the criticism, Jones argues, the Rosenwald Fund's Michael
    Davis set up meetings and sent Charles S. Johnson and his students into the county
    to study the communities and their views on health.

56 Ibid., 90.

57 Taliaferro Clark, *Control of Syphilis*, 53.

58 Noted syphilologist John H. Stokes argued that syphilis was "a medical and sanitary
    problem" whose "last line of defense crumbles before our attack"; Snow, Moore,
    Brown, and Parran, "Symposium on Research," 7.

59 Ibid., 17.

60 Taliaferro Clark to Dr. Michael M. Davis, Julius Rosenwald Fund, October 29, 1932,
    General Records of the Venereal Disease Division, 1918–36, Record Group 90, box
    239, Folder 1, PHS-NA.

61 E. Gurney Clark and Danbolt, "The Oslo Study," 311.

62 Joseph Earle Moore to Dr. Taliaferro Clark, September 28, 1932, in Reverby, *Tuske-*

gee's Truths, 80. Raymond Vonderlehr, who would go on to run the Study in 1933 in Tuskegee, told a meeting of the John A. Andrew Clinical Society that "our present information indicates definite biologic differences in the disease in Negroes and Whites"; Vonderlehr, "Comparison," 41. On the links between eugenics and the racial beliefs of the PHS venereal disease physicians, see Lombardo and Dorr, "Eugenics."

63 U.S. Public Health Service, *Annual Report*, 1933, 97. In his "Memorandum for Clinicians and Health Officers," an appendix to this final Rosenwald Fund Demonstration Project report, Clark warned: "REMEMBER. The older patients should not be treated with arsenicals unless they have only had their infection a comparatively short time, or have some definite lesion. Put these cases on potassium iodide and proto-iodide of mercury and gradually eliminate them from the clinic so as to have more time for the younger group." See also Taliaferro Clark, *Control of Syphilis*, 64.

64 Jones, *Bad Blood*, 78–83.

65 The idea that the PHS gave the men syphilis has been part of the Study's lore since 1972.

66 On the state of research at this time, see Marks, *Progress of Experiment*.

67 For a selection of the letters, see Reverby, *Tuskegee's Truths*, 73–115.

68 Taliaferro Clark to Dr. J. N. Baker, August 29, 1932, ibid., 74.

69 O. C. Wenger to Taliaferro Clark, October 10, 1932, box 239, Folder 1, PHS-NA.

70 On the importance of Joseph Earle Moore to the Study, see chapter 7.

71 O. C. Wenger to Taliaferro Clark, September 29, 1932, box 239, Folder 1, PHS-NA.

72 Clark told Dibble that the state's public health director opposed his officers giving treatments: "This policy quite naturally limits the utilization of Doctor Smith's services for treatment purposes as we had hoped to do." See Taliaferro Clark to Eugene H. Dibble, September 21, 1932, PHS-NA. For more detail on this, see Jones, *Bad Blood*, 91–150; and the letters in Reverby, *Tuskegee's Truths*, 73–88.

73 Taliaferro Clark to Michael M. Davis, October 29, 1932, box 239, Folder 1, PHS-NA.

74 Taliaferro Clark to Eugene H. Dibble, September 21, 1932, ibid.

75 Eugene H. Dibble to Dr. R. R. Moton, September 17, 1932, in Reverby, *Tuskegee's Truths*, 75–76.

76 H. S. Cumming to Dr. R. R. Moton, September 20, 1932, ibid., 77.

77 Dr. R. R. Moton to Surgeon General H. S. Cumming, October 10, 1932, box 239, Folder 1, PHS-NA.

78 Joseph Earle Moore to Taliaferro Clark, September 30, 1932, box 239, Folder 1, PHS-NA.

79 Ibid., 80.

80 For a longer discussion of what happened to the wives and children, see chapter 6. There were very few studies at the time that took homosexuality or male-to-male sex into account, and this kind of research did not happen in rural Alabama.

81 See, for example, Murray Smith to Taliaferro Clark, May 2, 1933, box 239, Folder 1, PHS-NA.

82 See chapter 9 on Eunice Rivers.

83 "The biggest obstacle to the program has been the necessity of including the remaining ¾ of Macon County, which was not touched by the Rosenwald Fund demonstration"; O. C. Wenger to Taliaferro Clark, January 7, 1933, box 239, Folder 2, PHS-NA.

84 R. A. Vonderlehr to Taliaferro Clark, February 23, 1933, ibid. Vonderlehr discusses the problem of getting consents for the blood testing as well, in a letter to Clark on February 11, 1933, ibid.

85 R. A. Vonderlehr to Dr. Carey, Tuskegee Veterans Hospital, February 16, 1933, Record 214, box 15, TMF.

86 Laurie, Deposition, *Pollard v. U.S.*, 20.

87 R. A. Vonderlehr to Taliaferro Clark, January 7, 1933, box 239, Folder 2, PHS-NA.

88 A few months later, Vonderlehr solved the syringe-tube problem "in the most efficient manner. We are using these tubes on selected cases only"; R. A. Vonderlehr to Taliaferro Clark, February 28, 1933, ibid.

89 R. A. Vonderlehr to Taliaferro Clark, October 26, 1932, ibid.

90 Taliaferro Clark to R. A. Vonderlehr, January 9, 1933, and O. C. Wenger to Taliaferro Clark, January 7, 1933, ibid.

91 Syphilis Control Demonstration, Macon County, January 1933, and February 1933, ibid.

92 R. A. Vonderlehr to Taliaferro Clark, February 6, 1933, ibid.

93 R. A. Vonderlehr to Austin Deibert, December 5, 1938, box 12, Folder Personnel General 1938–39, Tuskegee Syphilis Study Records, CDC-GA.

94 Eugene H. Dibble to R. R. Moton, March 28, 1933, box 239, Folder 2, PHS-NA. Dibble confided to Moton: "This however, is very confidential information which Dr. Vonderlehr will give to the public as research work in connection with the U.S. Public Health Service and our hospital"; Hugh Cumming to J. N. Baker, August 5, 1933, ibid.

95 O. C. Wenger to D. G. Gill, November 23, 1932, ibid.

96 O. C. Wenger to Taliaferro Clark, January 9, 1933, ibid. Rivers, in her deposition for the lawsuit after the Study ended, also agreed that the men from the Rosenwald Fund Demonstration Project were not the same men who were in the Study; see Laurie, Deposition, *Pollard v. U.S.*, 93.

97 Taliaferro Clark to Joseph Earle Moore, December 30, 1932, box 239, Folder 2, PHS-NA.

98 Smith, Taliaferro Clark, and Vonderlehr understood the financial problems. They all lost money when their banks closed in 1933.

99 R. A. Vonderlehr to Taliaferro Clark, January 22, 1933, in Reverby, *Tuskegee's Truths*, 82.

100 Taliaferro Clark to R. A. Vonderlehr, April 9, 1933, box 239, Folder 2, PHS-NA. Clark refused Vonderlehr's request to amend PHS regulations so that he could attend to subjects outside the county who might have complications from the spinal taps.

101 R. A. Vonderlehr to Taliaferro Clark, February 11, 1933; R. A. Vonderlehr to Taliaferro Clark, March 6, 1933; R. A. Vonderlehr to Taliaferro Clark, April 5, 1933, ibid.

102 R. A. Vonderlehr to Taliaferro Clark, March 8, 1933, ibid.

103 Crenner, "Tuskegee Syphilis Study," 9. I am grateful to Christopher Crenner for sharing his paper with me before it was published.

104 Taliaferro Clark to R. A. Vonderlehr, January 9, 1933, and January 16, 1933, box 239, Folder 2, PHS-NA.

105 I thank my unnamed reader for the press for assistance on this point.

106 R. A. Vonderlehr to Taliaferro Clark, February 11, 1933, box 239, Folder 2, PHS-NA.

107 O. C. Wenger to R. A. Vonderlehr, April 14, 1933, ibid.

108 Taliaferro Clark to R. A. Vonderlehr, February 16, 1933, ibid.

109 Crenner, "Tuskegee Syphilis Study."

110 Macon County Health Department to Dear Sir, April 1933, in Reverby, *Tuskegee's Truths*, 187. This letter in particular is used to show the PHS's deception. Although clearly a spinal tap was not a "special treatment," at this point in the Study the PHS was still providing drugs for syphilis.

111 R. A. Vonderlehr to Taliaferro Clark, April 21, 1933, box 239, Folder 2, PHS-NA.

112 Laurie, Deposition, *Pollard v. U.S.*, 129.

113 R. A. Vonderlehr to Taliaferro Clark, April 20, 1933; G. W. McCoy to R. A. Vonderlehr, May 10, 1933, box 239, Folder 2, PHS-NA.

114 O. C. Wenger to Taliaferro Clark, May 24, 1933, ibid.

115 See Eugene H. Dibble to Taliaferro Clark, June 22, 1933; Eunice Rivers to R. A. Vonderlehr, June 29, 1933; J. H. Ward, Manager of the Veterans Administration Hospital in Tuskegee, to Taliaferro Clark, June 19, 1933; Taliaferro Clark to Eugene H. Dibble, June 6, 1933, ibid.

116 R. A. Vonderlehr to Taliaferro Clark, April 8, 1933, in Reverby, *Tuskegee's Truths*, 82–83.

117 Ibid.

118 Joseph Earle Moore to R. A. Vonderlehr, August 15, 1933; R. A. Vonderlehr to U. J. Wile, Harold N. Cole, Paul O'Leary, August 18, 1933, box 239, Folder 3, PHS-NA.

119 R. A. Vonderlehr to O. C. Wenger, July 19, 1933, in Reverby, *Tuskegee's Truths*, 83–84.

120 O. C. Wenger to R. A. Vonderlehr, July 21, 1933, ibid., 85 (underlining in the original letter).

121 On the use of this kind of terminology as a hidden form of subjugation, see Hartman, *Scenes of Subjection*.

122 O. C. Wenger to R. A. Vonderlehr, July 21, 1933, and August 5, 1933, box 239, Folder 3, PHS-NA. The sinister-sounding nature of Wenger's cold reasoning, however, has to be read as a concern about postmortems inflected by his views on race and his understanding of how poor people worried their bodies would be used. Wenger would have known about this from his medical school training and his experiences as a clinician. See Blakeley and Harrington, *Bones in the Basement*; and Lederer, *Subjected to Science*.

123 Summary of Alabama State Board of Health Annual Reports, 1932 and 1933, box 2, MS C 264, HEW-NLM.

124 R. A. Vonderlehr to Murray Smith, August 29, 1933, box 239, Folder 3, PHS-NA.

125 On the importance of agreements for autopsies in the study, see Lederer, "Tuskegee Syphilis Study," 266–75.

126 H. M. Marvin to R. A. Vonderlehr, August 2, 1933, box 239, Folder 3, PHS-NA; Jones, *Bad Blood*, 139–40.

127 Vonderlehr's defense is clearest in Vonderlehr et al., "Untreated Syphilis," 857. Vonderlehr asked Peters for details, for example, on a cardiovascular case; see R. A. Vonderlehr to Eugene H. Dibble, August 12, 1936; and Peters to R. A. Vonderlehr, August 20, 1936, Record 519, box 34, TMF.

128 R. A. Vonderlehr to Dr. H. T. Jones, Tallassee, Alabama, November 20, 1933, in Reverby, *Tuskegee's Truths*, 86–87. As Vonderlehr acknowledged: "Hypertension and arteriosclerosis were frequent complications and a control group of 200 Negroes is now being examined with the idea of noting the prevalence of arteriosclerosis and hypertension in this non-syphilitic group."

129 R. A. Vonderlehr to Eugene H. Dibble, July 28, 1933, box 239, Folder 2, PHS-NA.

130 R. A. Vonderlehr to Michael M. Davis, October 30, 1933, box 239, Folder 3, PHS-NA.

131 R. A. Vonderlehr to Eugene H. Dibble, October 2, 1933; R. A. Vonderlehr to John R. Heller Jr., October 23, 1933, ibid.

132 R. A. Vonderlehr to John R. Heller Jr., November 25, 1933; Heller to R. A. Vonderlehr, November 20, 1933, ibid.

133 R. A. Vonderlehr to O. C. Wenger, October 24, 1933; Wenger to Vonderlehr, October 24, 1933, ibid.

134 John R. Heller to R. A. Vonderlehr, November 20, 1933, ibid.

135 R. A. Vonderlehr to J. J. Peters, February 27, 1934; R. A. Vonderlehr to Joseph Earle Moore, February 27, 1934; Moore to Vonderlehr, February 28, 1934; Peters to Vonderlehr, March 4, 1934, box 239, Folder 4, PHS-NA.

136 Eunice Rivers to R. A. Vonderlehr, January 3, 1934; Vonderlehr to Rivers, January 6, 1934, ibid.

137 R. A. Vonderlehr to John R. Heller, January 11, 1934, ibid.

138 John R. Heller to R. A. Vonderlehr, January 13, 1934, ibid.

139 "Patient X," Auburn, Alabama, to the PHS, June 4, 1934; R. A. Vonderlehr to Patient X, June 7, 1934, in Reverby, *Tuskegee's Truths*, 87–88.

140 R. A. Vonderlehr to John R. Heller, February 13, 1934, box 239, Folder 4, PHS-NA.

141 John R. Heller to R. A. Vonderlehr, March 9, 1934; Vonderlehr to Heller, March 12, 1934, ibid.

142 R. A. Vonderlehr to J. J. Peters, April 17, 1934; R. A. Vonderlehr to Eugene H. Dibble, April 17, 1934; R. A. Vonderlehr to Eunice Rivers, April 19, 1934, ibid.

143 R. A. Vonderlehr to Eugene H. Dibble, April 6, 1934, ibid.

144 Vonderlehr reminded Smith: "This old Negro, you will recall, walked all the way to town for his spinal puncture after he had failed to show up for his first appointment and had been scolded by one of us for his negligence"; R. A. Vonderlehr to Smith, May 2, 1934; Smith to Vonderlehr, May 7, 1934, ibid.

145 Eunice Rivers to R. A. Vonderlehr, November 17, 1934, ibid.

146 Eunice Rivers to R. A. Vonderlehr, August 14, 1934, ibid.

147 R. A. Vonderlehr to McMullen, August 13, 1934, ibid.

148 McMullen to Heller, September 20, 1934, ibid.

149 McMullen to O. C. Wenger, September 14, 1934, ibid.

150 John R. Heller and Bruyere, "Untreated Syphilis," 119–24.

151 Jones, *Bad Blood*, 154.

152 See Holloway, *Passed On*. There was a rumor after 1972 within the PHS that Rivers's husband, whom she married in the 1950s, was an undertaker in the county. He was not. Although there was an undertaker in the county named Rivers, he was no relation; personal communication with David Sencer, August 1, 2005.

153 Rivers et al., "Twenty Years of Follow-up," 127–28. Even during the Depression, men and women in the county kept up their burial insurance. Mrs. Rosa Lancaster, in Shorter, Alabama, told one of the researchers sent by Charles S. Johnson into the county in 1930: "I pay $1.25 a month to the Mosaics. You get a $50.00 burial, a tombstone, and your relatives get $300.00 when you die." Others had trouble keeping up their payments. Mary Stuart explained: "Didn't have nothing to keep hit up and they don't pay you nothing. A poor man died right over there whose been paying his dues for years and they didn't even bury him. Ain't nothing to some of these insurances"; box 526, Folder 5, RF-Fisk.

154 The article was published twice; see Vonderlehr et al., "Untreated Syphilis."

155 See Charles J. McDonald, "Contribution of the Tuskegee Study"; and Solomon, "Rhetoric of Dehumanization."

156 J. Lawton Smith, "Ad Hoc Committee — Tuskegee Study," box 15, Folder 1959, CDC-GA. Smith was an ophthalmologist, neurosurgeon, and neurologist at the Miami School of Medicine and a consultant to the PHS in the 1960s on the Study.

157 Vonderlehr et al., "Untreated Syphilis," 859.

158 Ibid., 858–59.

159 Laurie, Deposition, *Pollard v. U.S.*, 98.

160 Vonderlehr et al., "Untreated Syphilis." The word "Tuskegee" would become part of the Study's title in the published reports only in 1954 with the eighth article; see Olansky et al., "Environmental Factors," 691–98.

161 For further discussion of disputes on what actually was "read" at the autopsies, see chapter 6.

162 See Halpern, *Lesser Harms*.

163 Jones, *Bad Blood*, 147.

CHAPTER 3

1 Raymond Vonderlehr to J. Jerome Peters, October 28, 1937; Vonderlehr to Murray Smith, October 28, 1937; Vonderlehr to C. A. Walwyn, October 28, 1937; Vonderlehr to R. D. Lillie, NIH, November 6, 1937, box 7, Folder General Correspondence 1937, CDC-GA.

2 See chapter 6. The assumption is often made that the men were completely passive objects in the PHS's hands. On the complicated role of current subjects, see Elliott, "Guinea-Pigging."

3 There were no annual blood draws between 1933 and 1939; see Olansky, Harris, Cutler, and Price, "Untreated Syphilis," 516.

4 Brandt, *No Magic Bullet*, 122–60; Parascandola, *Sex, Sin, and Science*.

5 For a contemporary view of the project and the "wagon" in Glynn County, Georgia, see Davenport, "Bad-Blood Wagon," 9–10, 27–30. The photo showing a black woman reading a flyer that says "COLORED PEOPLE Do You Have Bad Blood?" comes from the Glynn County campaign, not from Macon County in Alabama, although it is often used as a visual on the Study.

6 Reginald James, "The Mobile Clinic and Syphilis in the Rural Areas of Macon County, Alabama," 8, TUA. James ran the mobile clinic in 1940 (see chapter 5). I am grateful to Cynthia Wilson for finding this document.

7 R. A. Vonderlehr to Doctor M. O. Bousfield, Rosenwald Fund, May 29, 1937, box 5, Folder Correspondence 1937, CDC-GA.

8 Perry, "Questionnaire."

9 Between December 1939 and December 1940, Reginald James treated 604 patients for syphilis in Macon County: 406 women and 198 men. He reported that a third had had previous treatment; Reginald James, "The Mobile Clinic and Syphilis in the Rural Areas of Macon County, Alabama," 6, 12, TUA.

10 Reginald James complained about having to drive the bus as well as provide the treatments. In a sarcastic aside, Vonderlehr wrote to the Rosenwald Fund's M. O. Bousfield, "I am very sorry to learn that one of the reasons why Doctor James left the Macon County mobile unit was because a chauffeur was not provided"; R. A. Vonderlehr to William B. Perry, July 25, 1941, box 220, Folder 4, RF-Fisk.

11 Thomas Parran to Doctor J. N. Baker, January 18, 1938; William B. Perry to R. A. Vonderlehr, June 24, 1938, box 12, Personnel General 1938–39, CDC-GA.

12 In her deposition in the legal case that followed the end of the Study, Rivers confused this program with the Rosenwald Fund Demonstration Project. When asked if she worked on the Rosenwald Fund Demonstration Project, she replied: "I don't know anything about the workings of it because there was a Dr. Perry who was doing this and I was not—I am not familiar with that"; Laurie, Deposition, *Pollard v. U.S.*, 10, 114.

13 On supplies sent to Tuskegee, see A. E. Russell to E. W. Norris, March 15, 1938; A. E. Aselmeyer to Norris, December 28, 1937; Norris to Russell, March 18, 1938, box 7, Folders General Correspondence 1937 and 1938, CDC-GA.

14 See Brandt, *No Magic Bullet*, on the continued moralizing and fearmongering by the syphilologists and public health officials despite the availability of treatment across the country.

15 Austin V. Deibert to R. A. Vonderlehr, November 26, 1938, in Reverby, *Tuskegee's Truths*, 89–90.

16 Ibid.

17 Austin V. Deibert to R. A. Vonderlehr, March 27, 1939, box 7, Folder 1939, CDC-GA.

18 R. A. Vonderlehr to Austin V. Deibert, November 16, 1938, box 7, Folder 1938, CDC-GA. Vonderlehr also once again checked with Moore at Hopkins; see further discussion in chapter 7.

19 See appendix. Seventy-four men in the Study do not have the date of their first exam noted on their records, and it is not possible to know when they were recruited.

20 R. A. Vonderlehr to Austin V. Deibert, February 8, 1939, box 7, Folder 1939, CDC-GA.

21 Ibid. Vonderlehr also thought examining those already treated was a waste of time since data of this sort was available through the Cooperative Clinical Group research.

22 R. A. Vonderlehr to Austin V. Deibert, November 6, 1938, box 7, Folder 1938, CDC-GA.

23 Since malaria was so widespread and malarial fevers were a "cure" for neurosyphilis, Deibert thought doing the taps was not worth the problems; Austin V. Deibert to R. A. Vonderlehr, March 20, 1939, in Reverby, *Tuskegee's Truths*, 91–92.

24 Austin V. Deibert to R. A. Vonderlehr, February 5, 1939, box 7, Folder 1939, CDC-GA.

25 R. A. Vonderlehr to Austin V. Deibert, February 8, 1939, ibid.

26 Deibert, "Notes on Cardiovascular Syphilis."

27 Deibert went on to become the chief of the Cancer Control Branch of the National Cancer Institute in the 1940s.

28 Dr. D. G. Gill at the Alabama Bureau of Preventable Diseases was not concerned, however, since he thought the Study's men were mostly too old for the military; Gill to R. A. Vonderlehr, July 3, 1942; Vonderlehr to Gill, July 10, 1942, in Reverby, *Tuskegee's Truths*, 95–96.

29 R. A. Vonderlehr to Murray M. Smith, April 30, 1942; Smith to Vonderlehr, June 8, 1942; Smith to Vonderlehr, August 6, 1942, ibid.

30 Using the published names of all those drafted in World War II in or near Macon County and comparing them to the names of the men in the Study, it is possible to estimate that less than ten of the men whose names were identified ended up in the army. Of course, perhaps they were drafted elsewhere or were indeed too old to serve. Ernest Hendon, for example, one of the controls in the Study and the last survivor to die, was drafted and served when he lived in Cleveland.

31 Murray Smith to R. A. Vonderlehr, August 6, 1942; Vonderlehr to Smith, August 11, 1942; Austin V. Deibert to Smith, August 22, 1942, HEW Ad Hoc Panel on the Tuskegee Syphilis Study, Bound Book 2, TUA. The August 6 and August 11 letters are reprinted in Reverby, *Tuskegee's Truths*, 95–96. There were legal issues as well. By 1943, Alabama had become the first state to require testing by county health departments of "all civilians between the ages of 14 and 50" for syphilis. In the piloted counties (not Macon), recommendations were then made to those who tested positive to go for treatment. The men in the Study, of course, already thought they were being treated. Even if they had questions, they would have had to find a private doctor or present themselves to the health department or to Tuskegee Institute where the Study was known. It is probable that the PHS, by trying to keep the men from treatment, violated Alabama law.

32 On the rapid treatment centers, see Parascandola, *Sex, Sin, and Science*, 79–80, 119–28.

33 Thomas Parran to Catherine A. Doran, Assistant Secretary, Milbank Memorial Fund, November 4, 1943, box 7, Folder 1941, CDC-GA.

34 On the racial discourse on sickle cell, see Wailoo, *Dying in the City of Blues*.

35 There is a large body of literature on the history of the Tuskegee Airmen, now given a National Historic Site in Tuskegee; see <www.tuskegeeairmen.org>.

36 Wenger, "Untreated Syphilis." In fact, claims that the follow-up was going well would be undermined two years later by data that showed that 26 percent of the syphilitics and 35 percent of the controls were lost to follow-up by 1948.

37 John R. Heller and Bruyere, "Untreated Syphilis."

38 On the rhetoric of the medical reports of the Study, see Solomon, "Rhetoric of Dehumanization."

39 Deibert and Bruyere, "Untreated Syphilis."

40 A. P. Iskrant to Miss Usilton and Dr. Bauer, July 30, 1948, box 1, Folder Working Documents, National Library of Medicine, Bethesda, Maryland; also in Jones, *Bad Blood*, 181.

41 Rosahn, "Studies in Syphilis VII." Rosahn's report appeared right before that of Deibert and Bruyere. Rosahn then published it in numerous other medical journals and, with the support of the PHS, all of them in a pamphlet, Rosahn, *Autopsy Studies*. By 1959, it was in its seventh printing and was clearly widely read.

42 Moore, "Unsolved Clinical Problems," quoted in Rosahn, *Autopsy Studies*, 1. Rosahn was interested in trying to standardize the ways the tissue changes were read and was critical of what had been done before; ibid., 10–11.

43 For a clear statement of these views in the immediate postwar period, see Reynolds and Moore, "Syphilis."

44 Rosahn, "Studies in Syphilis VII," 293. The report does not make clear why the patients who were autopsied were untreated for syphilis, but it suggests that in this retrospective study there was no attempt to keep anyone from treatment. For a more contemporary view of this as an immunological problem, see Scythes et al., "New Gold Standard." Scythes argues for the link between HIV/AIDS susceptibility and syphilis, something made much more conspiratorial early in the AIDS epidemic by medical writer Harris L. Coulter, in *AIDS and Syphilis*.

45 Rosahn, *Autopsy Studies*, 58.

46 Ibid., 40.

47 The story of penicillin has been told many times. See Parascandola, *Sex, Sin, and Science*; and Dowling, *Fighting Infection*, 125–57. Mahoney's initial reports can be found in Mahoney, Arnold, and Harris, "Penicillin Treatment of Early Syphilis," in *Venereal Disease Information*; and Mahoney, Arnold, and Harris, "Penicillin Treatment of Early Syphilis," in *American Journal of Public Health*.

48 Dowling, *Fighting Infection*, 146.

49 Shafer, Usilton, and Price, "Long Term Studies," 565.

50 Concern with the so-called Herxheimer reaction had appeared in connection with use of the heavy metals as well; see Benedek and Erlen, "Scientific Environment."

51 See chapter 7; and Moore, *Modern Treatment*, 173, 176, 195.

52 Moore, "Management of Syphilis," 21–23; Diseker et al., "Long-Term Results."

53 On the "Blue Star" multicenter approach supported by the PHS, see Bauer, "Evaluation"; and White, "Unraveling the Tuskegee Study."

54 See Benedek and Erlen, "Scientific Environment."

55 Kampmeier, "Late Manifestations," 695. Kampmeier never mentioned the Study in this review.

56 This position was taken by Vernal Cave, a venereal disease specialist who served on the HEW Ad Hoc Advisory Panel after the Study ended; Cave affidavit, *Pollard v. U.S.*; Benedek and Erlen, "Scientific Environment;" Reverby, "More Than Fact and Fiction."

57 The literature on the doctors' trials and Nazi medicine is extensive; see Proctor, *Racial Hygiene*; Annas and Grodin, *Nazi Doctors*; Schmidt, *Justice at Nuremberg*; and Weindling, *Nazi Medicine*.

58 Katz, "Nuremberg Code."

59 The Study was never named by the Nazi defendants as a parallel because the lack of any kind of consent by the men in the Study would not have been apparent in the one research report that was available at the time, nor was the parallel then made to Alabama as a prison camp.

60 Harkness, "Nuremberg and the Issue of Wartime Experimentation."

61 Ibid.

62 Katz, "Nuremberg Code," 1662. See also Fletcher, "Case Study."

63 See Jones, *Bad Blood*, 180, for the discussion on Heller's views. Jones's memory of this interview comes from James H. Jones interview, November 12, 1998.

64 Pesare, Bauer, and Gleeson, "Untreated Syphilis."

65 Wenger, "Untreated Syphilis."

66 Ibid.

67 Schuman et al., "Untreated Syphilis," 551; Mr. Lloyd Simpson, Field Investigator, to Dr. Stanley Schuman, Clinical Investigations, March 3, 1952, box 1, Folder 1952, CDC-GA. The major surveys were done in 1932–34, 1938–39, 1948, 1952–53, and 1968–70.

68 R. A. Vonderlehr to Stanley Schuman, February 5, 1952, box 1, Folder 1952, CDC-GA.

69 Peters et al., "Untreated Syphilis." This paper described the effect penicillin was having on venereal disease treatment and was published in the first issue of *Journal of Chronic Diseases*, the new name for *American Journal of Syphilis, Gonorrhea, and Venereal Diseases*. Joseph Earle Moore edited both journals. Historian/physician Benjamin Roy argued that the paper was published for political reasons in a less scientific journal but failed to understand that they were the same journal; see Roy, "Tuskegee Syphilis Experiment: Biotechnology and the Administrative State." The importance of Peters's work was also stressed by J. R. Heller when he wrote to the Milbank Memorial Fund asking for more money in 1947; see Heller to Catherine A. Doran, Milbank Memorial Fund, December 4, 1947, box 7, Folder 1947, CDC-GA.

70 J. J. Peters to John C. Cutler, February 14, 1955, box 7, Folder 1955, CDC-GA.

71 Ad Hoc Committee Meeting, April 5, 1965, p. 3, box 8, Folder 3, CDC-GA.

72 Stanley Schuman to James H. Peters, December 15, 1952; Schuman to Peters, December 30, 1952; Schuman to Eleanor Walker, February 10, 1952, box 2, Folder 1952, CDC-GA.

73 James H. Peers to J. Jerome Peters, November 12, 1952, ibid.

74 Peters et al., "Untreated Syphilis," 127.

75 Peters to Cutler, July 7, 1953, box 7, Folder 1953, CDC-GA. The suggestion for this research came from Dr. Peers, the PHS/NIH pathologist with whom Peters had long been collaborating.

76 Roy, "Tuskegee Syphilis Experiment: Biotechnology and the Administrative State," 310.

77 Stanley Schuman to Sidney Olansky, November 21, 1951, box 7, Folder 1951, CDC-GA; Eleanor Walker to Dr. John C. Cutler, December 4, 1952, in Reverby, *Tuskegee's Truths*, 101.

78 Sidney Olansky to John C. Cutler, November 6, 1951, in Reverby, *Tuskegee's Truths*, 99–101.

79 Stanley Schuman to Sidney Olansky, November 21, 1951, box 7, Folder 1951, CDC-GA.

80 Stanley Schuman to Sidney Olansky, January 29, 1952, box 7, Folder 1952, CDC-GA.

81 Cutler, "Study of Untreated Syphilis in the Negro Male," 1, *Symposium on Venereal Disease and the Treponematoses*, May 29, 1956, box 17, Folder Termination, CDC-GA. Peters also presented his paper on x-ray diagnosis of aortitis at this meeting; see C. A. Smith, Medical Director, Chief, Venereal Disease Program, PHS, to J. J. Peters, March 23, 1956, box 7, Folder 1956, CDC-GA.

82 Brandt, "Racism and Research," 27; Rivers et al., "Twenty Years of Follow-up," 125.

83 See Solomon, "Rhetoric of Dehumanization"; and Brandt, "Racism and Research," 27.

84 For a list of where the tests were being done, see "Public Health Service to Dear Sir," October 18, 1955, 102.

85 Count D. Gibson Jr. to Dr. Sidney Olansky, May 28, 1955. I am grateful to Dr. Irwin Schatz for sending me his copy of this letter. As far as I know, this is the earliest letter of criticism of the Study from within the medical profession that focuses on the ethics. Count Gibson, who died at eighty-one in 2002, was a southerner and a leader in the community health center movement who taught for decades at Stanford Medical School. He had a long-standing commitment to health care for the poor. Personal communication from H. Jack Geiger, April 24, 2003.

86 Sid[ney Olansky] to Count [Gibson], n.d., but presumably in 1955, and sent to Dr. Irwin Schatz by Count Gibson in 1972.

87 Schuman et al., "Untreated Syphilis," 557. Olansky is the second author on this paper.

88 Olansky, "Untreated Syphilis," 184. In describing the "159 surviving syphilitic patients," he wrote: "It is worth noting that the bulk of these patients were untreated."

89 Unfortunately, Dr. Gibson died before I could discuss this with him. Reports on the comments come from Dr. H. Jack Geiger interview, May 3, 2003, and from interview with John Hatch, Ward Kenan Professor of Public Health Emeritus at the University of North Carolina, May 13, 2003.

90 Gibson did talk to historian James H. Jones about this in the 1980s, after *Bad Blood* appeared, and Jones confirms that Gibson told him he always felt concerned about

the Study and his inability to do anything more. The Columbia Point Health Center in Boston that he and Geiger started was named the Geiger-Gibson Health Center in the early 1990s.

CHAPTER 4

1   Roy, "Tuskegee Syphilis Experiment: Biotechnology and the Administrative State," argues that they kept the Study going to use the men's blood to test against the new treponema pallidum immobilization serology test. Olansky told Cutler in 1951, "There is much valuable material here for aid in evaluation of the TPI procedure"; Sidney Olansky to John C. Cutler, December 6, 1951, in Reverby, *Tuskegee's Truths*, 101. But Don Millar, a PHS physician who was involved in the Study in the early 1970s, reported that this would have been unnecessary since there was enough syphilis-positive blood available; Don Millar interview, January 12, 2007.

2   "Initial Planning Conference—Tuskegee Study," November 21, 1957, box 4, Folder 1957, CDC-GA, 3. They ordered, in bulk: "12 gallons of I.Q.S. (Iron-quinine-strychnine, an iron elixir recognized by the U.S. national formulary of recognized drugs), 10,000 tablets A.P.C. (aspirin), 500 powder boxes, 6 cartons of 48 each, 4 ounce screw cap bottles, and vitamins."

3   Twenty-five-year certificate, in Reverby, *Tuskegee's Truths*, 187.

4   The new plan seems to have worked. As William J. Brown, the Venereal Disease Division chief, explained a few years later, the PHS officers were able to examine 171 "patients" in Macon County and "38 . . . elsewhere, principally in Cleveland, Chicago and Detroit." The autopsies continued as the men continued to die. By 1962, Brown concluded that "at the present time you might say we are marking time until the study is brought to a close and final results can be reported. This will probably be when the services of Nurse Rivers and Dr. Peters are no longer available"; William J. Brown, Chief, Venereal Disease Branch, to Dr. Stanley H. Schuman, July 16, 1962, box 1, Folder 1962, CDC-GA. Schuman was a former director of the Study and was then teaching epidemiology at the Public Health School at the University of Michigan.

5   Even after Rivers married Julius Laurie and her formal name became Eunice Laurie, she was still often referred to in the correspondence as "Nurse Rivers"; see further discussion in chapter 9; Eunice Laurie to Eleanor V. Price, CDC, Venereal Disease Division, September 12, 1963, box 19, Folder Nurse Rivers Correspondence, CDC-GA.

6   Quoted in Jones, *Bad Blood*, 169.

7   Fletcher, "A Study in Historical Relativism," in Reverby, *Tuskegee's Truths*, 276–98.

8   Anne R. Yobs to Eunice Laurie, May 18, 1964, box 8, Folder 1964, CDC-GA; James B. Lucas to William J. Brown, September 10, 1970, in Reverby, *Tuskegee's Truths*, 107–9.

9   Meeting Re: Tuskegee Study, Present: Dr. Schroeter, Dr. Olansky, Dr. Yobs, Mrs. Price, and Mr. Donohue, April 5, 1965, HEW materials noted as M22–8, I-B Basic, HEW-NLM. The Communicable Disease Center (now the massive Centers for Disease Control) was formed in 1946 as a small section of the PHS housed in Atlanta. It soon outgrew the PHS.

10 Anne R. Yobs to Eunice Laurie, November 6, 1963, box 8, Folder 1963, CDC-GA.

11 James Reeb was beaten to death in Selma, and Ku Klux Klan members shot Viola Liuzzo after the march. Charles Gomillion, a sociologist at Tuskegee University and the head of the Tuskegee Civic Association, was the plaintiff in the case; and Fred D. Gray, who became the lawyer for the Study's participants in their lawsuit, was the attorney; see Gray, *Bus Ride to Justice*. Gomillion reported that he knew nothing about the Study; see Reverby, *Tuskegee's Truths*, 114–15.

12 This letter, left in the National Archives (CDC-GA) rather than in private hands, is usually cited as the first medical criticism of the ethics rather than of the procedures of the Study; see Irwin Schatz to Donald H. Rockwell, June 11, 1965, in Reverby, *Tuskegee's Truths*, 103. There may have been other private correspondence and talks (other than those noted), but it is impossible at this time to know from whom unless the letters were left in archives or posted on the Internet.

13 Rockwell, Yobs, and Moore, "Tuskegee Study." Unfortunately, James H. Jones gives the date of this article as 1961, not 1964, and this mistake is carried forward in my *Tuskegee's Truths* in Susan Bell's timeline of the Study.

14 Irwin J. Schatz to Donald H. Rockwell, June 11, 1965, in Reverby, *Tuskegee's Truths*, 103–4; Dr. Irwin J. Schatz interview. I am grateful to Dr. Schatz for discussing his role in the Study with me.

15 Anne R. Yobs to Dr. E. J. Gillespie, June 15, 1965, in Reverby, *Tuskegee's Truths*, 104. Schatz never knew about this internal memo until I told him about it. He found out about Gibson's letter after the story of the Study broke in 1972.

16 Schatz did discuss the Study, in a letter to William B. Beam, editor of the *Archives of Internal Medicine*, in 1972 after the story of the Study broke. Beam wrote back to him, in a "gracious letter," Schatz recalled, writing that "in retrospect he had made an error in publishing it [the Study report]" and that the journal had "obligations to apply moral and ethical standards," which they had not done. Schatz thought this was an "interesting admission," reflecting slow acceptance of changing standards of morality; Irwin J. Schatz interview.

17 Ronald Wilson, "Eight Month Evaluation of Peter Buxtun," box 6, Folder Buxtun, 1965, CDC-GA. Buxtun's last name is often misspelled "Buxton."

18 Peter Buxtun, "January Narrative," City and County of San Francisco, January 29, 1965, box 4, Folder Buxtun, CDC-GA.

19 Peter Buxtun, "March Narrative," March 26, 1965; "July Narrative," July 21, 1965; "September Narrative," September 16, 1965, ibid.

20 Peter Buxtun interview, November 11, 1998. All quotes come from this interview unless otherwise noted. Parts of Buxtun's story also come from his testimony before the U.S. Senate in 1973; see Buxtun, "Testimony by Peter Buxtun." In the interview, Buxtun referred again and again to the version of the story in the Jones book. When he could not remember a detail, he asked me to look it up in Jones's book. His own telling of the story is, of course, inflected by the many times he has told it over the last three decades and by the ways Jones's book portrays his experience.

21 Buxtun, "A Means to an End," "December narrative," November 17, 1965, 3, Box 4, Folder Buxtun, CDC-GA.

22 Peter Buxtun interview, November 11, 1998.

23 "Volunteers with social incentives" comes from the article Rivers was supposed to have authored; see chapter 9.

24 Peter Buxtun to William Brown, November 9, 1966, box 6, Folder Buxtun, CDC-GA.

25 William Brown, Draft, December 7, 1966, ibid.

26 Peter Buxtun to William Brown, November 9, 1966, ibid.

27 Peter Buxtun to William Brown, November 24, 1968, in Reverby, *Tuskegee's Truths*, 105.

28 Report of telephone call from Dr. Brown to Dr. Eugene Stollerman, January 15, 1969, box 15, Folder 1969, CDC-GA.

29 Years later, Sencer agreed that a more community-minded physician might have made a different argument and might have pushed them to see the possible political consequences of what had been done; David Sencer interview, January 12, 2007. I am grateful to Dr. Sencer for his willingness to discuss the Study with me and to rethink it.

30 Ad Hoc Committee Minutes, February 6, 1969, box 15, Folder 1969, CDC-GA. Jones had a different read of the meeting's concerns; see Jones, *Bad Blood*, 193–98.

31 Yobs et al., "Do Treponemes Survive"; J. Lawton Smith, "Spirochetes," 623.

32 For more discussion of what happened in 1969 at this meeting, see chapter 7.

33 William Brown to Peter Buxtun, undated draft, box 6, Folder Buxtun, CDC-GA.

34 Peter Buxtun to William Brown, March 29, 1969, ibid.

35 Peter Buxtun interview, November 11, 1998.

36 Jenkins went on to found a number of organizations that did research on health disparities among African Americans. He worked at CDC for more than three decades and organized the public health program at Morehouse School of Medicine in 1992. In a final honor/irony, he served as the manager of the Participants Health Benefits program for the survivors and families of the Study.

37 Bill Jenkins, panel discussion, "Tuskegee: Could It Happen Again?" Applied Research Ethics National Association Conference, "Tuskegee: Can Past Lessons Guide Researchers and IRBs in the Future?" Boston, December 7, 1997, author's notes. Jenkins also relates this experience on the 1993 PBS *Nova* program, "Deadly Deception."

38 See, for example, Pesare, Bauer, and Gleeson, "Untreated Syphilis."

39 Jenkins's role did not appear in Jones's book on the Study because there were no papers by or about him in any of the archives, and his critique was not mentioned by any of the principals that Jones interviewed. Jenkins's role was first revealed in the *Nova* video, "Deadly Deception."

40 Jenkins, panel discussion, "Tuskegee: Could It Happen Again."

41 Ralph Featherstone, a former Student Nonviolent Coordinating Committee organizer and a leader of the group Jenkins was part of, was killed on March 9, 1970, by a car bomb in Maryland outside a courthouse where Black Panther H. Rap Brown was supposed to be on trial.

42 Arnold Schroeter interview; "Selections from the Final Report," 171.

43 Arnold Schroeter interview.

44 Dr. Caldwell to Dr. Schroeter, April 9, 1970, box 8, Folder 1970, CDC-GA; see also Caldwell to Schroeter, April 22, 1970, ibid.

45 Windell R. Bradford Field Report, June 1, 1970; Joseph G. Caldwell to Eunice Laurie, May 25, 1970, ibid.

46 Record 082, box 6, TMF.

47 James Lucas to William Brown, September 10, 1970, in Reverby, *Tuskegee's Truths*, 107–9.

48 Caldwell's report was not published until after the public revelations about the Study. But since his work was done in 1968–70, it is possible he was discussing his data with others inside CDC before the report was published; see Caldwell et al., "Aortic Regurgitation," 192.

49 Buxtun, "Testimony by Peter Buxtun"; Jean Heller, "Syphilis Victims"; Peter Buxtun interview, November 11, 1998.

50 Olansky et al., "Environmental Factors." This was the first time the word "Tuskegee" appeared in the Study title and was the eighth report on the Study published.

CHAPTER 5

1 The literature on the politics of health in the 1970s is vast. Good starting points for the critique from the left are Health-PAC, *American Health Empire*; and Sidel and Sidel, *Reforming Medicine*.

2 Heller, "Syphilis Victims."

3 Jean Heller interview, July 18, 2005.

4 Dr. Donald Printz, a CDC spokesman, was the first to link the rhetoric about the Study with the experimentation in Nazi death camps, and thus it was the CDC, not someone from the black public, that first used the word "genocide"; Dr. Donald Printz, quoted in James T. Wooten, "Survivor of '32 Syphilis Study Recalls a Diagnosis," *New York Times*, July 27, 1972, 18. More than three decades later, however, Printz did not recall using the term; Don Printz interview.

5 Gilbert, "Coming of a Prophecy," 53. See also newspapers in Clippings File, Tuskegee Syphilis Study Papers, TUA.

6 The defense of the Study came mainly from the researchers who were no longer at the CDC; see Jones, *Bad Blood*, 222; and "Ex-Chief Defends Syphilis Project," *New York Times*, July 28, 1972, 29. The story went out from the AP and was presumably done as follow-up by Jean Heller (no relation to John R. Heller).

7 A clipping from an unnamed newspaper in the Clippings File, TUA, shows that a longer version of this AP story went out under the headline "Syphilis Study Defended by Doctor in Charge." This story included John Heller's quotes about who was responsible and his comments about Millar.

8 Reverby and Sims, "Charlie Wesley Pollard."

9 Sikora, "'Got Headache for Two Weeks,' Recalls Syphilis Study Victim," *Birmingham News*, 1979, no date/month given, Clippings File, Tuskegee Syphilis Study Papers, TUA. Gray had been doing Charlie Pollard's legal work on the deeds for his farm for "a decade," Pollard told one journalist; see Cramer, "$10-Million Giveaway."

10 Peter Buxtun could not recall how he found Mr. Pollard when he and Jean Heller traveled to Tuskegee after the story broke. Heller does not recall meeting Pollard

in Montgomery. But Jean Heller remembers that Fred Gray provided the contact. Peter Buxtun interview, March 20, 2004; Jean Heller interview, July 18, 2005.

11 "Great Pox," *Time* 38 (October 26, 1936): 60–64.

12 James T. Wooten, "Survivor of '32 Syphilis Study Recalls a Diagnosis," *New York Times*, July 27, 1972, 18. Note that the headline makes it sound as if the Study took place only in 1932.

13 Stanley Schuman, Professor of Epidemiology, University of Michigan, to Broadus Butler, December 1, 1972, box 2, Folder Correspondence, HEW-NLM. From 1951 to 1953, Schuman had worked on the Study with Sidney Olansky in the CDC's venereal disease research lab. Schuman did assert, however, that anyone with a positive serology for syphilis was "assured that he carried serological, not infectious traces of the disease."

14 Johnson, "Shadow of the Plantation: Survival." Jones learned of the multiple meanings of "bad blood" from the Johnson book, his interviews with several of the survivors, and attorney Fred Gray; telephone interview, July 30, 2004. Dr. H. L. Harris, in writing to the Rosenwald Fund's Michael Davis on July 13, 1931, argued, "It would be interesting to discover the effect upon clinic attendance were the terminology of bad blood replaced by a term which would identify this disease with the bad disease which the patients know under a variety of local names"; box 526, Folder 2, RF-Fisk.

15 James T. Wooten, "Survivor of '32 Syphilis Study Recalls a Diagnosis," *New York Times*, July 27, 1972, 18.

16 "Interview #3," HEW-NLM, 1973, in Reverby, *Tuskegee's Truths*, 134.

17 Poster and flyer in author's collection.

18 Jones named his book, the first major book-length historical account of the Study, *Bad Blood*, and the power of this metaphor has multiplied because his book grounds other accounts; see chapter 10.

19 Syphilis is actually quite difficult to pass on except through direct contact with the sores because the bacteria cannot survive in the air.

20 Although the report made it clear later, in quotes from the CDC's J. D. Millar, that the men were not infectious, although their wives might have been, the elements that would paint the PHS white doctors as death-dealing infectors were in place; Jeanne Fox, "Doctors Victimize Blacks," *Watts Star Review*, August 3, 1972, n.p.

21 Richard Little, "Doctors Say Pencillin [*sic*] More Risk Than Cure," *Birmingham News*, n.d., Clippings File, TUA. Since Fred Gray is quoted as representing the men, this was probably written about August 1972. The report makes clear that the statement was drafted by Dr. Edward Lammons, Walter Pack, and Nurse Eunice Laurie.

22 Jeanne Fox, "Tuskegee Reports: Profile of Black 'Guinea Pig,'" n.d., no newspaper, Clippings File, TUA. For more on the link between the Study and other medical research seen as unethical, see chapter 10.

23 Jean Heller, "Participating Doctor Says Syphilitics Not Told of Experiment," *Birmingham News*, July 27, 1972, n.p, Clippings File, TUA. Harriet Washington, in *Medical Apartheid*, between pages 342 and 343, has a 1953 picture of a PHS physician doing a blood draw on a Study subject in Macon County. The man has visible

rubber tubing on his arm, which would indicate a blood draw, but Washington writes: "Study subject receives an injection from a PHS physician." Then she adds: "The men were not injected with syphilis, but they were administered injections and underwent other procedures that maintained the illusion that they were undergoing treatment for syphilis." To a casual reader, this could be quite confusing. The injections were treatment at the beginning of the Study.

24 Jean Heller, "Participating Doctor Says Syphilitics Not Told of Experiment," *Birmingham News*, July 27, 1972, n.p, Clippings File, TUA.

25 "U.S. Health Experiment Kills 126 Black Men," *Los Angeles Herald-Dispatch*, August 3, 1972, n.p., Clippings File, TUA. The article states directly: "Of the 600 men, the AP declared, 126 Black men were allowed to die because the government refused to give them penicillin treatments." The newspaper was very direct. It called the Study "genocide" and concluded: "Hence, the government of the U.S. are quietly murdering Blacks. Are Blacks safe in the U.S.?"

26 "At least 28 Died in Syphilis Study, Reports on Tuskegee Tests Indicate Much Higher Toll," *New York Times*, September 12, 1972, 23. Allan M. Brandt, in his widely cited article "Racism and Research," uses the figures "at least 28, but perhaps more than 100." Jones uses the same numbers; see *Bad Blood*, 2. For further discussion of the deaths, see chapter 6.

27 Richard Little, "Doctors Say Pencillin [*sic*] More Risk Than Cure," *Birmingham News*, n.d., Clippings File, TUA. See also "Aide Questioned Syphilis Study, Age Called Reason for Not Treating Men in Program," *New York Times*, August 9, 1972, 43. This is an AP story, probably written by Jean Heller.

28 John R. Heller, quoted in Jack Slater, "Condemned to Die for Science," *Ebony* 38 (November 1972): 184.

29 Richard Little, "Doctors Say Pencillin [*sic*] More Risk Than Cure," *Birmingham News*, n.d., Clippings File, TUA.

30 "The VD Treatment Program," no newspaper, n.d., Clippings File, TUA. In the file, the story was pasted on a page with another article that was clearly dated July 27, 1972.

31 For differing views on this and the ways the Study does—or should—resonate, see Gamble, "Under the Shadow"; Stephen B. Thomas and Quinn, "Tuskegee Syphilis Study"; and Fairchild and Bayer, "Uses and Abuses."

32 "NAACP Condemns 'Criminal' US Agency Study of Syphilis," *New Courier*, August 12, 1972, n.p., Clippings File, TUA.

33 For details on the legislative and policy history surrounding human experimentation in this period, see Frankel, "Public Policy." I am grateful to Marc Frankel, now director of the Scientific Freedom, Responsibility, and Law Program at the American Association for the Advancement of Science, for sending me a copy of his dissertation. See also Fletcher, "Case Study."

34 Panel members were Ronald H. Brown, general counsel, National Urban League; Vernal Cave, M.D., director of Venereal Disease Control, New York City Health Department; Jean L. Harris, M.D., executive director of the National Medical Association Foundation; Seward Hiltner, professor of theology at Princeton; Jay Katz, M.D., professor of law and psychiatry at Yale; Jeanne C. Sinkford, D.D.S., associate dean,

College of Dentistry at Howard; Fred Speaker, Harrisburg, Pa., former attorney general of Pennsylvania and prominent Republican; and Barney Weeks, president of the Alabama Labor Council. Broadus Butler, president of Dillard University, was the chair.

35 Broadus N. Butler to Charles C. Edwards, assistant secretary for health and scientific affairs, HEW, April 23, 1973, box 8, Folder Tuskegee Syphilis Study General III, General V, CDC-GA; "Report on HEW's Tuskegee Report," *Medical World News*, n.d., ca. April–May 1973, ibid. See also Mervin DuVal to Marc Frankel, n.d., quoted in Frankel, "Public Policy," 310; and "Selections from the Final Report." For major critiques of the panel, see Brandt, "Racism and Research"; and Washington, *Medical Apartheid*.

36 Warren Brown, "A Shocking New Report on Black Syphilis Victims," *Jet Magazine* 43 (November 9, 1972): 28. Cave had also been president of the National Medical Association. He had worked closely with Senator Robert Kennedy on economic development in Brooklyn. A dermatologist by training, Cave had been the director of the Venereal Disease Control Bureau in New York City for many years. Born in Panama to Barbadian parents, Cave worked in New York City from the 1950s until his death on May 6, 1997, ten days before the federal apology; see Robert McG. Thomas, "Dr. Vernal G. Cave, 78, Dies; Led in Medical and Civic Issues," *New York Times*, May 12, 1997, A15.

37 "Selections from the Final Report," 158.

38 Brandt, "Racism and Research"; Washington, *Medical Apartheid*, 157–85.

39 Washington, following the positions taken by Jay Katz and Vernal Cave, argues that the panel was too weak and that it provided a "cover-up"; see Washington, *Medical Apartheid*, 169–75; see also Reverby, "Inclusion and Exclusion."

40 Jones, *Bad Blood*, 211.

41 This problem was cited by panel member Dr. Jay Katz and by historian Allan M. Brandt. Katz (1922–2008), a psychiatrist from Yale Law School, was considered one of the key national figures in the crafting of concepts of informed consent; see Katz, Capron, and Glass, *Experimentation*; Katz, *Silent World*; and Clayton and Levine, *Collected Writings*. In response to Brandt's article and a query from Senator Edward Kennedy, CDC officials in 1980 argued that they had not hidden anything, that it was perhaps "an oversight not to resort to the Archives as a source of information," and that the Ad Hoc Advisory Panel had much of this information already. "If," the official noted, "HEW's staff . . . had been engaged in a 'cover up,' [they] would not have supplied other information almost as damaging"; Joel M. Mangel to Charlie Miller, "Note to Charlie Miller," September 12, 1980, box 20, Tuskegee Working File, CDC-GA.

42 William Watson for David Sencer to Executive Secretary of HEW Panel, December 5, 1972, box 2, Katz Folder, HEW-NLM.

43 Historians Allan M. Brandt and James H. Jones found the correspondence and records, which were at that time scattered in the thousands of old PHS files in the National Archives.

44 This argument is made by Brandt, "Racism and Research"; and by Jones, *Bad Blood*.

45 Washington, *Medical Apartheid*, 174. Katz made a similar argument—that Butler was protecting Rivers—to me; Jay Katz interview.

46 Dr. Robert H. Story to Dr. Broadus N. Butler, December 4, 1972, box 2, Folder Correspondence, HEW-NLM; David Sencer interview, August 1, 2005.

47 Jay Katz interview.

48 Ibid.

49 "Statement of Fred Gray," U.S. Congress, Senate, *Quality of Health Care*, 1033.

50 "Probe of Syphilis Study Limited, Panelist Claims," *Birmingham News*, May 1, 1973, n.p., Clippings File, TUA.

51 Eleanor Price to Broadus Butler, December 9, 1972, box 2, Folder Correspondence, HEW-NLM.

52 "Statement of Leonard J. Goldwater," ibid. In his book, *Mercury*, Goldwater argues that mercury should never be used to cure syphilis and that its dangers outweighed its usefulness; see, especially, 215–30.

53 Cobb, "Tuskegee Syphilis Study," 347. Cobb and Eugene Dibble, who had died four years before the Study was made public in the newspapers, had been close friends. It is impossible to know if Cobb was protecting his friend or expressing his views and those of the panel's chair, Broadus Butler.

54 Arnold Schroeter interview.

55 Stanley Schuman, testimony before the HEW Panel, December 1, 1972, box 2, HEW-NLM. Schuman had worked on the Study with Sidney Olansky at the Venereal Disease Research Laboratory between August 1951 and February 1953.

56 Previous histories emphasize the divisions among the panel members. I am interested here in the divisions among those who provided testimony because of the insight it gives to understandings of the Study.

57 Joshua W. Williams, testimony before the HEW Panel, February 23, 1973, 1–22, box 2, HEW-NLM.

58 Arnold Schroeter, testimony before the HEW Panel, February 23, 1973, 22–49, ibid.

59 Arnold Schroeter interview.

60 Caldwell et al., "Aortic Regurgitation," 192.

61 Reginald James, testimony before the HEW Panel, February 23, 1973, 50–77, box 2, HEW-NLM.

62 Rivers claimed in her own testimonies to her friends that Dr. James was lying. The entire HEW panel never heard her claims because she never provided testimony except in an interview with Vernal Cave, which was destroyed. See Reverby, "Rethinking"; and chapter 9.

63 The Carver website at Tuskegee University, where Carver taught for decades, provides a "list of products made from peanuts by George Washington Carver." Under Medicines is "Oils, Emulsified w/mercury for Venereal Disease" (2). When and why Carver did this, I have not been able to discover. See <http://www.tuskegee.edu/global/story.asp?s=1107158&ClientType=Printable>, accessed July 13, 2005. Schroeter told the same story about Carver but may have heard this from Heller; Arnold Schroeter interview.

64 John R. Heller, testimony before the HEW Panel, February 23, 1973, 80–122, HEW-NLM.

65 Reginald James, ibid., 104.

66 Reginald James, Joshua Williams, and John R. Heller, ibid., 109–10.

67 Ibid., 120. See also "Ex-Chief Defends Syphilis Project: Says Alabama Plan Was Not Unethical or Unscientific," *New York Times*, July 28, 1972, 29. This was a filed AP story that would also have gone out to other newspapers.

68 Schroeter, in his interview, recalled that James had agreed with him, off record, at the end of their exchange. But there is no written evidence to corroborate this possibility.

69 "Selections from the Final Report," 166. Brandt emphasizes this point, in "Racism and Research." For more on the debates on research at this time, see chapter 10.

70 Jay Katz interview.

71 Advisory Committee on Human Radiation Experiments, *Final Report*, 14–15, 20. Katz would continue to argue for such a national board throughout his career; see Katz, "Regulation of Human Experimentation."

72 Broadus Butler to Charles C. Edwards, April 23, 1973, box 8, Folder General III, CDC-GA.

73 This viewpoint is argued most strongly in Frankel, "Public Policy," 235. Washington accepts Katz's view that Butler was protecting Rivers (*Medical Apartheid*, 174). I argue that as a black college president and former Tuskegee Airman he was protecting the Tuskegee Institute; see Reverby, "Inclusion and Exclusion," 109. Unfortunately, Butler died before either Washington or I could interview him, and he left no papers that would help explain his actions.

74 Frank Miller and Russ Haviak, public health advisers with the CDC, "Summary of First and Second Meeting with Lawyer, Fred Gray," Draft, 5/15/73, box 20, Folder Venereal Disease, CDC-GA. The meetings were held on April 15, 1973, and May 14, 1973. Gray claimed that the HEW panel had been a "whitewash" since no compensation was recommended (7).

75 Frankel, "Public Policy," traces this history. The Study is covered in Parts 3 and 4, in U.S. Congress, Senate, *Quality of Health Care*.

76 Treatment paid for by the federal government wherever the remaining men wanted it was not offered until April 14, 1973, even though the Study had been made widely public beginning on July 26, 1972, and even though HEW Ad Hoc Advisory Panel members had demanded termination and care at a press conference on October 25, 1972.

77 Statement of Henry F. Simmons, M.D., Deputy Assistant Secretary for Health and Scientific Affairs, HEW, July 10, 1973, U.S. Congress, Senate, *Quality of Health Care*, 1446–85; David Sencer interview, August 1, 2005.

78 C. L. Hopper to David J. Sencer, January 10, 1973, box 8, Tuskegee Study General V, CDC-GA.

79 The CDC's David Sencer predicted that care for the remaining family members might run between "22.8 and 127.5 million dollars over a projected 38-year period"; David J. Sencer to the Assistant Secretary for Health, September 12, 1973, ibid. By

2004, the program was caring for nineteen widows, children, and grandchildren from the Study at a cost of $4 million that year. It would prove to cost more to the government than the survivors and families would win in their lawsuit.

80 For Gray's view of the hearings, see Gray, *Tuskegee Syphilis Study*.

81 See further discussion in chapter 6.

82 "Testimony by Four Survivors," in Reverby, *Tuskegee's Truths*, 147–48. Three seconds of Charlie Pollard and Fred Gray can be seen on the short video made to commemorate the twenty-fifth anniversary of the Belmont Report; see "Belmont Report Educational Video," <http://www.hhs.gov/ohrp/belmontArchive.html#histReport>, accessed July 18, 2005.

83 Cave, "Statement." I tried repeatedly to interview Dr. Cave before he passed away but was unsuccessful.

84 U.S. Congress, Senate, *Quality of Health Care*.

85 William O. Hosking to Mrs. Elizabeth Kennebrew, June 25, 1973, box 12, Personnel Assignment Folder, CDC-GA.

86 See chapter 11.

87 Gray, "The Lawsuit"; Gray, *Tuskegee Syphilis Study*.

88 Gray, *Tuskegee Syphilis Study*. See also Edgar, "Outside the Community."

89 *Pollard v. U.S.* The records of the lawsuit are in the Frank M. Johnson Jr. Federal Courthouse in Montgomery. See J. J. Cramer, "The $10-Million Giveaway," *American Lawyer* (October 1979): 22–24. Gray originally agreed with Pollard that he would get half of any compensation (not an uncommon percentage in this kind of case). In the end, Judge Frank Johnson awarded him 10 percent, or $1 million. He continued to track down heirs and would be involved in the case for the next three decades.

90 Fred D. Gray interview.

91 Jack Slater, "Condemned to Die for Science," *Ebony* 38 (November 1972): 184.

92 Nancy Hicks, "Reparations Are Asked for Men Who Survived Study on Syphilis," *New York Times*, August 16, 1972, 14.

93 When Allan M. Brandt made the early documents he had found in the National Archives available to Jay Katz, Katz asked Kennedy for new hearings. Kennedy wrote to HEW about this, hinting about a cover-up. CDC officials were adamant that they had not hidden anything. Jones was working in the records beginning in 1970; Brandt was there in 1976–77. Jones was aware of the HEW panel but not of its failure to get the early records (email from James H. Jones, July 7 and 25, 2005; email from Allan M. Brandt, July 22, 2005). See "Plaintiffs Are Narrowed in Syphilis Research Suit," *New York Times*, July 14, 1974, 40. Both Jones and Gray acknowledge Jones's role.

94 James H. Jones, telephone interview, July 25, 2005.

95 Harold Edgar, "Memorandum, Tuskegee Syphilis Study," November 18, 1972, 11, TMF-Edgar. I am grateful to Hal Edgar and David Rothman for allowing me to see these. See also Edgar, "Outside the Community."

96 Harold Edgar, "Memorandum, Tuskegee Syphilis Study," November 18, 1972, 17, TMF-Edgar.

97 The CDC's J. Donald Millar agreed on this point with Gray. Speaking to the *Ebony*

reporter, he said, "Would it have been conceivable to do such a study on whites? My feeling is that the study would not have been done on whites"; Slater, "Condemned to Die for Science," 190.

98 *Pollard v. U.S.*, "Allegations of Facts," 21.

99 Harold Edgar, "Memorandum, Tuskegee Syphilis Study," November 18, 1972, 16, TMF-Edgar; Robert D. McFadden, "Frank M. Johnson Jr., Judge Whose Rulings Helped Desegregate the South, Dies at 80," *New York Times*, July 24, 1999, A15; Howell Raines, "Judge Frank Johnson Goes Home to the Hills," Editorial, *New York Times*, July 26, 1999, A18. See also Gray, *Bus Ride to Justice*.

100 Harold Edgar, "Memorandum, Tuskegee Syphilis Study," November 18, 1972, 12, TMF-Edgar.

101 Gray, "The Lawsuit," 477; Fred D. Gray interview.

102 In 1998, while taking historian James Jones and me to dinner in a fancy Montgomery restaurant, Gray looked around at the elegantly attired white waiters, smiled, and remarked how he remembered when it would have been impossible for him to eat there—and with us.

103 Palmer worked with Cornell playwright/physician David Feldshuh on the video study guide for *Miss Evers' Boys*. See chapter 11; and Palmer, "Paying for Suffering."

104 Affidavit of Ira Myers, July 3, 1974, *Pollard v. U.S.*, volume 3. Myers's and Olansky's positions were countered by Vernal Cave; see Affidavit of Vernal Cave, ibid.

105 On Cave's position, see Cave, "Proper Uses and Abuses."

106 The judge's opinion is in his dismissal of the defendants' filing for summary judgment; see *Pollard v. U.S.*, October 31, 1974.

107 Caldwell et al., "Aortic Regurgitation," 192.

108 Harold Edgar, "Memorandum, Tuskegee Syphilis Study," November 18, 1972, 12, TMF-Edgar.

109 "Plaintiffs Are Narrowed in Syphilis Research Suit," *New York Times*, July 14, 1974, 40. Roger W. Rochat, Office of Program Planning and Evaluation, to Assistant Director, Bureau of State Services, CDC, June 14, 1974, box 2, Folder 1974, CDC-GA. Rochat's examination of the mortality data suggested that there was higher mortality among the men with syphilis prior to 1944, but not between 1944 and 1954 and between 1954 and 1964. Rochat recalls that he was compiling this data in preparation for providing medical care for the men; Robert Rochat interview.

110 Caldwell argued for treatment during late syphilis, based on the Study data; see Caldwell et al., "Aortic Regurgitation," 193. However, on an individual basis, some cases made it clear that even large amounts of penicillin may not have saved patients whose heart damage was too advanced. For an example from outside the Study, an African American man with syphilitic aortitis and bacterial endocarditis died despite being given massive amounts of penicillin, in Mokotoff et al., "Treatment of Bacterial Endocarditis." The lead author on this report, a cardiologist, was my late father, and the research was done at Michael Reese Hospital in Chicago. The man in this case was not part of the Study.

111 James H. Jones interview, July 25, 2005; Harold Edgar interview.

112 Gray makes clear that he had hoped for more money in the settlement and that

more would have been given in a case today; see Gray, "The Lawsuit." In the end, Gray would get about 12½ percent in legal fees. He was given 10 percent to start, and the rest was held back over the years as he searched for the men's heirs and families. In 1994, Gray was still searching for "105 people scattered across the nation, who are entitled to a share of the interest accumulated in the case," he told a reporter, Matt Smith. Smith's story says the money went to 9,000 people, but Gray uses the figure 6,000 in his book *The Tuskegee Syphilis Study*. Matt Smith, "Interest Payments to Wrap Up Controversial Study on Syphilis," *Montgomery Advertiser*, August 21, 1994, B1. CDC officials and Gray often disagreed on a number of issues — such as who would find the families and when the women and children would be treated. For the CDC's side of this, see Richard H. Bruce to Kenneth Vines, February 5, 1975, box 5, Correspondence 74–75 File, CDC-GA.

113 Robert Rochat interview.

CHAPTER 6

1 Herman Shaw interview. All quotes from Mr. Shaw are from this interview unless otherwise noted. See also Reverby, "Herman Shaw"; and Junod, "Deadly Medicine," 509.

2 Other men interviewed for the Rosenwald Fund Demonstration Project cited the problem of paying for the license tags. Green Adair, from Hardaway, told his interviewer that he could not afford the price of a license tag, but that if he had been white he could have put a "lost tag" on his car and gotten away with it, as he had seen whites do. Mose Graves, of Chesson, reported that there was a way around the tag problem: "Right now you will find one tag running some three or four cars. Jest like I want to go to town I would go and borrow the other fellow's tags." See interviews with Green Adair and Mose Graves, box 526, Folders 6 and 8, RF-Fisk.

3 Fred Gray picked Mr. Shaw as the spokesman for the men; see Gray, *Tuskegee Syphilis Study*, 153–54.

4 Individual names were used when the story of the Study first broke in 1972, in the 1990s in a series of videos, and at the federal apology in 1997 (see chapter 11). The National Archives released their medical records in 2004 (see note 7).

5 Ayers, *What Caused the Civil War*, 180.

6 There are now two ongoing oral history projects at Tuskegee University to interview family members and women connected to the university and its health work.

7 Boxes 1–39, TMF. Simmons College historian/librarian Tywanna Whorley filed a Freedom of Information Act request and made possible the opening of the entire archive of the men's medical records in 2004; see Whorley, "Tuskegee Syphilis Study." I am grateful for Professor Whorley's prodigious efforts and our conversations about what these records mean. I expect that her continued work on the records will provide even more insights.

8 Although not about medical records, see this problem discussed in Portelli, *Death of Luigi Trastulli*.

9 Before the TMF opened up, the only access I had to participant medical files was to ones originally held by Harold Edgar, one of the attorneys in the lawsuit; see TMF-Edgar. For privacy reasons per my agreement with Harold Edgar, I kept no

records of the men's names and used the coding number given by the PHS. This collection had seventy-one records.

10 I appreciate Evelynn M. Hammonds's discussions with me about why I should do this. I thank Dr. Robert White for raising the medical questions so distinctly, even if I have disagreed with him about his analysis of the problems.

11 My research assistant, Rachel Stern, and I recorded selected information from all the medical records of the Study's participants in the National Archives onto a form. Joan Huang provided stellar data management and the initial sorting into the programs Epi-Info and Excel. Donna Stroup, of Data for Solutions, ran the statistical calculations. The date of entry into the Study for 74 of the 624 men was not given in the medical records and could not be determined. See appendix for detailed tables. Further tables are available on the website: <http://www .examiningtuskegee.com/>.

12 The men's names have been listed on the website by the National Archives (see <http://www.archives.gov/southeast/finding-aids/tuskegee.html>) and by attorney Fred Gray (*Tuskegee Syphilis Study*). Fred Gray had their names printed on the floor of the Tuskegee Human and Civil Rights Multicultural Center in Tuskegee; see chapter 12. Their names are also used in this book, although they are not linked to their record numbers; see appendix. The National Archives website gives the numbers for the Study of 425 syphilitics and 209 controls. But there are mistakes in this count (some listed in each category belong in the other category), and at least ten of the records are missing or have been withdrawn. In his book on the Study, attorney Fred Gray lists the men's names and comes up with the figure of 624. Jones uses the figures of 399 and 201, which are usually the ones quoted (*Bad Blood*, 1).

13 Comments of Ernest Hendon, on *Voices of the Tuskegee Syphilis Study* (DVD). Bill Jenkins, of the Morehouse School of Medicine, provided me with a copy of this DVD, which was funded by the CDC.

14 See appendix tables.

15 "Last Known Addresses," *Pollard v. U.S.* I am grateful to Katie Seltzer for compiling the numbers from the raw data.

16 Herman Shaw interview; Charlie Wesley Pollard interview; Fred Simmons interview; Fred Simmons obituary, *Tuskegee News*, February 2000, <http://dollsgen .com/special_obituary_tribute.htm>, accessed July 25, 2002; "Deadly Deception," *Nova*; Charles G. Gomillion to Susan M. Reverby, October 12, 1994, in Reverby, *Tuskegee's Truths*, 114–15; Mike Harden, "Breaking Silence: Tuskegee Study Survivor Can Forgive, but Not Forget," *Columbus Dispatch*, October 10, 1999, 11; Gray, *Tuskegee Syphilis Study*, 106–7; Dennis McLellan, "E. Hendon, Part of Infamous Study," *Philadelphia Inquirer*, January 26, 2004, <http://www.philly.com>, accessed January 31, 2004.

17 In the PHS's survey of 220 controls and subjects, 19.5 percent of the controls and 15 percent of the subjects reported schooling beyond seventh grade; see Olansky, Simpson, and Schuman, "Environmental Factors," 695.

18 Elizabeth Sims interview, January 17, 2007.

19 Reverby, "More Than Fact and Fiction."

20 Affidavits of Leorie Berry, Sam Doner, and Archie Foster, *Pollard v. U.S.*

21 "Cotton Yields Fall Short of Assuring Profit on Crops," June 18, 1931, 8; "One Hundred and Twenty-five Barrels of Flour Arrives in City," May 26, 1932, 1; "All Public Schools in Macon County Are Closed Indefinitely," November 24, 1932, 1; "Alabama's Cotton Crop Smallest in Ten Years," December 5, 1932, *Tuskegee News*, 1.

22 Herman Shaw interview; Gray, *Tuskegee Syphilis Study*, 107. On the sharecroppers union, see Litwack, *Trouble in Mind*, 433; and Rosengarten, *All God's Dangers*.

23 Gray, *Tuskegee Syphilis Study*, 106–7.

24 Charlie Wesley Pollard interview; Reverby and Sims, "Charlie Wesley Pollard." Pollard also met Rivers and was recruited into the Study at the Rosenwald School next to the Shiloh Church. When school was in session, he was examined in his cousin's front yard; see Laura Parker, "'Bad Blood' Still Flows in Tuskegee Study," *USA Today*, April 28, 1997, 6A.

25 Parran, *Shadow on the Land*, 165.

26 This point is made clearly in Susan L. Smith's discussion of Rivers's role in the Study; see Susan L. Smith, *Sick and Tired*, 112; and Susan L. Smith, "Neither Victim nor Villain."

27 See Record 472, box 31, TMF; and Records 522 and 527, box 35, TMF.

28 Shafer, Usilton, and Gleeson, "Untreated Syphilis," 273.

29 Data comes from analysis of TMF. All subsequent data comes from the analysis of these files. Earlier deaths are also confirmed in Siddique, "Life Expectancy." For the PHS summary, see Caldwell et al., "Aortic Regurgitation."

30 Stokes, *Modern Clinical Syphilology*, 1019.

31 Christopher Crenner explores theories for neurological complications that differentiated between the idea of "internal resistance" to the disease and possibly differing strains of the bacteria. Joseph Earle Moore of Johns Hopkins held to the former belief. Crenner, "Tuskegee Syphilis Study," 9.

32 Siddique ("Life Expectancy") finds 23 who were switched between 1938 and 1970; my count found only 12.

33 For examples of uncertainty of the syphilitic diagnosis, see Record 168, box 13; Record 188, box 14; Record 254, box 18; Record 351, box 23; Record 404, box 27, TMF.

34 Record 003S, box 1; Record 187, box 14; Record 537, box 35, TMF.

35 See appendix tables.

36 I am grateful for Dr. Beth Fisher's discussions with me for this formulation. For example, Karen Sutton, the biographer of Sam Doner, writes about his death, without autopsy, at age 90 in 1998. She concludes: "His cause of death is not listed as syphilis, but rather myocardial infarct (heart attack), hypertension (high blood pressure), and diabetes, all complications of syphilis"; Sutton, "Sam Doner," 27.

37 "At least 28 Died in Syphilis Study," *New York Times*, September 12, 1972, 23; "Condoms in Africa Are Infected with HIV Says Archbishop," *Ligali: Equality for African People*, September 29, 2007, <http://www.ligali.org>, accessed September 30, 2007.

38 Dick Bruce Report, 1974, box 3, Dick Bruce Folder, 13, CDC-GA. Bruce examined the medical records and autopsy reports to come to his conclusions. He also noted: "The similarity of the clinical symptoms of syphilitic and atherosclerotic aortitis reduces the efficiency of clinical methods in the detection of syphilitic aortitis."

39 James Jones, for example, implies that Rivers was successful at getting the autopsies,

quoting her 1954 report that "she approached 145 families and all but one granted permission" for the procedure (*Bad Blood*, 152). But the data from the medical records gives a more complete number: 228 were autopsied and 396 were not. This includes, of course, the men who died after 1973.

40 Eunice Rivers to Dr. Sidney Olansky, August 17, 1953, Record 566, box 37, TMF.

41 Record 001S, box 1, TMF. He was one of the few men who were clearly in both the Rosenwald Fund Demonstration Project and the Study, and he received 30 to 40 heavy metals treatments at the Macon County Health Department in 1932, the year he entered the Study but after the Rosenwald Fund Demonstration Project had closed.

42 The rate of risk of autopsy by case status before 1973 was 65.1 percent for the syphilitics versus 73.6 percent for the controls.

43 Stokes, *Modern Clinical Syphilology*, 1027–29, 1036, 1068–69; Moore, *Modern Treatment*, 52. Radiologist J. T. Driskell, for example, wrote on one man's report in 1963: "The heart is enlarged and of a hypertensive or aortic configuration"; Record 187, box 14, TMF. The man was a control.

44 Royster et al., "Anatomic Findings," 66.

45 Record 386, box 26; Record 299, box 33, TMF.

46 Stokes, *Modern Clinical Syphilology*, 1019.

47 Record 007, box 1, TMF. The man died from pneumonia in 1962, but the record notes that "permission is not granted to examine the brain."

48 Record 187, box 14; Record 502, box 33, TMF.

49 Record 427, box 29, TMF.

50 The records do not always make it clear what the major cause of death was. That syphilis would have affected other diseases is to be expected, but how in each case is not always specified.

51 Record 051, box 4, TMF.

52 Charlie Wesley Pollard interview.

53 Record 520, box 35, TMF.

54 There continued to be a debate on whether even a few shots made a difference. This might, at the least, have affected whether the men were still contagious.

55 Moore, *Modern Treatment*, 258.

56 The case of one man is suggestive. CDC physician Robert Rochat wrote to the man's physician at a VA Hospital on July 8, 1974, after the Study closed and after the men were supposed to have been treated, suggesting the patient be given "a full course of penicillin treatment for syphilis" (Rochat to G. R. Watts, July 8, 1974, Record 574, box 38). Although the man was labeled a syphilitic, his PHS Venereal Disease Research Laboratory blood tests were normal. The doctors thought that he had arteriosclerosis and pulmonary emphysema. He received five to six shots of neoarsphenamine in the 1930s, one shot of penicillin from Murray Smith at the Health Department in 1952, antibiotic treatments for other conditions, and a report in 1968 of penicillin "for years" from Dr. Smith. He died after the Study closed, and no autopsy report exists.

57 Cynthia Wilson interview. Wilson described the hospital's doctors in the 1950s and 1960s.

58 Wenger, "Untreated Syphilis"; Don Printz interview, PHS retired, July 12, 2005. There was at least some evidence, however, that those lost to follow-up had the same experiences as those who were followed; see Bauer et al., "Do Persons Lost to Long Term Observation?"

59 C. A. Walwyn to Doctor Thomas Parran, January 21, 1938; Austin V. Deibert to Dr. R. A. Vonderlehr, June 12, 1939, box 12, Folder General 1938–39, CDC-GA.

60 Record A6S, box 1, TMF.

61 Reginald James, "The Mobile Clinic and Syphilis in the Rural Areas of Macon County, Alabama," 15–16, TUA; Reginald James, "Transcript 1973," 67, 108–9, HEW-NLM. James does not say what film he was showing, although it was probably either *Three Counties against Syphilis*, the film the PHS made on its rural campaigns in Georgia, or *Know for Sure*, which was produced for male audiences with "explicit depictions of male organs." See Parascandola, "VD at the Movies"; and Lederer and Parascandola, "Screening Syphilis."

62 Rivers claimed that James was "lying"; see chapter 9.

63 See chapter 3.

64 Walls, "Hot Springs Waters," especially 437. For more on the rapid treatment centers, see White, "Misrepresentations of the Tuskegee Study." Dr. White's article is, in part, an attack on my earlier work. I have answered him in a letter, in *Journal of the National Medical Association* 97 (August 2005): 1180–81. White is correct that the heavy metals were used in most of the rapid treatment centers, but at the Birmingham center, set up in 1945, penicillin was given in addition; see Denison and Smith, "Mass Venereal Disease Control." For more of an overview on rapid treatment centers, see Parascandola, *Sex, Sin, and Science*, 79–80, 119–28.

65 Denison and Smith, "Mass Venereal Disease Control," 197.

66 Affidavit of Charles Pollard, *Pollard v. U.S.* The affidavit does not make clear if Mr. Pollard knew the name of his disease or why he was supposed to go to Birmingham at the time or if he just learned about this after the story of the Study became public.

67 "Interview with Four Survivors," in Reverby, *Tuskegee's Truths*, 144.

68 Herman Shaw interview.

69 Denison and Smith, "Mass Venereal Disease Control," 197. This argument is more fully developed by White, "Misrepresentations of the Tuskegee Study."

70 Record 478, box 32, TMF. In 1958, Dr. Bunche, on fluoroscopic evidence, wrote that Shaw suffered from "syphilitic aortitis." Mr. Shaw died in 1999. His wife, examined in 1934, was deemed negative.

71 Record A12S, box 1; Record 540, box 36; Record 534, box 35, TMF.

72 Records A6S, A1S, box 1; Record 592, box 38, TMF.

73 Affidavit of Fred Simmons, *Pollard v. U.S.*; Record 482, box 32, TMF.

74 Rockwell, Yobs, and Moore, "Tuskegee Study," 797.

75 Joseph G. Caldwell et al., "Aortic Insufficiency," paper presented at American Venereal Disease Association Annual Meeting, June 22, 1971, 1, box 9, CDC-GA.

76 Termini and Music, "Natural History of Syphilis." This was published just five months before the AP story on the Study broke.

77 See appendix on cause of death by infection status.

78 Benedek and Erlen, "Scientific Environment"; Schamberg and Wright, *Treatment of Syphilis*. Whether or not penicillin, or even the earlier use of the heavy metals, might have helped those with advanced aortitis, aneurysms, or neurological deficits in the late stages of syphilis was certainly debated in the literature.

79 Robert Story interview. Dr. Story told the exact same story on the ABC *Primetime Live* segment on the Study that aired on February 6, 1992.

80 For example, Record 477, box 31, TMF: This man living in Florida was treated by the company doctor; and Record 254, box 18, TMF: This man, with no address given, was provided penicillin in Birmingham. With Medicare and Medicaid becoming available in 1966, it is possible that those who could not previously afford care finally could access private physicians, or that they continued to use city and county health departments. But, in 1972, Vernal Cave was still appalled by the poverty; see the report by Cave, "Report of Delegation II, November 2, 1972," box 17, HEW-NLM.

81 Records 284, A7, and 480, TMF-Edgar.

82 Records 204 and 137, TMF-Edgar; Record 329, box 22, TMF. In addition, this man received penicillin for other ills in 1957, 1960, and 1964, all in Macon County. The PHS also saw him in 1934, 1948, 1952, 1958, 1963, 1968, and 1970, and he passed away in August 1972, just a few weeks after the Study's history was made public.

83 Caldwell et al., "Aortic Regurgitation," 189, 192–93. This paper was originally given at the American Venereal Disease Association Annual Meeting in 1971 and was submitted for publication in January 1972 (that is, before the Study was publicly revealed). In the mid-1960s, the PHS's Anne R. Yobs, Sidney Olansky, and Donald Rockwell (all of whom had also published articles on the Study) joined other researchers in a study of 46 "inmate volunteers" designed to explore the question of whether the spirochetes survived even adequate treatment. Their conclusion: adequate penicillin treatment made a difference. Yobs et al., "Do Treponemes Survive."

84 Record 261, box 18; Record 239, box 17; Record 18, box 2; Record 488, box 32, TMF.

85 Record 611, box 39, TMF. The cause of death at autopsy was given as generalized arteriosclerosis and "tabes dorsalis from history."

86 Records 219 and 108, TMF-Edgar; Record 194, box 14, TMF.

87 Record 194, box 14, TMF.

88 William J. Brown to Dr. Ruth Berrey, June 17, 1970, box 1, Folder 1970, Laurie Papers.

89 Ibid. This man had been given "shots" for bad blood in 1933 and 1938 by Dr. Murray Smith at the health department. There was also some indication that he had syphilitic aortitis; Record 355, TMF-Edgar.

90 Record A6S, box 1, TMF. For more on McRae's role, see chapter 11.

91 Record 289, TMF-Edgar.

92 Affidavit of Carrie Bell Griffin, October 11, 1974, *Pollard v. U.S.*

93 Fred Gray asserts this forcefully: "They were in the secondary stage [actually they were supposed to be in the tertiary stage] of the disease and were not contagious to others." Gray also argues that the wives "did not permit the disclosure of this information to affect [their] relationship"; Gray, *Tuskegee Syphilis Study*, 106.

94 As the CDC's director, David Sencer, admitted after the Study ended: "While the

study was designed so that only individuals having syphilis for more than two years [actually five years] should have been included, our records do not permit us to state with absolute confidence that errors in the selection of participants did not occur"; David J. Sencer, Director, CDC, to Mark S. Frankel, March 23, 1976, box 4, Folder Controlled Correspondence 1976, CDC-GA.

95 For example, Vonderlehr's notes on one man's 1933 record read: "Married 2 weeks before examination; wife's wass. [Wassermann test for syphilis] neg. before marriage. Has she been infected. No blood test since marriage"; Record 091, box 7, TMF. On another, he wrote: "Wife's wass checked. Yes, negative." A later note read that wife was "examined repeatedly while in Tuskegee thru 1946, no treatment"; Record 320, box 22, TMF.

96 Record A13S, box 1, TMF. "Jones" owned his own farm, was a local preacher, and was treated with penicillin for skin infections and pneumonia by Dr. Smith at the Macon County Health Department in 1963, 1966, and 1968. He died after the Study closed. "Harrison" also received penicillin for "bad blood" in the 1940s; Record A04S, box 1. "Houston" was treated with penicillin in 1963 in Ohio; Record 018, box 1. "Green"; Record 053, box 1.

97 James T. Wooten, "Survivor of '32 Syphilis Study Recalls a Diagnosis," *New York Times*, July 27, 1972, 18; Charlie Wesley Pollard interview.

98 Record 425, box 29, TMF.

99 Richard Bruce, "Status of Wives of Tuskegee Study," October 31, 1977; Richard H. Bruce to Assistant Director, Bureau of State Services, November 17, 1977, box 7, Follow-up Folder, CDC-GA.

100 Richard Bruce, "Telephone Conversation with Mrs. Eunice Laurie regarding treatment of infected spouses and children of the Tuskegee Study participants," June 6, 1974, ibid.

101 Richard Bruce, "Status of Wives of Tuskegee Study," October 31, 1977, ibid.

102 Ibid.

103 Affidavit of Plaintiff Catherine Brown, *Pollard v. U.S.* In August 1974, the judge denied separate claims for the wives on their own behalf, arguing that they had to get administrative relief first but that they could sue as claimant heirs.

104 David J. Sencer, Director, CDC, to Assistant Secretary for Health, "Recommended Course of Action for Follow-up of Spouses and Children of Tuskegee Syphilis Study (TSS) Participants—ACTION," September 12, 1973, box 8, Folder TSS General V, 1–3, CDC-GA. Sencer estimated that this would cost the government between $22.8 million and $127.5 million for the next nearly four decades.

Nor is it possible to tell if the untreated men infected their wives or vice versa. When the first Rosenwald survey and treatment program for syphilis swept through Macon County in the early 1930s, it was actually black women rather than black men who had a higher percentage of serological positive cases (29.35 percent of the women tested versus 26.98 percent of the men). Although this program was an effort to treat, only 1 percent of the 921 men and women who were positive received what Parran and Vonderlehr would have considered adequate treatment. "Table 1: Results of a Serological Survey on Rural Negroes in the Untreated Syphilis Study in Macon County, Alabama," and "Table 11: Amount of Arsphenamine and Heavy

Metals Given Negroes Found to be Serologically Positive in the Untreated Syphilis Study in Macon County, Alabama," attached to a memo from Eugene H. Dibble to Ralph Davis, Research Department, Tuskegee Institute, September 9, 1933, Dibble Papers. The numbers make it clear that this is the Rosenwald Fund Demonstration Project and not the Study.

105 Motion to Reconsider, *Pollard v. U.S.*, July 16, 1974.

106 The testing, however, showed more reaction to the blood tests—as "50 wives were tested" and "27 were found to be positive for syphilis," and a total of 20 children had the disease. Yoon, "Families Emerge"; Dick Bruce, "Memo to the Record," June 26, 1978, box 7, Follow-up Children Folder, CDC-GA.

107 David J. Sencer to Honorable Richard Schweiker, n.d. The drafted letter was in response to a letter to Senator Schweiker from Earline Cofield of the Prisoners' Rights Council of Philadelphia, "Re: Experiments Conducted in Conjunction with the 'Tuskegee Report (Syphilis Study),' but Only on Black Women," January 6, 1975, box 4, Folder Correspondence 1974–75, CDC-GA.

108 Yoon, "Families Emerge." The CDC's 1974 statistics showed that they had reached 112 men (68 with the disease and 44 controls) and that only 10 of those with the disease and 8 controls had not sent the CDC their medical bills for payment; "TSS Participant Status of 5/15/74," TMF-Edgar.

109 Alondra Nelson interview; Bryan Lindsey interview; Lloyd Clements, "Bioethics and African-American Health: A Personal and Historical Account of One Family's Experience with the Tuskegee Syphilis Study," speech given at Florida Community College, February 15, 2006. I am grateful to Mr. Clements of Tuskegee for informal discussions about his family and the Study and for the records and photographs he provided.

110 Herman Shaw quoted in Curtis L. Taylor, "Mistakes in the Past, Fears in the Present," *Newsday*, December 4, 1998, A-08. In my interview, Mr. Shaw used a similar phrase and called himself and the others "real American men"; Herman Shaw interview; Albert Julkes Jr. interview.

111 Comments of Albert Julkes Jr., *Voices of the Tuskegee Syphilis Study* (DVD).

112 Comments of Ernest Hendon, ibid.

113 Amy and Walter Pack interview; Johnny Ford interview; Jean Heller interview, August 16, 2006.

114 Junod, "Deadly Medicine," 522.

115 For a discussion of how hard it was to find the men and the role of attorney Fred Gray and his tensions with the CDC, see Richard H. Bruce to Kenneth Vines, February 5, 1975, box 5, Folder Correspondence 1974–75, CDC-GA.

116 Ibid.; Record 204, box 15, TMF; Jones, *Bad Blood*, 217–18.

117 Gray, *Tuskegee Study*, 106. Gray argues that such a small population in Macon County meant that many of the hundreds of men involved were related. But in what is probably a typing error, he lists the county's population as 2,000. It was 22,810 in 2005; see "Macon County, Alabama," *U.S. Census, State and County Quick Facts*, <http://quickfacts.census.gov/qfd/states/01/01087.html>, accessed June 29, 2006.

118 Vernal Cave, "Report of Delegation II," 4, HEW-NLM; Howard Settler Jr. interview. On contemporary issues of stigma in Alabama, see Lichtenstein, "Stigma."

119 Johnny Ford interview.

120 See *Alabama Stories* (DVD).

121 Comments of Albert Julkes Jr., *Voices of the Tuskegee Syphilis Study* (DVD).

122 Family members made these comments in an open discussion at the Shiloh Community Restoration Program, January 17, 2007, Notasulga, Alabama.

123 Shaw, "Comments"; Charlie Wesley Pollard interview.

124 Stephen B. Thomas and Curran, "Tuskegee: From Science to Conspiracy to Metaphor."

125 Comments of Albert Julkes Jr., *Voices of the Tuskegee Syphilis Study* (DVD).

126 Johnson, *Soul by Soul*, 207.

127 Associated Press, "State Honors Study Victims," *Columbus Ledger-Enquirer*, May 9, 2001. I am grateful to Albert Julkes Jr. for sending me this clipping and for working for the Alabama apology.

128 Comments made by family members, Shiloh Community Restoration Program, January 17, 2007, Notasulga, Alabama.

129 Shaw, "Comments." On the shift in language from victim to survivor in another context, see Alcoff and Gray, "Survivor Discourse," 260–90.

CHAPTER 7

1 Liel Schillinger argues that in writings about the South, in particular for outsiders, "transgressions appear more archetypal"; see his "Hot Zones," *New York Times*, August 27, 2006, Book Review, 17.

2 Stokes and Beerman, "Fundamental Bacteriology," 18. Gjestland, *Oslo Study* (11), repeated this phrase to explain why the reinvestigation of the Oslo data was needed in 1955.

3 Moore's World War I experience motivated him to make this switch from psychiatry to a specialty in syphilis. Adolph Meyer, Hopkins's leading psychiatrist, was clearly upset to lose one of his best students to another division of medicine; see Joseph Earle Moore to Dr. Meyer, July 6, 1917; Meyer to Moore, July 26, 1917; and Moore to Meyer, November 18, 1917, Correspondence Moore Folder, box 1, Meyer Papers, Chesney Archives.

4 Moore, "Venerology in Transition," 217.

5 Henry M. Thomas Jr., "Memorial," xlix.

6 His view on the morality of research is discussed in Marks, *Progress of Experiment*, 105. Moore chaired the National Research Council's Committee on Medical Research during World War II, and Marks discusses his role extensively. See also Jones, *Bad Blood*, particularly chapter 7.

7 Alan Chesney, "Joseph Earle Moore," typescript of obituary, Moore Folder, box 17, Chesney Papers, Chesney Archives.

8 Hahn, "Obituary for Joseph Earle Moore, 1892–1957."

9 Joseph Earle Moore to Clark, September 28, 1932, in Reverby, *Tuskegee's Truths*, 78–80. See also Benedek and Erlen, "Scientific Environment."

10 Thomas B. Turner, "Race and Sex Distribution," 159–84.

11 Moore, *Modern Treatment*, 256.

12 Gjestland, *Oslo Study*, 364.

13 Moore, *Modern Treatment*, 249, 256, 570.

14 John H. Stokes to Alan Chesney, July 12, 1928, Committee on Research on Syphilis Folder, box 17, Chesney Papers, Chesney Archives.

15 Henry M. Thomas Jr., "Memorial," 1.

16 "Report of the Activities of the Lab of Experimental Syphilis of the Department of Medicine of Johns Hopkins University, July 1, 1929–June 30th, 1930," 2–5, Committee on Research on Syphilis Folder, box 17, Chesney Papers, Chesney Archives.

17 Moore, "Relation of Neuroreoccurrences," 117–36.

18 Moore, Cole, and O'Leary, "Cooperative Clinical Studies," 317–31.

19 Moore, *Modern Treatment*, 283.

20 On the need for more information and repeat studies for another venereal disease, see Benedek, "Gonorrhea." Urban patients were notoriously hard to keep track of, and the assumption that rural subjects would not move as often must have been alluring. On the difference between urban and rural subjects, see Dowling, *Fighting Infection*, 102; see also Lederer, "Tuskegee Syphilis Study."

21 Moore to Clark, September 28, 1932, in Reverby, *Tuskegee's Truths*, 78–80.

22 On the importance of Moore's role in training younger doctors, see Vonderlehr and Heller, *Control of Venereal Disease*, 169. "In 1952 or 53, Peters wrote a paper for publication. Dr. Earle Moore tore it to shreds and it was never published," a report on the study at the PHS noted in 1965; see "Meeting Re: Tuskegee Study," April 5, 1965, Ad Hoc Folder 3, box 6, CDC-GA. However, Moore did publish the paper by Peters in the first year after his journal, *American Journal of Syphilis*, changed its title to *Journal of Chronic Diseases*; see Peters et al., "Untreated Syphilis."

23 See Moore, *Modern Treatment*; and Moore, *Penicillin in Syphilis*. Similarly, two urban Buffalo, N.Y., researchers in 1946 argued for the need for a study on African Americans with treated and untreated latent syphilis. They cited the problems with Oslo and with two other studies (including one from Hopkins that Moore worked on) and never mention Tuskegee. See Jordon and Dolce, "Latent Syphilis."

24 Marks, *Progress of Experiment*, 102–3. I am grateful to Harry Marks for discussing Moore with me.

25 Moore seems to have some difficulties with quick therapy programs; see Reuben Kahn to Rear Admiral Harold W. Smith, October 15, 1942, box 1, Folder 1, Kahn Papers.

26 "Meeting Re: Tuskegee Study," HEW materials noted as M22–8, I-B Basic, HEW-NLM; Moore et al., "Treatment of Early Syphilis." "Dr. Moore believed that the precise and extended studies which had yield[ed] important information concerning the natural history of syphilis and its management could be applied to a number of other long-term diseases, knowledge about which was meager"; David Seegal, "In Memoriam," 93.

27 See Niedelman, "Penicillin in Late Latent Syphilis." For an earlier argument opposing the use of arsenicals in latent syphilis, see Kenney, "A Plea for Conservatism." For more discussion of the medical thinking that informed this argument at the time, see Benedek and Erlen, "Scientific Environment"; and White, "Misinformation and Misbeliefs."

28 Moore, *Penicillin in Syphilis*, 147; Moore, "Venerology in Transition," 218. In Great Britain, syphilologists were called venerologists.

29 Moore, "Impending Loss."

30 Wenger did not expect to be in the Alabama countryside, but he could never be sure where the PHS might need him. H. S. Cumming to Surgeon O. C. Wenger, April 20, 1933; O. C. Wenger, "Questionnaire for Applications for Appointment in the Reserve of the PHS," 3, n.d.; and R. A. Vonderlehr, "O. C. Wenger Confidential Efficiency Report," November 22, 1937, 2; Official Personnel Folder of Oliver C. Wenger, PHS Commissioned Corps, National Archives and Records Administration, Civilian National Personnel Record Center, St. Louis. I am grateful to John Parascandola, former historian of the PHS, who obtained these records for me.

31 O. C. Wenger to R. A. Vonderlehr, July 21, 1933, in Reverby, Tuskegee's Truths, 85.

32 For example, Carley and Wenger, "Prevalence of Syphilis."

33 Official Personnel Folder of Oliver C. Wenger, PHS Commissioned Corps, National Archives and Records Administration, Civilian National Personnel Record Center, St. Louis. Wenger appears to have been given lower grades for "tact" on a consistent basis. Jones, in Bad Blood, argues that the PHS doctors were racial "liberals" who cared about providing health care in black communities. Despite his language, Wenger fits this description.

34 "The campaigns of the Philippine Constabulary . . . constituted America's first experiment in warfare in the jungle"; Hurley, Jungle Patrol, 1.

35 Audrey Wenger McCully, "United States Public Health Service Venereal Disease Clinic and Government Free Bath House (1919–1936)," The Record: Annual Publication of the Garland County Arkansas Historical Society, Hot Springs, Arkansas, 1981, 95–105.

36 Ibid., 99. Wenger did have some typical doctor humor. When he took time out to go fishing, his boat was called "The Spirochete."

37 O. C. Wenger, n.d., quoted in ibid., 103.

38 For an example of the contemporary debate on research in the developing world and its parallels to the Study, see the debate on the AZT trials for AIDS between New England Journal of Medicine editor Marcia Angell and Harold Varmus and David Satcher, then heads of the NIH and the CDC, respectively, in Reverby, Tuskegee Truths, 578–88; see also Rothman, "Shame of Medical Research." And see the rebuttals between Dr. Barry Bloom and David Rothman, New York Review of Books 48 (March 8, 2001); and between John F. Murray and David Rothman, New York Review of Books 48 (May 17, 2001).

39 On the history of rapid treatment centers, see Parascandola, Sex, Sin, and Science.

40 De Kruif, Fight for Life, 493.

41 J. F. Pilcher quoted in Reynolds and Moore, "Progress," 666.

42 De Kruif, Fight for Life, 298. De Kruif, known for being the idea man behind Sinclair Lewis's famed novel Arrowsmith, did not always report accurately, and we do not know for sure if Wenger actually said this.

43 Herman Bundesen to R. A. Vonderlehr, February 22, 1937, Official Personnel Folder of Oliver C. Wenger, PHS Commissioned Corps, National Archives and Records Administration, Civilian National Personnel Record Center, St. Louis.

44 De Kruif, Fight for Life, 285.

45 Parran, "Syphilis: A Public Health Problem," 149.

46 Parran, "Syphilis: The White Man's Burden," 62, 65.

47 See Wenger and Ricks, "Public Health Aspect of Syphilis."

48 For those receiving the full treatment, Parran reported in 1937, a 40 percent goal was reached: "An average of 8.4 arsphenamines and 72.6 mercury rubs"; Parran, "Syphilis: The White Man's Burden," 62, 65.

49 See Fee, "Sin versus Science." Fee, *Disease and Discovery*, 211, states that in 1933 they were only giving out four arsphenamine shots. See also Poirier, *Chicago's War on Syphilis*. O. C. Wenger was the PHS's key leader in the Chicago antisyphilis campaign.

50 See Kampmeier, "Comments," for a history of treating and some of the problems involved in it. Kampmeier's clinic for the indigent at Vanderbilt in Nashville was able to get 50 percent of its black patients and 80 percent of its white patients to stay in treatment for a year. But most clinics reported treatment rates more in the range of 10 percent, up to 50 percent at the most.

51 Schuman et al., "Untreated Syphilis," 544. This is in a discussion of the earlier expectations of the Study.

52 The assumption that individuals would get the diseases anyway occurred in other research; see Bean, "Walter Reed"; and Howell and Hayward, "Writing Willowbrook."

53 See Lombardo and Dorr, "Eugenics"; and Pernick, "Eugenics and Public Health." Such views were also supported by Dr. J. N. Baker, Alabama's state health officer in the 1930s, who approved Alabama's participation in the Study and fought to give the state the right to sterilize those seen as unfit; see Larson, *Sex, Race, and Science*, 33, 140, 146, 148.

54 O. C. Wenger to R. A. Vonderlehr, July 21, 1933, 84–87; R. A. Vonderlehr to Dr. H. T. Jones, Tallassee, Alabama, November 20, 1933, in Reverby, *Tuskegee's Truths*. As Wenger would write in 1950, looking back on his participation, the Study was organized to follow "the syphilitic process when uninfluenced by treatment and to compare those findings with results after treatment had been given." It was clear that the comparative group that was treated was not in Macon County; Wenger, "Untreated Syphilis," 97.

55 Ibid., 98.

56 Wenger was corresponding with Reuben Kahn, of the Kahn test for syphilis, in an effort to set up a conference on false positives. He sent Kahn a copy of his letter to Vonderlehr. Wenger to Vonderlehr, November 28, 1941, box 1, Folder 1, Kahn Papers.

57 Poirier, *Chicago's War on Syphilis*, 200–201; Brandt, *No Magic Bullet*. Poirier makes clear the struggle on the part of Chicago's African American leadership to fight the assumptions about syphilis as a racialized disease. This did not happen in quite the same way in Tuskegee; see the chapters on Dr. Dibble and Nurse Rivers. On Wenger's work in Trinidad, see Wenger, *Caribbean Medical Center*.

58 Schuman et al., "Untreated Syphilis," 545. In 1972, Schuman repeated this position by telling the Ad Hoc Committee: "After a complete and negative examination (in 1952), a man with positive serology for syphilis was assured that he carried serological, not infectious traces of the disease"; Stanley H. Schuman to Broadus N. Butler,

December 1, 1972, Folder Correspondence, box 2, HEW-NLM. The possibility that some of the men who switched from control to syphilitic might be contagious did not seem to trouble Wenger. Rather, it is possible he thought that it was merely that they had older cases, which had not been picked up on earlier serologies and history-takings. And, as a public health man, he would not have been focused on those who could in all probability no longer infect others.

59 See Goodman, McElligott, and Marks, "Introduction: Making Human Bodies Useful."

60 Ibid., 10.

61 *Jacobson v. Massachusetts*, 197 U.S. 11 (1905); *Buck v. Bell*, 274 U.S. 200 (1927). See Colgrove and Bayer, "Manifold Restraints."

62 Lederer, *Subjected to Science*, 21–23; Bean, "Walter Reed"; Guiteras, "Experimental Yellow Fever." Rivers's caregiving and the Milbank Memorial Fund promise of money for burial in Tuskegee are eerily similar, even if the lack of written consent is of course a major difference.

63 Katz, "Reflections on Informed Consent."

64 Herzig, *Suffering for Science*, 43.

65 O. C. Wenger to R. A. Vonderlehr, July 21, 1933, in Reverby, *Tuskegee's Truths*, 85.

66 Goodman, McElligott, and Marks, "Introduction: Making Human Bodies Useful," 12.

67 Mahoney, Arnold, and Harris, "Penicillin Treatment"; Hobby, *Penicillin: Meeting the Challenge* (New Haven: Yale University Press, 1985), 155–56, quoted in Parascandola, "John Mahoney and the Introduction of Penicillin." On the cheering, see the report by two of the physicians who ran the Study: Vonderlehr and Heller, *Control of Venereal Disease*, 55. On the history of concerns about treatment and morality, see Brandt, *No Magic Bullet*.

68 Stokes, *Modern Clinical Syphilology*, 1256; John C. Cutler, "Experimental Studies on Human Inoculation with Syphilis, Gonorrhea and Chancroid," 1946–48, Pan American Health Organization under the direction of the Venereal Disease Research Laboratory of the PHS, Guatemala, 4, box 1, Folder 1, Cutler Papers. Cutler was involved in PHS-sponsored studies in Guatemala in 1946–47.

69 Jan Ackerman, "Obituary: John Charles Cutler/Pioneer in Preventing Sexual Diseases," *Pittsburgh Post Gazette*, February 12, 2003, 3. From 1960 on, Cutler worked in Pittsburgh, with time out at the Pan American Health Organization in Washington. He headed the Pittsburgh Public Health School's population division and was the acting dean in 1968–69. After he passed away in 2003, a lecture series was established in his honor at the school, and he is remembered as compassionate, gentle, and gentlemanly; see <www.publichealth.pitt.edu/imagescontent/publichealthmag/2004_1spring/Cutler-SP04.pdf>, accessed December 8, 2006.

70 Junod, "Deadly Medicine"; "Dr. Sidney Olansky," Olansky Dermatology Associates, <http://www.olanskydermatology.com/profile_sidney.php>, accessed August 6, 2005. Olansky was the author of more than 140 articles on dermatology. He died on December 28, 2007.

71 Olansky appeared on the ABC *Primetime Live* segment on the Study, which aired February 6, 1992, and is explored in Junod, "Deadly Medicine." Cutler is in the *Nova*

film, "Deadly Deception." When he was criticized in the pages of the *American Journal of Public Health* for not mentioning the Study or his role in it in an article on venereal disease control, Cutler replied in part, "I hope we can apply the knowledge gained from our past errors as well as our past successes"; see John C. Cutler, "Dr. Cutler's Response," in Reverby, *Tuskegee's Truths*, 508.

72 Olansky, Harris, Cutler, and Price, "Untreated Syphilis."

73 Friedman and Olansky, "Diagnosis."

74 Schuman et al., "Untreated Syphilis," 551, 553.

75 Ibid.; Olansky et al., "Untreated Syphilis," 177.

76 Olansky, Simpson, and Schuman, "Environmental Factors."

77 "Transportation to and from the hospital was provided. Incentives in the form of free, hot lunches and free medicine [for diseases other than syphilis] were given"; see Schuman et al., "Untreated Syphilis," 545.

78 Ibid., 544.

79 Cutler, "Venereal Disease," 616.

80 Shafer, Usilton, and Gleeson, "Untreated Syphilis," 689. For an argument that the debate on whether to give penicillin in latent syphilis continued well into the 1950s, see Benedek and Erlen, "Scientific Environment."

81 Chester, Cutler, and Price, "Serologic Observations"; Curtis et al., "Penicillin Treatment"; Yobs et al., "Do Treponemes Survive." This last study, done in a prison, showed both that treponemes might persist after treating and that penicillin should be given, "regardless of stage or duration of infection at the time of adequate therapy (387)." See also J. Lawton Smith, *Spirochetes*, especially 303–15. Smith argues several differing theories to explain the persistence of the spirochetes and suggests the need for more studies to understand the phenomenon.

82 Harkness, "Research behind Bars"; Hornblum, *Acres of Skin*; Ian Urbina, "Panel Suggests Using Inmates in Drug Trials," *New York Times*, August 13, 2006 (on current reconsiderations of using prisoners).

83 Magnuson et al., "Inoculation Syphilis." Olansky and Cutler both worked on this research and are coauthors of the article. See also Olansky, "Syphilis — Rediscovered"; and Brunham, "Insights."

84 Olansky, "Syphilis — Rediscovered," 6.

85 Radolf and Lukehart, "Immunology of Syphilis," in *Pathogenic Treponema*, 305.

86 Cutler et al., "Local Herxheimer Reaction."

87 Collart, "Persistence of *Treponema Pallidum*," 291. Syphilis, it was concluded, should be seen as similar to any other "long-term infectious disease."

88 Friedman, "Syphilitic Aortic Insufficiency," 17. Friedman also concluded: "Once the disease has reached the stage of clinical recognition there is no conclusive evidence that specific treatment improves longevity." For a longer discussion of the medical climate, see Benedek and Erlen, "Scientific Environment."

89 Schuman et al., "Untreated Syphilis," 556.

90 The analysis here is based on writings from the 1970s and interviews done with several of the surviving physicians between 2005 and 2007.

91 There was no real discussion of the neurological problems. Perhaps this followed from the assumptions of the earlier period that since African Americans were

not likely to get neurosyphilis or had been exposed to protective malarial fevers, such worries were not part of their concern; see Austin Deibert to Doctor Vonderlehr, March 20, 1939, in Reverby, *Tuskegee's Truths*, 91–92. Kampmeier, "Tuskegee Study," and Kampmeier, *Essentials of Syphilology*, argue for lack of treatment for older patients with cardiovascular complications, although these were written before penicillin was widely available. For a brief critique of Kampmeier, see Brandt, "Racism and Research."

92 Jones, *Bad Blood*, 282. Jones interviewed the PHS/CDC's William J. Brown, John R. Heller, Sidney Olansky, and David Sencer in 1977.

93 Auchmutey, "Ghosts of Tuskegee."

94 Peter Buxtun interview, November 11, 1998.

95 Cutler also repeated these positions on video in interviews with playwright/physician David Feldshuh in 1994; see *Susceptible to Kindness* (VHS); and Auchmutey, "Ghosts of Tuskegee."

96 "The Tuskegee Study," *Primetime Live*, ABC News, aired February 6, 1992.

97 Auchmutey, "Ghosts of Tuskegee"; Junod, "Deadly Medicine." In fact, Olansky's obituary made no mention of his role in the Study.

98 Dr. Sidney Olansky, Olansky Dermatology, <http://www.olanskydermatology .com/profile_sidney.php>, accessed August 6, 2005.

99 Dr. J. Don Millar interviews, August 8, 2005, and January 12, 2007.

100 David Sencer interviews, August 1, 2005, and January 12, 2007; Don Printz interview, July 12, 2005. Alfonso Holguin, one of the PHS physicians who had gone to talk to the Macon County Medical Society in 1969, similarly recalled that the PHS believed that it had not harmed those who had survived thus far with the disease. Given that, and because the Medical Society seemed to give the PHS the black imprimatur it wanted, Holguin thought the PHS should have kept the Study going because it provided the men with the exams and the death benefits, which would stop when the Study did; Alfonso Holguin interview.

101 Jordon and Dolce, "Latent Syphilis." In the discussion after the paper was given, Jordon stated, "We have probably in the past over-treated patients with bismuth. Moore has expressed the belief that bismuth therapy has been overemphasized in the treatment of latent syphilis. . . . Howe found that the amount of cellular infiltrate in the aortic wall of patients who died after having syphilis bore an inverse relationship to the amount of arsenical therapy the person had received. He found there was almost no relationship to the amount of bismuth. This confirms from the pathologic standpoint what we have observed from the clinical standpoint."

CHAPTER 8

1 Eugene H. Dibble Jr. to Dr. R. R. Moton, September 17, 1932, in Reverby, *Tuskegee's Truths*, 75–76. Tuskegee Institute became Tuskegee University in 1985, seventeen years after Dibble's death.

2 Jones (*Bad Blood*) discusses Dibble's role throughout his book but not his motives. Fred Gray barely mentions Dibble, claiming that Tuskegee Institute's "cooperation" was sought and that Dibble and Moton "permitted the government to use the facilities of the hospital for the Study"; Gray, *Tuskegee Study*, 46.

3 Martin, "In Search of Booker T. Washington," 43.

4 Eugene H. Dibble Jr., M.D., "Biographical Data," Dibble Finding Aid File, Dibble Papers; "Eugene Heriot Dibble," n.d., Howard University citation, box 22, Folder 8, ibid.; Schafer, "Eugene Heriot Dibble, Jr." Dibble's father owned a store and land in Camden, was educated at Bridgewater Normal School in Massachusetts, and was in the South Carolina House of Representatives between 1876 and 1878. Dibble attended Howard University just as it was trying to upgrade its facilities but receiving little or no support from white philanthropists; see Savitt, *Race and Medicine*, 260, 265.

5 His family claimed to trace its lineage back to an African princess who married an English seafarer marooned on islands off Sierra Leone's coast, through a daughter or granddaughter of this couple who arrived at the port of Charleston in 1764 as a free black woman; Bond, *Black American Scholars*, 44–47. Bond, in a letter to Tuskegee's librarian in 1968, explained, "The Dibbles were never slaves"; Horace Mann Bond to Tuskegee librarian, March 7, 1968, box 1A, Dibble Papers.

6 Weiss, "Robert R. Taylor."

7 Tuskegee Institute, Release of the Convocations Committee, Moton Memorial, vol. 1, December 2, 1963, box 1, untitled folder, Dibble Papers.

8 Irving Harris, box 526, Folder 7, RF-Fisk; Mae Basey, April 4, 1963, box 22, Folder 14, Dibble Papers.

9 Irene Beavers interview.

10 "Alabama lynchings," <http://users.bestweb.net/~rg/lynchings/Alabama%20Lynchings.htm>, 6, accessed June 28, 2003.

11 See discussion in chapter 1.

12 George I. Davis, "Negro's Story of Tallapoosa Revolt Differs from Account by Creditor," *Montgomery Advertiser*, December 24, 1932, 2, box 12, Clippings Folder, Dibble Papers. For more on the shoot-out, see Rosengarten, *All God's Dangers*; and clippings from *Tuskegee News*, December 22–29, 1932, box 12, Clippings Folder, Dibble Papers. Dibble kept the clippings in his files.

13 For more on these statues, which were ubiquitous in the South, see Savage, *Standing Soldiers*.

14 Guy Rhodes, "Tuskegee Square Gets Facelift Courtesy Federal Funding," *Tuskegee News*, March 20, 2008, A-3.

15 "Cabaret Minstrels a Big Success," *Tuskegee News*, February 18, 1932, 1.

16 Richard Robbins, "Pittsburgh Charity Lauded for History of Helping Those in Need," *Pittsburgh Tribune-Review*, February 3, 2008. Robert Hingson, a famed white anesthesiologist who was running the trip, held his ground, and Dibble went to Africa funded by a charity still known today as Brother's Brother Foundation.

17 "The Negro academic strata Washington created and inspired could not exist without key compromises in politics to the white establishment"; Marable, "Tuskegee and the Politics of Illusion," 13. The phrase "politics of deference" comes from Paul L. Puryear and is quoted in Carmichael and Hamilton, *Black Power*, 124.

18 Eugene H. Dibble to Robert R. Moton, April 5, 1933, box 57, Dibble Folder, Moton Papers, TUA.

19 See Eugene H. Dibble to Dr. James T. Montgomery, Chair, Alabama State Medical

Association, May 28, 1963; Dibble to Dr. F. J. L. Blassingame, May 15, 1958, box 17, Folder 16, Folder Alabama State Medical Association, box 12, Dibble Papers.

20 Eugene H. Dibble to Moton, March 23, 1933, box 57, Local Correspondence Folder, Moton Papers, TUA; see also boxes 40, 45, 50, 53, 57, Local Correspondence Folders, ibid.

21 Moton to Mrs. H. I. Balderston, December 5, 1932, box 166, Folder 1360, ibid.

22 Louis Mike Rabb interview.

23 Naomi Rogers, "Race and the Politics of Polio."

24 Nicholson J. Eastman to Joe Mitchell, April 27, 1951; "Summary of the Findings and Recommendations of the Committee of the Obstetrics and Pediatric Divisions," ca. 1953, box 27, Folder 6, Dibble Papers.

25 See Ward, *Black Physicians*; Cobb, "Special Problems."

26 Dibble, "Statement of Dr. Eugene Dibble," 189. I am grateful to Karen Kruse Thomas for access to this document.

27 Eugene H. Dibble to Harold Klinger, April 14, 1961, box 29, Folder 8, Dibble Papers.

28 Eugene H. Dibble to Patterson, February 21, 1936, 2, box 32, Folder 9, ibid.

29 John A. Andrew Memorial Hospital was closed in the fall of 1987. There is still no hospital in Tuskegee.

30 Beardsley, *History of Neglect*, 383.

31 See Savitt, *Race and Medicine*. I am grateful to Todd Savitt for discussing the problem of continuing medical education for African American physicians with me. The National Medical Association formed in 1895, when the American Medical Association barred black doctors from membership through its local societies; see Baker et al., "African American Physicians and Organized Medicine."

32 Eugene Heriot Dibble," n.d., Howard University citation, box 22, Folder 8, Dibble Papers.

33 John A. Andrew Clinical Society Program, April 5–11, 1936.

34 Dibble to Patterson, February 21, 1936, 2, box 32, Folder 9, box 22, Folder 8, Dibble Papers.

35 Dibble, Rabb, and Ballard, "John A. Andrew Memorial Hospital."

36 Louis Mike Rabb interview.

37 Vonderlehr, "Comparison"; Deibert, "Notes on Cardiovascular Syphilis"; Olansky, "Diagnosis and Treatment."

38 W. Montague Cobb, "Nomination of Eugene H. Dibble, Jr." box 1, Folder 1, Dibble Papers.

39 See Callis, "The Need for Training of Negro Physicians"; Cobb, "Special Problems"; Beardsley, "Making Separate, Equal."

40 Russell W. Brown and Henderson, "Mass Production." On the racial aspects of the HeLa cell line, see Landecker, "Immortality"; and Landecker, *Culturing Life*. The Carver Research Center now does work in biomedical research. The link between agricultural and biomedical research is a long-standing one.

41 Thomas S. Hosty, Director, Bureau of Labs, Alabama Department of Public Health, to Eugene H. Dibble, December 10, 1959; Donald Bogue to Dibble, June 2, 1964, box 20, Folder 9, box 20, Folder 4, Dibble Papers.

42 There is much literature on the question of "fair benefits," the standard of care, and social justice in international research. See Angell, "Ethics of Clinical Research"; Varmus and Satcher, "Ethical Complexities"; Wendler, Emanuel, and Lie, "Standard of Care Debate"; London, "Justice"; and Wasunna, "Researchers Abroad."

43 Eugene H. Dibble to W. H. Y. Smith, October 10, 1957, asking for his opinion on the current state of the "venereal disease problem" before Dibble gave a talk on it; box 19, Folder 9, Dibble Papers.

44 As Dibble explained to Tuskegee's president, Frederick D. Patterson, in 1936, "The Clinic also gives the people in this section of the South an opportunity to see the finest specialists in America, whom these people would not otherwise have an opportunity to come in contact with for the treatment of their conditions"; Eugene H. Dibble to Patterson, February 21, 1936, 2, box 32, Folder 9, ibid.

45 Eugene H. Dibble to Moton, January 11, 1933, box 57, Local Correspondence, Folder Dibble, Moton Papers, TUA. Everyone was asking Tuskegee to help. Even the venerable W. E. B. Du Bois, then editor of the NAACP paper *The Crisis*, was pleading with Moton to renew his "advertising contract" with the paper and send ten subscriptions to his friends; Du Bois to Moton, January 11, 1932, box 179, General Correspondence Folder 1496, ibid.

46 Eugene H. Dibble to Clay H. Dean, March 22, 1960, box 19, Folder 10, Dibble Papers.

47 Eugene H. Dibble to Dr. Reuben L. Kahn, June 20, 1957, box 28, Folder 15, ibid.

48 Eugene H. Dibble to Moton, January 11, 1933, box 57, Local Correspondence Folder, Moton Papers, TUA.

49 J. W. Williams, M.D., to Dr. F. D. Patterson, September 25, 1936, box 32, Folder 9, Dibble Papers.

50 Anne R. Yobs to Alexander Robertson, Milbank Memorial Fund, August 18, 1965; Yobs to Robert B. Adams, Montgomery Baptist Hospital, October 28, 1965; Yobs to Eugene Dibble, November 3, 1965, box 8, Folder 1965, CDC-GA.

51 Dibble, Rabb, and Ballard, "John A. Andrew Memorial Hospital," 9.

52 Mike Rabb, the institute's comptroller and later the hospital's professional administrator, was accepting the checks for the autopsies from the Milbank Memorial Fund. It is not clear, however, that he knew what the checks were really for. On surgeon general nominee Henry Foster's lack of knowledge of the Study when he was at the John A. Andrew Memorial Hospital, see chapter 12.

53 For an example of how W. E. B. Du Bois struggled with these concepts at the beginning of the twentieth century, see Bay, "World Was Thinking Wrong about Race."

54 Wilson, *Jim Crow Joins Up*, 10.

55 Dibble is listed as the fifth author on Hosty, "Human Anti-Rabies Gamma Globulin."

56 See Tapper, "An 'Anthropathology'"; and Julian Herman Lewis, *Biology of the Negro*.

57 In his files, Dibble kept reports, for example, on racial differences with respect to the hemolysis of red blood cells; see Childs, "Primaquine Sensitivity."

58 Callis, "Comparative Therapy"; Callis, "Primary Syphilis." The articles reported on a "symposium on syphilis by the Medical Officers' Study Club of the United States

Veterans Administration Hospital at Tuskegee, Alabama," held in 1929, three years before the Study began. Taliaferro Clark followed the research as well, telling Raymond Vonderlehr that he was interested in "the related problem of the relative susceptibility of Negroes of varying degree of white mixture to certain inoculation"; Clark to Vonderlehr, February 9, 1933, box 239, Folder 2, PHS-NA.

59 See Braslow, "Influence of Biological Therapy"; and Whitrow, "Wagner-Jauregg."

60 Fong, "Therapeutic Quartan Malaria"; Boyd and Kitchen, "Observations"; Humphreys, *Malaria*.

61 Schamberg and Wright, *Treatment of Syphilis*, 525. This belief is repeated in the second edition of Moore, *Modern Treatment*, 374.

62 "Address of Dr. Eugene H. Dibble, Jr., Manager, Veterans Administration, Tuskegee, Alabama, at the State Service Office School of Instruction, Veterans Administration, Atlanta, Ga., May 23, 1940," 4, unpublished paper, box 23, Folder 3, Dibble Papers.

63 Black pathologist Julian Herman Lewis, writing just two years later in 1942 in his more exhaustive compendium, *The Biology of the Negro*, argued that there was dispute in the literature over whether there was less or even more neurosyphilis in blacks. He posited socioeconomic factors as affecting the extensiveness of syphilis and that what he saw as the shorter historic time that black people had been exposed to syphilis meant that they had not yet developed "tissue immunity" as a people (182–83).

64 "Address of Dr. Eugene H. Dibble, Jr., Manager, Veterans Administration, Tuskegee, Alabama, at the State Service Office School of Instruction, Veterans Administration, Atlanta, Ga., May 23, 1940," 4, unpublished paper, box 23, Folder 3, Dibble Papers. George C. Branche was also sending the quartan blood to Dr. Raymond Vonderlehr; Branche to Vonderlehr, January 26, 1933, Record 234, box 17, TMF.

65 Branche to Vonderlehr, January 26, 1933, Record 234, box 17, TMF. George C. Branche also did research on the use of the quartan strain while he was at the Tuskegee VA Hospital. See also Julian Herman Lewis, *Biology of the Negro*, 180–83; and White, "Unraveling the Tuskegee Study."

66 "Address of Dr. Eugene H. Dibble, Jr., Manager, Veterans Administration, Tuskegee, Alabama, at the State Service Office School of Instruction, Veterans Administration, Atlanta, Ga., May 23, 1940," 4, unpublished paper, box 23, Folder 3, Dibble Papers, 5–6.

67 On this development as a researcher, see Kahn, "Inspiration of Research." On his Wenner-Gren–funded trip, see Kahn, "A Serologist Abroad (August 24 to October 7, 1953), typescript, box 28, Folder 15, Kahn Papers. One of Dibble's sons worked in Kahn's Michigan laboratory, and Kahn visited Tuskegee. The men kept up a lively correspondence, reported on their research efforts to one another, and asked after each other's wives. Kahn also worked closely with the PHS. See letters in box 1, Folder Correspondence 1939–43, Kahn Papers.

68 Donald Bogue to Eugene H. Dibble, June 2, 1964, box 20, Folder 9, Dibble Papers. Other letters in this file give more details on the research. In 1964, the first Helsinki Declaration from the World Medical Association focused on the importance of

consent in research; see Faden, Beauchamp, and King, *History and Theory of Informed Consent*.

69 Record 181, box 13; Record 323, box 23; Record 399, box 27, TMF.

70 Laurie, Deposition, *Pollard v. U.S.* Administrator Mike Rabb recalled that Dibble often forgot names but remembered diagnoses; Louis Mike Rabb interview.

71 Eugene H. Dibble to D. G. Gill, September 22, 1955, box 17, Folder 9, Dibble Papers.

72 For a view of the divisions in Tuskegee and at Tuskegee Institute over civil rights, see Norrell, *Reaping the Worldwind*; Forman, *Sammy Younge*; and Patton, "Insurgent Memories," <http://www.crmvet.org/nars/gwen.htm>, accessed August 17, 2008.

73 Susan L. Smith, "Neither Victim nor Villain," 355; see also Cobb, "Tuskegee Syphilis Study."

74 Forman, *Sammy Younge*; "2001 Interview with Jimmy Rogers," Veterans of the Civil Rights Movement, <http://www.crmvet.org/vet/rogers/htm>, accessed June 30, 2004.

75 For discussion of the legacy of Booker T. Washington from this perspective, see Norrell, "Understanding the Wizard"; and Leverenz, "Booker T. Washington's Strategies." On the role of black professionals behind the scenes in the civil rights movement, see Hine, "Black Professional Class"; and Hine, "Rehearsal for Freedom."

76 "Memorandum for Honorable David K. Niles from Phileo Nash, March 12, 1946, 2, box 56, Folder Minorities-Negro-General-VA Hospitalization 1946, Papers of Phileo Nash, Harry S. Truman Presidential Library, Independence, Missouri. Karen Kruse Thomas provided this to me.

77 Johnny Ford interview.

78 Thomas J. Ward Jr. (*Black Physicians*, 263) argues that black doctors' need to prove themselves to whites explains in part their acceptance of the Study. He explains Dibble's role but does not consider whether this generalization applied to him.

79 I am grateful to Cynthia Wilson at Tuskegee University for discussions on this point.

80 Marable, "Tuskegee and the Politics of Illusion." The term comes from existentialist Jean-Paul Sartre and is about bad faith. The quote for the definition is from Philosophy Pages, <http://www.philosophypages.com/dy/m2.htm>, accessed October 20, 2008.

CHAPTER 9

1 Sedwick, *Women of Courage*, cover photograph. The Oveta Culp Hobby medal she wears in this photograph functions almost as if it were a *punctum*, what French theorist Roland Barthes, in *Camera Lucida*, suggests is a place in a photograph that reaches out to us almost unawares as an ironic and subjective point. Rivers says very clearly that of all her awards the Hobby medal was the one that mattered the most to her; see Thompson, "Eunice Rivers Laurie Interview," 20.

2 Ibid. Rivers claimed she retired from the Study in 1965, but she continued to help on occasion through 1972; see Laurie, Deposition, *Pollard v. U.S.*, 120.

3 Ruth Hill, the organizer of the black women's oral history project at the Schlesinger Library at Radcliffe, the project upon which the photography was based, provided me, on January 24, 1994, with the quote on Rivers's hands and why she was chosen for the cover and poster. As Hudita Mustafa has argued: "Portraits are strategic presentations of partial truths: women work on themselves as canvases of representation, navigating the relative risks of display and concealment to forge their social selves"; Mustafa, "Portraits of Modernity," 188.

4 Historian Joan Scott, in her influential article "The Evidence of Experience," concluded: "Experience is at once always already an interpretation and is in need of interpretation" (37).

5 Rivers is often seen as the only "woman," other than the men's wives, in the story. There were other (white) women who worked on the Study—Anne R. Yobs (physician and researcher), Geraldine A. Gleeson, Eleanor V. Price, Lida J. Usilton, Eleanor N. Walker, Martha Bruyere, and Dorothy S. Rambo (statisticians or epidemiologists). On the ignoring of these women, see White, "Sociocultural Issues."

6 Quoted in Laura Parker, "'Bad Blood' Still Flows in Tuskegee Study," USA Today, April 28, 1997, 6A. Frank Cooper, Emma Cooper's father, went blind.

7 Laurie, Deposition, Pollard v. U.S., 109.

8 Herman Shaw interview, Washington D.C., May 15, 2007.

9 On "Nurse Rivers syndrome," see Thornton, "African Americans Moving into the 21st Century." For one of the best critiques of the "Tuskegee" way, see the first one hundred pages of Ralph Ellison's magnificent novel, Invisible Man.

10 Brandt, "Racism and Research," 24.

11 National League for Nursing, Critical Thinking in Nursing (VHS).

12 For a critique of the blame heaped upon her, see Hammonds, "Your Silence Will Not Protect You," 345.

13 In the play and film, Miss Evers' Boys, the Rivers character is seen giving testimony at the fictional equivalent of the Kennedy Senate hearings. This never happened; see chapter 11.

14 A Conversation on Moral Intuition at the National Bioethics Center (DVD).

15 Rev. Charles Noble interview. In her deposition, she reports on going to Atlanta to meet with CDC officials a year after the story of the Study broke: "I came back and had to go in the hospital after fooling with all of those things up there"; Laurie, Deposition, Pollard v. U.S., 79.

16 Her notoriety is in part because she is the only person to whom historian James H. Jones devotes an entire chapter in Bad Blood and because she became the central character in the play and then the film Miss Evers' Boys. For more on Jones's view, see chapter 10; on the play/film, see chapter 11.

17 Interview with Vanessa Northington Gamble in Susceptible to Kindness (VHS).

18 She is buried in the Greenwood Cemetery in Tuskegee. I try, every time I go there, to clear the gravestone.

19 The 1953 article on the Study, which lists Rivers as the first author, provides a contradiction. "The nurse was a native of the county," it reports, "who had lived near her patients all her life, and was thoroughly familiar with their local ideas and customs."

Yet a page or two later the article states that she was "born in Georgia"; Rivers et al., "Twenty Years of Follow-up," 125, 128.

20 "In Loving Memory of Mrs. Eunice Verdell Laurie," Funeral Program, September 1, 1986, box 1, Laurie Papers; Thompson, "Eunice Rivers Laurie Interview"; "Salaries," box 18, Salaries Folder, CDC-GA. The pre-1930 census records place her birth at "abt 1900."

21 Smith, "Neither Victim nor Villain," 352.

22 Early County, 1920 Census Records. Rivers reports on the deaths of the two older children in Thompson, "Eunice Rivers Laurie Interview," 3.

23 Kittie Harvin is in the 1900 census but not the 1910 census. After his wife died, Albert Rivers remarried and raised two more children in the household; 1920 U.S. Federal Census Record, Jakin, Early, Georgia, roll T625–245, page 4A, Enumeration District 74, image 474.

24 Thompson, "Eunice Rivers Laurie Interview," 4.

25 Ibid., 5.

26 Ibid., 10.

27 Ibid., 11. For a longer description and analysis of this kind of work, see Smith, "Neither Victim nor Villain," 348–64.

28 Smith, "Neither Victim nor Villain."

29 Jones, interview with Eunice Rivers Laurie, May 3, 1977, tape 1, 10. I am grateful to James H. Jones for providing me with this copy of his interview. My assessment is based on reading her reports and on correspondence in the Tuskegee University archives and in the public health department records in the Alabama State Archives in Montgomery.

30 Thompson, "Eunice Rivers Laurie Interview," 14.

31 Laurie, Deposition, *Pollard v. U.S.*, 12.

32 See Lederer, "Tuskegee Syphilis Study," 266–75.

33 Dibble and Williams, "Interview with Eunice Rivers Laurie." There was no transcription of the tape. I made my own transcription with the assistance of Carmen Bryant; see Dibble and Williams, "Interview with Nurse Rivers." Williams was the Tuskegee University archivist at the time, and Helen Dibble, Dr. Eugene Dibble's widow, was a librarian.

34 Thompson, "Eunice Rivers Laurie Interview," 15–16.

35 Dibble and Williams, "Interview with Nurse Rivers," 337.

36 Eunice R. Laurie to Miss Eleanor V. Price, September 12, 1963, box 8, Correspondence Folder, CDC-GA.

37 Thompson, "Eunice Rivers Laurie Interview," 16.

38 Elizabeth Sims interview, July 29, 2008.

39 Kimmelman, "Therapeutic Misconception."

40 Jones, interview with Eunice Rivers Laurie, tape 1, 10.

41 Laurie, Deposition, *Pollard v. U.S.*, 28.

42 John C. Cutler to Mrs. Eunice R. Laurie, May 6, 1958, Laurie Papers.

43 Eunice Rivers to Jessie Marriner, Director of the Bureau of Child Hygiene and Public Health Nursing, September 9, 1932, Alabama Department of Public Health,

Folder Macon County Miscellaneous 1930–33, Alabama Administrative Files, 1928–35, State Archives, Montgomery; Irene Beavers interview.

44 Dibble and Williams, "Interview with Nurse Rivers," 321. In Thompson, "Eunice Rivers Laurie Interview" (14), Rivers makes this position even clearer: "And they never took anybody with early syphilis. And early syphilis was about three years or two years, that's considered early. After that, it was supposed to be late syphilis. What it was doing, it was doing it to you, you weren't transmitting it." In her deposition, she also says that the men in the early and secondary stages would have chancres and rashes; Laurie, Deposition, *Pollard v. U.S.*, 29.

45 Dibble and Williams, "Interview with Nurse Rivers," 326.

46 This theme of caring, not diagnosing, is a constant in all of her interviews.

47 Laurie, Deposition, *Pollard v. U.S.*, 33.

48 Record 388, box 26, TMF.

49 Anne R. Yobs to Eunice Rivers Laurie, November 6, 1963; Laurie to Yobs, November 18, 1963, Record A12, box 1, TMF. It is possible, of course, that Yobs was lying about the treatment, but the medical record shows penicillin treatment being given in 1951.

50 Dibble and Williams, "Interview with Nurse Rivers," 322, 323, 331. All the quotes in this paragraph are from this interview unless otherwise noted.

51 This view of what she was doing comes out most strongly throughout her deposition (Laurie, Deposition, *Pollard v. U.S.*) and in her interview with historian James Jones.

52 Thompson, "Eunice Rivers Laurie Interview," 23.

53 On this dilemma, see Wilkerson, *False Dawn*.

54 Dibble and Williams, "Interview with Nurse Rivers," 326; Laurie, Deposition, *Pollard v. U.S.*, 86.

55 For a more theoretical discussion of some of these issues of power and empathy/caring (although primarily for medicine, not nursing), see More and Milligan, *Empathic Practitioner*.

56 Dibble and Williams, "Interview with Nurse Rivers," 325.

57 Rev. Charles Noble interview.

58 Laurie, Deposition, *Pollard v. U.S.*, 98.

59 Rivers et al., "Twenty Years of Follow-up." In the article, "she" claims to have lost only one autopsy case. Jay Katz, who served on the Ad Hoc Advisory Panel, thought she had not written this (Jay Katz interview). It is possible she was interviewed for the article rather than wrote it herself. Physicians Stanley Schuman and Sidney Olansky were the coauthors, as was field organizer Lloyd Simpson. The conclusion of the article, emphasizing cooperation and the need for the follow-up worker, reads as if it were almost an internal argument for the PHS to keep funding such nonmedical work if long-term studies were to succeed.

60 This is, of course, my "reading" of her voice on the Dibble and Williams, "Interview with Nurse Rivers," tape.

61 Laurie, Deposition, *Pollard v. U.S.*, 102.

62 When I presented my first talk on Nurse Rivers to a nursing audience at Fitchberg State College in 1992, many of the older nurses in the audience responded with

stories of their own "research" experiences at major teaching hospitals. They voiced
their clearly troubled sense that they often had no idea what they were giving to the
patients. One nurse had an insightful comment when she told me: "The only person
who is blind in a double blinded research study is the nurse."

In using these two voices, Rivers speaks in what Mae Henderson describes as
"the internal dialogue with the plural aspects of self"; see Henderson, "Speaking in
Tongues," 17.

63 Laurie, Deposition, *Pollard v. U.S.*, 95.

64 Ibid., 122–24. Gray's questions are leading and show how he was trying to protect
her.

65 This is the view most clearly articulated by Jones, *Bad Blood*—that by the 1940s the
Study's nontreatment rationale was so strong that even the presence of penicillin
did not change the thinking of those in charge of the Study.

66 Laurie, Deposition, *Pollard v. U.S.*, 118–30. Gray later said that she should have had
counsel. He suggests that she defended herself without this kind of legal support.
See Gray's discussion about her in *A Conversation on Moral Intuition at the National Bioethics Center* (DVD).

67 Thompson, "Eunice Rivers Laurie Interview."

68 Francis Johnson interview.

69 Peters et al., "Untreated Syphilis," 147–48.

70 Laurie, Deposition, *Pollard v. U.S.*, 68–69.

71 Jones, interview with Eunice Rivers Laurie, tape 1, 31.

72 Darlene Clark Hine uses the term "super moral" to describe women like Rivers; see
her "Rape and the Inner Lives of Black Women," 915.

73 Thompson, "Eunice Rivers Laurie Interview," 9.

74 Helen Taylor Dibble and Daniel Williams, "Interview," 325.

75 Clarke, "Professional Commitment," 125. All of the women Clarke interviewed
worked in Tuskegee and were about a decade younger than Rivers. Many of them
knew her.

76 Irene Beavers interview.

77 Ibid.

78 Hine, "Rape and the Inner Lives of Black Women," 915.

79 Higginbotham, "Beyond the Sound of Silence," 58–59. For further discussion of this
differentiation within the black community, see Carby, *Reconstructing Womanhood*;
Higginbotham, *Righteous Discontent*; and the essays in Hine, *Black Women's History*. On health in particular, see Susan L. Smith, *Sick and Tired*.

80 Jones, interview with Eunice Rivers Laurie, tape 1, 15–16.

81 Hammonds, "Black (W)holes," 137.

82 Etter-Lewis, *My Soul Is My Own*, 186.

83 Reginald James, Testimony before the HEW Panel, February 23, 1973, 50–77, box 2,
HEW-NLM.

84 Rivers's time sense here and her views are at odds with Jones's reading of Dr. Reginald G. James's comments from a *New York Times* interview published on July 27,
1972, the day after the Tuskegee story broke. Jones wrote: "Between 1939 and 1941 he
had been involved with public health work in Macon County—specifically with the

diagnosis and treatment of syphilis." In his interviews, James claims it was Rivers who kept him from treating some of the men in the Study and that this left him "distraught and disturbed." He claims to have treated a man who never returned, presumably fearful over the loss of his benefits (Jones, *Bad Blood*, 6).

85 Dibble and Williams, "Interview with Nurse Rivers," 329. In her deposition, she says the same thing about her advice to the men: "I said go find your doctor"; Laurie, Deposition, *Pollard v. U.S.*, 117.

86 See also Jones, interview with Eunice Rivers Laurie, tape 1, 19.

87 This is the point of view taken by both Jones and Gray.

88 Irene Beavers interview.

89 Ibid.

90 Seward Hiltner to Broadus Butler, October 29, 1972, Ad Hoc Advisory Papers, Container 2, 5, HEW-NLM.

91 Joseph G. Caldwell to Dr. William J. Brown, May 4, 1970, Tuskegee Syphilis Study, box 8, Folder 1970, CDC-GA.

92 Eleanor N. Walker to Dr. John C. Cutler, December 4, 1952, box 1, Folder 1952, ibid.

93 Jones, interview with Eunice Rivers Laurie, tape 1, 36.

94 Interview with James H. Jones in *Susceptible to Kindness* (VHS).

95 Dibble and Williams, "Interview with Nurse Rivers," 331–32.

96 I am grateful to the late Dick Newman of the Du Bois Institute, Harvard University, for suggesting this parallel to Oskar Schindler, the German man whose "list" saved countless Jews from the Nazis.

97 Linda Williams, *Playing the Race Card*, 8. On moral rage and social change, Williams (308) quotes Bill Nichols, *Blurred Boundaries*, 39.

98 For this kind of analysis of Arendt's "banality of evil," see Neiman, *Evil in Modern Thought*, 301–3.

99 See Nelson, "Ethical Expertise," 69–87.

100 Amy and Walter Pack interview.

101 Laurie, Deposition, *Pollard v. U.S.*, 91.

102 Auchmutey, "Ghosts of Tuskegee."

103 James H. Jones to Susan M. Reverby, Personal Communication, July 7, 2004. This quote can be read as either her cold assessment of the situation or her sense that she was no longer able to care. I thank Kenneth Hamilton, Riggins Earl, and Cynthia Wilson for our lively debate over this in Tuskegee on July 30, 2008.

104 Smitherman, *Talkin and Testifyin*, 58.

105 Allen, *Without Sanctuary*. Cynthia Wilson at Tuskegee University reports that she is constantly asked why the men were examined in such deplorable conditions (interview with Cynthia Wilson, July 30, 2008). The assumption that the Tony Hooker photo montage reflects the condition of the hospital *before* it closed is often made.

CHAPTER 10

1 On the link between the Study and other abuses, see King, "Reflections on Race"; and Gamble, "Under the Shadow."

2 On the linkage of medical experimentation with medical encounters and education, see Washington, *Medical Apartheid*; and Reverby, "Inclusion and Exclusion." See also Holloway, "Accidental Communities."

3 Berlin, "American Slavery," 1265.

4 The exception here is White, "Unraveling the Tuskegee Study."

5 Rosenberg, "Meanings, Policies, and Medicine," 27.

6 Angell, "Ethics of Clinical Research"; Fairchild and Bayer, "Uses and Abuses."

7 Lederer, *Subjected to Science*; Jones, *Bad Blood*, 98–99; Veressayev, *Memoirs of a Physician*, 333–67.

8 For example, see the debate on the experimental surgeries of J. Marion Sims, in Schwartz, *Birthing a Slave*, 227–56; and Wall, "Medical Ethics of J. Marion Sims."

9 Edelstein, *Hippocratic Oath*. On the distinction between an oath and a code, see Robert Baker et al., *American Medical Ethics Revolution*.

10 James Jones argues that there was a "formless relativism" in medical ethics during the time of the Study, but subsequent historical research has questioned this. See, in particular, Fletcher, "Case Study"; and Freidenfelds and Brandt, "Commentary."

11 There are numerous histories of bioethics. See for example, Rothman, *Strangers at the Bedside*; Jonsen, *Birth of Bioethics*; and Halpern, *Lesser Harms*. In the postwar period, the term "biomedicine" began to be used to refer to the realm of biological research that increasingly informed medical research, practice, and medicine. In turn, bioethics replaced the concept of medical ethics alone.

12 For an excellent historical and visual guide to postwar ethics, see the historical sections of the Human Radiation Studies report, available through the website: <http://www.eh.doe.gov/ohre/index.html>, accessed July 9, 2006; and Katz "The Consent Principle of the Nuremberg Code," 228.

13 Moreno, "Protectionism in Research."

14 Halpern, "Constructing Moral Boundaries"; Halpern, *Lesser Harms*.

15 Moreno and Lederer, "Revising the History," 235.

16 Carol Levine, quoted in Childress, "Nuremberg's Legacy," 357. Moreno, "Protectionism in Research," uses the Tuskegee changes all as a subtitle to his article. Jonathan D. Moreno, "Protectionism in Research Involving Human Subjects," <http://www.onlineethics.org/cms/10153.aspx>, accessed October 20, 2008; Cooter, "Bioethics."

17 For recent rereadings of these scandals, see Howell and Hayward, "Writing Willowbrook"; and Lerner, "Sins of Omission."

18 Beecher, "Ethics and Clinical Research"; "Letters to the Editor"; Rothman, *Strangers at the Bedside*, 70–84, 263–65. See also Freidenfelds, "Recruiting Allies for Reform."

19 Jon Harkness, "Henry Knowles Beecher," *American National Biography Online*, <http://o-www.amb.org.luna.wellesley.edu/articles/12/12-01168.html>, accessed July 18, 2006; Harkness, Lederer, and Wikler, "Laying Ethical Foundations." I am grateful to Lara Freidenfelds and Martin Pernick for their discussions with me about Beecher.

20 The book was published in August 1972 but clearly had been finished the year before; Jay Katz interview.

21 Solomon, "Rhetoric of Dehumanization."

22 Advisory Committee on Human Radiation Experiments, *Final Report*, 74.

23 See Maschke, "Human Research Protections."

24 Richard Wright, *White Man, Listen!*, 109.

25 "Interview with Robert Levine," May 12, 2004, 5, *Oral History of the Belmont Report*, <http://www.hhs.gov/ohrp/belmontArchive.html>, accessed July 20, 2006.

26 Childress et al., *Belmont Revisited*. On the history of the report, see Jonsen, "Birth of the Belmont Report"; and Jonsen, "Belmont Report." This latter website also includes a video on the twenty-fifth anniversary of the report and oral history interviews with a number of the commissioners.

27 Jonsen, "Birth of the Belmont Report."

28 Moreno, "Protectionism in Research," 23; Brandt and Freidenfelds, "Commentary."

29 Goodman, McElligott, and Marks, "Introduction: Making Human Bodies Useful."

30 Halpern, "Constructing Moral Boundaries," 77, 86.

31 Arthur Caplan, quoted in Wolinsky, "Steps Still Being Taken."

32 Interview with Robert Levine, twenty-fifth anniversary of the Belmont Commission Report, 2004, Oral Histories of Commission Members, <http://www.hhs.gov/ohrp/belmontArchive.html/#hisArchive2>, accessed July 31, 2006.

33 See Roger Brown and Kulik, "Flashbulb Memories."

34 Fairchild and Bayer, "Uses and Abuses." Letters in response to this article's original publication can be found in *Science* 285 (July 2, 1999): 47–50.

35 These methodological debates are covered in many bioethics texts. See, for example, Jonsen, *Birth of Bioethics*; Bondeson et al., *New Knowledge in the Biomedical Sciences*; and Jonsen and Toulmin, *Abuse of Casuistry*.

36 Cooter, "Bioethics;" Jonsen, *Birth of Bioethics*; Beauchamp, *Principles of Biomedical Ethics*. On the problem this creates for "communities" as other, see Holloway, "Accidental Communities."

37 Jonsen, *Birth of Bioethics*, 335.

38 Goodman, McElligott, and Marks, "Introduction: Making Human Bodies Useful," 4–5.

39 See Kahn, Mastroianni, and Sugarman, "Introduction: Changing Claims about Justice in Research."

40 When the Belmont commissioners began to look at prisoners and research, they discovered that being in a research study was seen as an "extra," more often offered to white than to black prisoners. For this history, see Harkness, "Research behind Bars." On this move from exclusion to inclusion, see Epstein, *Inclusion*; and Reverby, "Inclusion and Exclusion."

41 King was put on the commission because of her civil rights background and also, in all probability—along with Dorothy Height, the longtime president of the National Council of Negro Women—to be the African American voices. King had served as both the acting director and the deputy director of the Office of Civil Rights within HEW, now HHS.

42 Belmont Oral History Project, 7, LeRoy B. Walters Oral History Interview with

Patricia King, September 9, 2004, <http://www.hhs.gov/ohrp/belmontArchive/html>, accessed July 10, 2006.

43 King, "Race, Justice, and Research."

44 King, "Dangers of Difference"; King, "Dangers of Difference, Revisited"; Wolf, "Erasing Difference," 65.

45 Brandt, "Racism and Research"; Jones, *Bad Blood*.

46 Johansson, "Food for Thought," 101. For example, Yale law professor Harlan L. Dalton, in "AIDS in Blackface," 220, cites both Brandt and Jones in footnotes but then goes on to claim that the Study was one "in which the government purposely exposed black men to syphilis."

47 When I typed (on February 21, 2009) the words "Tuskegee syphilis" into Google, 84,600 hits resulted, as compared to 3,870 for "Willowbrook hepatitis" and 10,500 for "Jewish Chronic Disease Hospital and injection of live cancer cells."

48 James H. Jones interview, November 12, 1998. All quotes are from this interview unless otherwise noted. More than a decade after *Bad Blood*, Jones published his definitive *Alfred Kinsey: A Public Private Life*.

49 For more on white southerners and their families on race, see Curry et al., *Deep in Our Hearts*.

50 Jones refers to himself in the third person in connection with Gray in *Bad Blood*. He writes of himself as a "young historian" who provided Gray with "mounds of materials he had uncovered" and "helped with subsequent research on the case" (216). Jones's archival materials did in fact allow Gray to continue his lawsuit. Gray in turn has acknowledged the importance of their relationship; see Gray, *Tuskegee Syphilis Study*, 90. Jones remembers sitting in on the depositions, working with Columbia University law professor Harold Edgar to make the history meaningful and counter the claims the PHS doctors were to make. Gray also called in a group of the men who had been the subjects and controls to meet Jones in his office in Tuskegee, although Jones said laughingly that Gray introduced him as "Dr. Jones from Washington, D.C., who wants to interview you," before he realized that this would be a dreadful way to get any of the men from the Study to talk. And once the lawsuit ended in 1974 and the threat of the legal retribution no longer "hung over the researchers' heads," Jones found that several of them were only too willing to "testify" in their interviews with him to what they thought had happened.

51 Gray argues: "I felt the same about Tuskegee Institute as I did about Nurse Rivers — that the Institute and its officials were misled, betrayed, and taken advantage of as she had been"; Gray, *Tuskegee Syphilis Study*, 86.

52 Brandt, "Racism and Research." His book on venereal disease is *No Magic Bullet*.

53 For example, while it is true that men in the control group who got the disease were sometimes switched into the nontreatment program, Dr. Vonderlehr wrote to Murray Smith on August 11, 1942, to tell him that the controls who got syphilis "have lost their value to the study. There is no reason why these *patients should not be given appropriate treatment* [italics added]." Vonderlehr suggested that the only caveat might be objections from the PHS's man in Tuskegee, Dr. Deibert, but there is no evidence that this occurred, and Vonderlehr told Smith not to expect

it (Vonderlehr to Smith, August 11, 1942), in Reverby, *Tuskegee's Truths*, 96. Brandt uses the letters between Vonderlehr and Smith from earlier that summer that the Ad Hoc Advisory Panel had, but not the August letter, because this was then at CDC.

54 Brandt's article is reprinted in at least six collections in ethics, sociology, and history of medicine. Brandt would go on to a position in medical ethics and medical history at Harvard.

55 Shick, "Race, Class, and Medicine"; Chet Raymo, "Look Ahead, but Don't Forget the Shameful Past," *Boston Globe*, October 22, 1990, 24. I suspect that Raymo's comment about "many Americans" does not extend to African Americans. Similarly, physician playwright David Feldshuh (see chapter 11) had heard nothing about the Study until he read Jones's book; David Feldshuh interview, August 16, 2006.

56 The characterization of the reviews of *Bad Blood* in the footnotes of Capshew, *Kinsey's Biographers*, 471, is completely disingenuous and cherry-picks the quotes. See, for example, for reviews, H. Jack Geiger, "An Experiment with Lives," *New York Times*, June 21, 1981, 9; Brandt, "Infernal Medicine"; and Rosenkrantz, "Non-Random Events."

57 Jones would spend the rest of his career as a historian at the University of Houston and then at the University of Arkansas before retiring to continue writing.

58 Caplan, "James H. Jones, *Bad Blood*."

59 For an effort to provide a wide range of views on the Study and some of the primary documents, see *Tuskegee's Truths*, which has a preface by Jones and is in a series edited by Brandt. I, too, used Brandt's article as the introductory summary of the story of the Study.

60 My student assistant, Jacqueline Mahendra, searched the *New York Times* and ethnic news indexes for the Study from 1972 to 2004. I am grateful for this work.

61 On Tuskegee's layering on other historical experiences, see Gamble, "Under the Shadow." See also Love, *One Blood*.

62 Wil Hagood, "True or False, Rumors Spread," *Boston Globe*, December 15, 1996, A1.

63 U.S. Department of Health and Human Services, *Report of the Secretary's Task Force*. The report is referred to as the Heckler Report, after HHS secretary Margaret M. Heckler.

64 Auchmutey, "Ghosts of Tuskegee."

65 Epstein, *Inclusion*; Reverby, "Inclusion and Exclusion," 111.

66 Mastroianni and Kahn, "Swinging on the Pendulum," 21.

67 See Garber and Arnold, "Promoting the Participation of Minorities."

68 Epstein, *Inclusion*, 195. See also Gamble, "Trust," 437–38; and Jacobs et al., "Understanding African Americans' Views."

69 U.S. Department of Health and Human Services, *Prevention and Beyond*, 6, quoted in Quinn, "Belief in AIDS," S6–7.

70 Pickle, Quinn, and Brown, "HIV/AIDS Coverage in Black Newspapers."

71 Kwame Nantambu, "The Real Origin of AIDS and U.S. Tuskegee Experiment," November 15, 2001, <http://www.trinicenter.com/kwame/2001/nov/12001.htm>, accessed August 16, 2006. This claim is based on work done by Dr. Jack Felder. It

spread throughout the Black Muslim community and on the web. See, for example, Felder's self-published "AIDS-US Germ Warfare at Its Best with Documents and Proof" (1986) and "White People Want to Wipe Us Out," *The Final Call*, <http://www.finalcall.com/perspectives/interviews/dr_felder07-30-2000>, accessed August 17, 2006. See also Cantwell, *AIDS and the Doctors of Death*. This belief gained some momentum during the presidential bid of Barack Obama. Jeremiah Wright, Obama's former pastor, expressed this view during his now-infamous "God Damn America" sermon. Once again, the Internet was filled with statements about a conspiracy to infect African Americans, associating the Study with AIDS.

72 Freimuth et al., "African Americans' Views," 800. For example, an episode of the undercover cop show *New York Undercover*; see <http://epguides.com/NewYork Undercover/>, accessed August 18, 2006.

73 Stephen B. Thomas and Quinn, "Tuskegee Syphilis Study"; Stephen Thomas, quoted in M. A. J. McKenna, "Study in Shame," *Atlanta Journal-Constitution*, February 21, 1997, 01D; Carl Rowan, "Years Later, Ghosts of Tuskegee Still Haunt Blacks," *Chicago Sun-Times*, May 4, 1997, 30.

74 Gamble, "Under the Shadow."

75 Brandon, Isaac, and LaVeist, "Legacy of Tuskegee."

76 Gamble and Stone, "U.S. Policy on Health Inequalities."

77 As Lee later told a *Newsweek* reporter, "And given the history of African-Americans in this country, from slavery to the Tuskegee Experiment, it's not that farfetched"; transcript of Bill Maher, Michel Martin, Spike Lee, and Tucker Carlson exchange, on *Real Time with Bill Maher*, October 21, 2005; "Spike Lee: 'Not Far-Fetched' to Say New Orleans Levees Deliberately Destroyed," *NewsBusters*, <http://newsbusters.org/node/2441>, accessed August 18, 2006. This link also provides a video of the exchange. "Katrina Survivor to Spike Lee," *Newsweek*, August 13, 2006, <http://www.prenewswire.com/cgi-bin/stories.pl?ACCT+109&STOR>, accessed August 18, 2006.

78 On rumors and their role in the black community, see Patricia Turner, *I Heard It through the Grapevine*. Wil Haygood, "True or False, Rumors Spread," uses the phrase "rumor turned to gospel." It is a common expression, but the argument here is that this belief is not just in black communities.

79 I have given up trying to keep track of all the times this falsehood is repeated. I have tried repeatedly to correct this—by calling television news stations and writing back when newspaper reporters or bloggers misreport it and correcting it when I get asked about it at lectures, on radio shows, and at talks both academic and public. In regard to the Airmen, I was told this directly when I did a talk radio show on the Study in Chicago in the mid-1990s. I suspect part of this is a "February" problem: that is, actor Laurence Fishburne starred in both of the HBO movies, *Miss Evers' Boys* and *The Tuskegee Airmen*, which have been re-aired for more than a decade during Black History Month. On *Miss Evers' Boys*, see the next chapter. In regard to the students, comedian and activist Dick Gregory lectured in 1974 that the students would then return home to infect their communities; see Weisbord, *Genocide*, 37.

80 For this interpretation of the photograph, see Gamble, "The Enduring Legacy of

the Tuskegee Syphilis Study," Fifth Annual LeNoir NMA Pediatric Allergy, Asthma, and Immunology Lecture," March 27, 2003, University of California, San Diego, <http://www.uctv.tv>, accessed August 13, 2006.

81 I am grateful to my mother, Gertrude Fox Mokotoff, for assistance on this question. She was a bacteriologist and medical technician and did syphilis serologies at the Bedford Hills Tuberculosis Hospital in New York in the late 1930s.

82 Wendy Dingel, "Syphilis," Bacteriology at University of Wisconsin at Madison website, <http://www.bact.wisc.edu/Bact330/lecturesyphilis>, accessed August 14, 2006. See also Beerman, "Future Research Needs."

83 Magnuson et al., "Inoculation Syphilis." Two of the authors of this study were Sidney Olansky and John C. Cutler, both of whom directed the Study in the 1950s; see chapter 7. I thank Paul Weisner for help on this section.

84 Part of this argument was made in Reverby, "More Than Fact and Fiction."

85 See chapter 11 on the documentaries and play that appeared around the same time as the Human Radiation Experiment reports.

86 Portelli, *Death of Luigi Trastulli*, 2, 15.

87 Stephen B. Thomas and Quinn, "Tuskegee Syphilis Study." Vanessa Northington Gamble argues that Thomas and Quinn have put too much emphasis on "Tuskegee" itself. She writes that the black community's "mistrust [of the institutions of medicine and public health] predated public revelations of the Tuskegee Study"; see "Under the Shadow."

88 Patricia Turner, *I Heard It through the Grapevine*, 3. For an argument about the link between black bodies and citizenship, see Long, *Doctoring Freedom*.

89 Homi K. Bhabha uses the phrase "ideological construction of otherness"; see "The Other Question: The Stereotype and Colonial Discourse," *Screen* 24 (1983): 4, quoted in Mercer, *Welcome to the Jungle*, 176. Bhabha sees this fixity as "an important fixture of colonial discourse." But it is also true for "internal colonial" discourses as well.

90 Jill Lepore, "Just the Facts, Ma'am: Fake Memoirs, Factual Fictions, and the History of History," *New Yorker*, March 24, 2008, 80.

CHAPTER 11

1 The television references to "Tuskegee" are now too numerous to count. For examples, see the *House* episode that aired on February 2, 2007, and the *Saturday Night Live* version on October 28, 2006; see epilogue. I heard Peter Jennings on ABC and Tom Brokaw on NBC announce on the evening news broadcasts that the government gave the men syphilis.

2 In what would become the last chapter for the revised edition of *Bad Blood* in 1993, Jones used the work by Stephen B. Thomas and Quinn ("Tuskegee Syphilis Study") to make the AIDS/"Tuskegee"/trust link. See Jones, "The Tuskegee Legacy"; and the revised paperback edition of *Bad Blood*, which appeared in 1993. Numerous studies since then have tried to measure, through telephone surveys and focus groups, whether it is specifically "Tuskegee" that makes the difference in whether or not individuals will trust doctors or rather, as I am arguing here, that "Tuskegee" becomes a vocabulary word for a larger set of concerns. See also Gamble, "Under the Shadow of Tuskegee."

3 Linda Williams, *Playing the Race Card*, 4.

4 Gates, *Thirteen Ways*, 121.

5 On trauma and identity, see Eyerman, *Cultural Trauma*. On the "racial passion play," see Patricia Williams, "American Kabuki."

6 Byron, *Tuskegee Experiments*, CD, Nonesuch Records, 1991; Don Byron interview. Byron's music often reflects both race and class issues in historical perspective.

7 See <www.donbyron.com> for a full list of his recordings. Byron's albums range in style from Mickey Katz's klezmer music to Duke Ellington's big band sounds to Junior Walker's R&B.

8 Sadiq Bey often uses just his first name, as on this album; see W. Kim Heron, "The Story of Griot Galaxy and a Renaissance for Faruq Z. Bey," *MetroTimes*, June 25, 2003, <http://www.metrotimes.com/editorial/story.asp?id=5001>, accessed February 9, 2007.

9 Peter Watrous, "Music with Morality," *New York Times*, Arts and Leisure, February 23, 1992, 32.

10 Sadiq [Bey], "Tuskegee Experiment."

11 Byron expresses this view again on the track "Tuskegee Strutter's Ball," also on this album.

12 Steingroot, "Lauding Byron," 78, uses this term to describe Byron and also Mickey Katz's klezmer music and its place in American culture.

13 By contrast, the sound track for the *Nova* film on the Study, "Deadly Deception," used blues, and the ABC *Primetime Live* segment used gospel.

14 *Bad Blood* was filmed by the BBC and shown on A&E television in 1994. The National League for Nursing did a video entitled *Critical Thinking in Nursing: Lessons from Tuskegee*, which included interviews with historians and nursing leaders and a fictional dialogue written for an actress playing Rivers, which is called "a re-enactment of Eunice Rivers' thoughts."

15 Jay Schadler interview. For longer discussion of this segment, see chapter 7.

16 My own small involvement with the making of the segment highlights this problem. I had spoken briefly to the *Primetime* researcher as the broadcast was being planned. About an hour before the show went on live, an operator cut into a telephone conversation I was on (this was before call waiting) to announce an emergency call from ABC news. Correspondent Diane Sawyer had walked into the studio, read the script that introduced and closed the segment, and asked if penicillin would have made any difference. The researchers who had written her lines did not know. New to research on the Study, I scrambled to find the answer for them and wondered why they had not asked Dr. Tim Johnson, ABC's physician reporter. I called them back. "Not to worry," the young voice at the other end of the phone announced, "we looked up the answer in a medical book." And so, in front of millions of viewers, Sawyer intoned the safest vague answer possible: "We may never know how many from that research group could have been saved."

17 Sidney Olansky, quoted in Tom Junod, "Deadly Medicine," 513.

18 George Strait interview. All subsequent quotes from George Strait are from this interview. Strait had done other films with *Nova* and knew that ABC would not do something this long.

19 "Deadly Deception," *Nova*. The show first aired on January 26, 1993.

20 The documentary is *Three Counties against Syphilis*. See Parascandola, "Syphilis at the Cinema."

21 George Strait interview; Denise DiIanni interview.

22 Auchmutey, "Ghosts of Tuskegee."

23 David Sencer, CDC director in the late 1960s and early 1970s, believes that Cutler would never have done this because he was too straitlaced and polite a person; David Sencer interview, January 12, 2007.

24 There was a financial settlement in the *Pollard v. U.S.* lawsuit, but none of the doctors still alive at that time were ever punished. The question of why they were not seen as violating any laws is a continuing one raised about the Study.

25 Feldshuh, *Miss Evers' Boys*; Feldshuh and Bernstein (directed by Joseph Sargent), *Miss Evers' Boys*, HBO films.

26 James H. Jones, quoted in Auchmutey, "Ghosts of Tuskegee"; James H. Jones interview, November 12, 1998.

27 Feldshuh instead had to rely upon his own artistic craft, Jones's interpretation, and two of the interviews done with the real Rivers in the late 1970s.

28 Palmer, "Paying for Suffering." Palmer produced a video based on Feldshuh's play called *Susceptible to Kindness: "Miss Evers' Boys" and the Tuskegee Syphilis Study*.

29 Quoted in Jones, *Bad Blood*, 68.

30 Feldshuh made up the term "jilly" for the dance but later discovered that there is a term close to it that means a form of jazz dancing.

31 On jury films as a particular kind of American popular form, see Clover, "Law."

32 David Feldshuh interview, June 5, 1992. All quotes from Feldshuh are from this interview unless otherwise noted.

33 Bernstein, *Inside Out*. Bernstein wrote for the *New Yorker* and *Yank*. He was blacklisted in 1950 and wrote under other names. He is responsible for scripts for such films as *Fail-Safe*, *The Molly Maguires*, and *The Front*. Walter Bernstein interview. See also Dan Georgakas, "Bad Art Makes Bad Politics, An Interview with Walter Bernstein," *New Labor Forum* (Spring/Summer 1999), <http://qcpages.qc.cuny.edu/newlaborforum/old/html/4_books.html>, accessed February 10, 2007.

34 Walter Bernstein interview. Rivers is always shown with her hair pinned up in braids in most of the known photographs, and members of the community who knew her remember her this way; Elizabeth Sims interview, January 17, 2007.

35 Feldshuh, *Miss Evers' Boys*. In the HBO film version, the lines about racial burden are given to Ossie Davis, who plays the fictional nurse's father and is seen living with her in her "hometown" of Tuskegee.

36 Sam Martin, quoted in Edward Wyatt, "Classic Book about America's Indians Gains a Few Flourishes as a Film," *New York Times*, May 9, 2007, B4.

37 Physician and anthropologist Melvin Konner critiqued the film by arguing: "The perpetrators were not faceless or nameless as depicted in 'Miss Evers' Boys,' which shifts blame to an African American nurse and doctor"; Melvin Konner, "'Miss Evers' Boys': A Bad Start to a Very Important Discussion," *First Person: Emory Report*, <http://www.emory.edu/EMORY_Report/erarchive/1997/April/erapril.21/4_21_97FirstPerson.html>, accessed November 18, 2002.

38 "Laurence Fishburne and Alfre Woodward Star in HBO Movie about Tuskegee Experiment on Syphilis," *Jet* (February 24, 1997): 60.

39 Tom Teepen, "Play Redeems Tuskegee Study Victims," *Atlanta Journal Constitution*, October 18, 1990, A13.

40 Johnny Ford interview, Tuskegee, Alabama, January 9, 1995. Larry Palmer, "Comments on 'Miss Evers' Boys,'" Cornell Reunion Weekend, June 1992, Ithaca, New York. Palmer worked with Feldshuh on the video *Susceptible to Kindness* about the play and the Study and was critical of the Brotus character's tensions between "his personal identity as a professional with his identity as a black man" and the distance between him and the Study's subjects.

41 Levi, *The Drowned and the Saved*.

42 James Jones had been negotiating with Spike Lee's film company to do a fictional version of the Study, but when the HBO film appeared to be in production, Lee dropped his project.

43 Kenny Leon interview.

44 Scott Glasser interview. The problem of the historical drama is often the weight it must carry about what "really happened." I experienced this when I called the HBO legal department to inquire about obtaining still photographs from the film. The legal assistant I spoke with asked if I knew these "were actors and not the real men." I explained that I did, but clearly she was not sure everyone would.

45 Gray's timing may have had more to do with the federal apology that was about to be announced. He had not protested the play—when it was staged in Montgomery, Birmingham, and Tuskegee—which the men are shown attending in the "Deadly Deception" video.

46 *Conversation on Moral Intuition* (DVD).

47 As with the federal apology in 1997, Gray reminded Feldshuh that "Mr. Shaw had told the nation they were not boys"; see chapter 12.

48 Denzin, *Reading Race*, 21.

49 See parallel argument in Rocchio, *Reel Racism*.

50 See Levinson, "Obstinate Forgetting."

51 HBO, *The Tuskegee Airmen* (New York: HBO Films, Robert Markowitz, director, 1995).

52 Reverby, "History of an Apology," 6.

CHAPTER 12

1 This is the advice Howells gave to novelist Edith Wharton.

2 The surgeon general serves as the nation's chief health educator and as head of the PHS Commissioned Corps.

3 For a discussion of the process from Foster's viewpoint, see Foster with Greenwood, *Make a Difference*.

4 Foster worked at John A. Andrew Memorial Hospital from 1965 to 1973. He was often the only obstetrician serving poor black women in the eight-county area around Tuskegee.

5 Jones, *Bad Blood*, 209; "Foster Addresses New Questions," *New York Times*, February 25, 1995, 9.

6 Foster had some success in explaining his medical procedures in the face of botched abortions, lack of prenatal care, and the problems of families of mentally retarded young women in the segregated South, but the Study proved harder to explain away.

7 "Foster Addresses New Questions."

8 Neil A. Lewis, "Ex-Colleague Says Clinton Nominee Knew of Syphilis Study in 1969," *New York Times*, February 28, 1995, A19. McCrae, who passed away in 2005, moved out of Tuskegee to rural Georgia in the early 1970s. He was indicted for the illegal prescribing of pain medication in 1997 but argued that his indictment was "revenge" in a "government sting" for his comments on Foster and as part of the "New World Order" conspiracy; see "Revenge Alleged as Motive for Government Sting!," <http://www.thewinds.org/1997/08/luther_mcrae.html>, accessed January 1, 2006; Howard Settler Jr. interview, Tuskegee, Alabama, August 2, 2006. See also Foster, *Make a Difference*, 103.

9 I know that such phone calls were made to James Jones, Allan M. Brandt, Vanessa Northington Gamble, Jay Katz, and Hal Edgar, and to me. The order of the callers explains much about how the media-driven aspects of the confirmation process worked. I was called first by National Public Radio, then by HHS general counsel, and then by the White House Counsel's Office. Could I supply evidence, each caller asked me, that Foster was or was not at the medical society meeting? And could he have known about the Study before 1972? In addition, because I was writing on Nurse Rivers at the time, I was asked in particular if it was possible for Foster to have known her and if he could have learned about the Study as well from Dr. Dibble, who had hired him for the position at the hospital.

10 Telephone interview with Andrew Hyman and Anna Durant, General Counsel's office, HHS, March 10 and March 13, 1995. By the second phone call, it was clear that there was concern that this was going to reach up higher into the HHS hierarchy, because they had awarded Rivers the department's Oveta Culp Hobby award. I was asked who had recommended Rivers for the award. We also discussed the kinds of questions that might come up about the Study in Foster's hearings.

11 U.S. Congress, Senate, Committee on Labor and Human Resources, *Henry W. Foster, Jr., of Tennessee*. Sections of these hearings that are specifically on the Study are reprinted in Reverby, *Tuskegee's Truths*, 443–56. "Dr. Foster and the Syphilis Study," *Washington Post*, March 1, 1995.

12 Foster, *Make a Difference*, 161–64.

13 U.S. Congress, Senate, Committee on Labor and Human Resources, *Henry W. Foster, Jr., of Tennessee*, 242–44.

14 Foster, *Make a Difference*, 164. Dr. Foster reiterated the same position when we discussed it; interview with Dr. Henry Foster Jr., Nashville, Tennessee, December 13, 2005.

15 Foster was also caught up in the presidential aspirations of Republican senators Phil Gramm and Robert Dole, who engineered the parliamentary maneuver.

16 For details on the symposium, see <http://www.healthsystem.virginia.edu/internet/library/historical/medical_history/bad_blood>, accessed October 20, 2008. I spoke at this conference and served on the Legacy Committee that lobbied for the federal apology.

17 Fletcher, "Case Study," 295. My notes taken at the conference are on his brief history of the ethics of the Study and the one sentence about the apology. It was not central to his speech.

18 This conclusion is based on my notes and discussion with James H. Jones, who also spoke.

19 Rueben Warren interview.

20 A. Cornelius Baker to Susan Reverby, April 22, 2007. Baker was the executive director of the National Association of People with AIDS. I am grateful to Cornelius Baker for speaking to me and for sending me the "Syphilis in the South" agenda.

21 Weyeneth, "Power of Apology," 38.

22 A. Cornelius Baker interview.

23 For more on how inclusion became an issue in the 1990s, see Epstein, *Inclusion*.

24 Don E. Detmer to Susan Reverby, April 13, 2007; Don Detmer interview; Dixie Snider interview; Rueben Warren interview.

25 Ralph Katz interview. Katz is now at the dental school at New York University and continues to write on the question of the Study's impact on minority fears of medicine. Warren is the director of the National Bioethics Center at Tuskegee University.

26 James A. Ferguson, Dean of the School of Veterinary Medicine at Tuskegee University, to Dr. Velma Blackwell, Associate Provost for Continuing Education, January 12, 1996, author's collection. I was already in Tuskegee doing research when the meeting happened, and I joined the committee.

27 See <http://www.tv.com/new-york-undercover/show/377/summary.html>. Vanessa Northington Gamble interview. It was Gamble who brought up the importance of the TV show's view at the second meeting. "Tuskegee" would appear again and again in other TV shows. The description of the events at the meetings are from my notes taken at the time.

28 "Notes Taken by RVK (Ralph Katz) at Workshop," faxed to workshop members, January 22, 1996.

29 See Legacy Committee, "Legacy Committee Request," 566, for list.

30 "Memo," Ralph V. Katz to Vanessa Gamble, April 23, 1996, author's collection.

31 Susan M. Reverby to Anthony T. Winn, "Comments on the Tuskegee Study Draft," April 18, 1996. I raised the question of the larger community and was concerned about some of the complexity of the history.

32 Legacy Committee, "Legacy Committee Request," 559–60.

33 Vanessa Northington Gamble to Susan Reverby, December 19, 2006: "Although we made additional recommendations, I think that at this time we must concentrate on obtaining a Presidential apology. If you have any other suggestions about how we should proceed please contact me or John Fletcher," she wrote to members of the Legacy Committee; author's collection.

34 Rueben Warren interview; "Black Caucus Urges U.S. to Apologize for Deceiving Syphilis Victims 60 Years Ago," *Jet* (March 10, 1997). This article makes it sound as if only the Congressional Black Caucus was responsible for the apology.

35 Dixie Snider interview.

36 A. Cornelius Baker to Ferdette West, Legislative Assistant to the Honorable Louis

Stokes, U.S. House of Representatives, April 24, 1997, is an example. Baker provided a copy of the letter to me. At the same time, Baker was contacted by HBO representatives because they were interested in getting community involvement in the roll-out to the television premiere of *Miss Evers' Boys*, which was due to air on February 22, 1997. HBO actually considered trying to get the film launch to be at the White House but was worried that White House officials might want to "edit." As Baker would later tell a reporter, "'The Tuskegee story is a central part of childhood lore' in many black communities. . . . It is 'one of the definite things we were told by our grandparents.'"

37 Sandra Crouse Quinn and Stephen Thomas interview. Thomas also told a reporter that Black Muslims were keeping the Study's story alive in communities; see Jeff Stryker, "Tuskegee's Long Arm Still Touches a Nerve," *New York Times*, April 13, 1997, 4:4.

38 Louis Stokes and Maxine Waters to The Honorable William Jefferson Clinton, February 7, 1997. I am grateful to Cornelius Baker for providing me with a copy of this letter.

39 Reverby, "History of an Apology."

40 Shaw, "Herman Shaw's Remarks." I was at the apology, and the description is from my notes and memory of the event.

41 Clinton, "President William J. Clinton's Remarks." Clinton also extended the charter of the National Bioethics Advisory Commission to October 1999.

42 Harter, Stephens, and Japp, "President Clinton's Apology." This analysis links the apology to the Clinton Race Commission and the AZT debate (see next chapter). But both came after, not before, the apology.

43 "White House Apology on Tuskegee," *CNN Live*.

44 Martin Kasindoft, "Tuskegee Survivors Make Trek to Capital for Apology," *USA Today*, May 15, 1997, 6A. The interview was done before the apology.

45 Schoen, *Choice and Coercion*, 248.

46 Fairchild and Bayer, "Uses and Abuses."

EPILOGUE

1 The term "counter-narrative" comes from Shweder, "Tuskegee Re-Examined."

2 The letters are available at the Public Citizen website, <http://www.citizen.org/publications>. The original letter was sent April 22, 1997, and was signed by Lurie and Wolfe, four other ethicists, an AIDS medical care director, and pediatrician George Silver. See also Audrey Addison, "Placebos, Ethics and Women," *Vibe Magazine* (Fall/Winter 1997): 22; and Angell, "Ethics of Clinical Research." For a case study of the debate, see "The Debate over AZT Clinical Trials," Harvard University Kennedy School Case Study, <http://www.ksg.harvard.edu/case/azt>, accessed June 20, 2007.

3 Varmus and Satcher, "Ethical Complexities."

4 Marcia Angell, "Tuskegee Revisited," *Wall Street Journal*, October 28, 1997, 1.

5 The "gold standard" in drug trials in the United States is a randomized, double-blind test of a new drug against a placebo. In cases where this is seen as unethical,

the new drug is to be tested against the standard drug for the particular disease or condition.

6 Personal communication, Daniel Wikler, Harvard School of Public Health, April 28, 2008.

7 Dr. Maina Kahindo, quoted in Gitau Warigi, "African AIDS Study Generates Anger, Bitter Exchanges," *Africa News Online*, <http://www.africanews.org>, accessed June 21, 2007.

8 See the quotes and argument in "Debate over AZT." See also Studdert and Brennan, "Clinical Trials."

9 World Medical Association, Revised Declaration of Helsinki Number 29, <http://www.wma.net.e/policy>, accessed June 22, 2007; Lie et al., "Standard of Care Debate"; Schuklenk, "Standard of Care Debate." I am grateful to Daniel Wikler for assistance on this issue.

10 "FDA Scraps Helsinki Declaration on Protecting Human Subjects," *Integrity in Science Watch Week of 5/05/2008*, <http://www.cspinet.org/integrity/watch/index .html>, accessed July 6, 2008.

11 One letter responding to Angell's editorial in the *Wall Street Journal* argued that there was a difference between scientists and doctors. "For the scientist," John Staddon, from the Department of Psychology at Duke University, wrote, "the only ethical question is whether any individual volunteer in the study would be worse off if the study were done than if it were not done"; "Letter to the Editor," *Wall Street Journal*, November 11, 1997, <http://o-proquest.umi.com.luna.wellesley.edu>, accessed June 9, 2007.

12 See Reverby, "Tuskegee: Could It Happen Again?"

13 For a parallel argument about the circulation of feminist ideas in the transnational setting, see Davis, *Making of Our Bodies, Ourselves*.

14 Benedek, "'Tuskegee Study' of Syphilis." The article was originally published in 1978.

15 The major "counter-narratives," in addition to the Benedek article, are Benedek and Erlen, "Scientific Environment"; White, "Unraveling the Tuskegee Study"; and Shweder, "Tuskegee Re-Examined." Shweder's article was picked up by *Arts and Letters Daily* and widely circulated on the Internet. Robert White has also written numerous other articles on the Study, including critiques of my work, in particular in *Journal of the National Medical Association*.

16 St. John, "Treatment of Cardiovascular Syphilis," 149.

17 In 1973, the federal investigating committee made an effort to thoroughly investigate the medical literature on treatment for late latent syphilis and concluded that the men should have been treated, especially after penicillin became widely available.

18 See H. Jack Geiger to the American Public Health Association's "Spirit of 1848" Listserv, "Re: Shweder article on Tuskegee," January 24, 2004, <http://www.spiritof 1848@yahoogroups.com>. See also Reverby, "More Than Fact and Fiction"; and Reverby, "Misrepresentations of the Tuskegee Study," 1180–81.

19 Robert White's and Richard Shweder's articles were both debated on the "Spirit

of 1848" Listserv when they appeared. On conservative use, see Jonah Goldberg, "Tall Tales about Tuskegee," May 2, 2008, National Review Online, <http://article .nationalreview.com>, accessed February 25, 2009.

20 Robert White has been untiring in his efforts to get the "facts" about the Study out. Although we have disagreed in and out of print, I do appreciate his efforts to counter much of the mythology.

21 Reverby, "More Than Fact and Fiction," 27.

22 Sheryl Gay Stolberg, "The Biotech Death of Jesse Gelsinger," *New York Times Magazine*, November 28, 1999, 136–40, 149–50.

23 Kampmeier, "Tuskegee Study," 200.

24 Gieryn, "Boundary-Work," 781. For a longer and contemporary discussion of this, see Epstein, *Inclusion*, 14, 111.

25 Shweder, "Idea of Moral Progress," 54.

26 In 2008, for example, opponents of a proposition favoring stem cell research in Michigan used photographs from the Study and a frightened and apparently black male voice to argue that unregulated medical research was too dangerous; see <http://www.2goes2far.com/in-the-name-of-good.html>, accessed October 23, 2008.

27 For a longer discussion of the politics of BiDil's approval and the "Tuskegee" link, see Reverby, "Special Treatment." See also Jonathan Kahn, "How a Drug Becomes Ethnic"; and Jonathan Kahn and Sankar, "BiDil."

28 Dr. Steven Nissen interview.

29 Quoted in Eric Wolff, "Professors Defend Tuskegee Study," *New York Sun*, January 28, 2004, 5.

30 *Saturday Night Live*, October 26, 2007.

31 Reverby, "More Than Fact and Fiction."

32 Holloway, "Accidental Communities," 9.

33 Macon County, Alabama, <http://www.ecanned.com/AL/2007/01/income-and-poverty-in-macon-county.shtml>, accessed June 12, 2008.

34 The history of the fight over the Thomas Reed Ambulatory Care Center can be tracked through the pages of the weekly *Tuskegee News*.

35 Jeff Thompson, "Hospital Study Dissected," *Tuskegee News*, October 4, 2007, 1.

36 Tuskegee University National Bioethics Center, <http://www.tuskegee.edu/Global/category.asp?C=35026>, accessed May 12, 2008.

37 See *Alabama Stories* (DVD).

38 On the Shiloh Community Restoration Project, see <http://www.shilohcommfound .com>, accessed October 26, 2008.

Bibliography

UNPUBLISHED SOURCES

Alabama Department of Archives and History, Montgomery, Ala., Administrative Files, Department of Public Health

Columbia University, Mailman School of Public Health, David Rothman Office, New York, N.Y.

  Tuskegee Medical Files, medical and legal records from *Pollard v. United States*, Harold Edgar Papers

Fisk University, John Hope and Aurelia E. Franklin Library, Special Collections, Nashville, Tenn.

  Rosenwald Fund Papers

Frank M. Johnson Jr. Federal Building and U.S. Courthouse, Montgomery, Ala.

  Pollard v. United States Filings and Papers

Johns Hopkins Medical School, Alan M. Chesney Archives, Baltimore, Md.

  Alan M. Chesney Papers

  Adolph Meyer Papers

  Joseph Earle Moore Papers

James H. Jones, private collection, Washington, D.C.

  Interview with Eunice Rivers Laurie, Tuskegee, Ala.

National Archives and Records Administration, College Park, Md.

  U.S. Public Health Service, General Records of the Venereal Disease Division, 1918–36

National Archives and Records Administration, Civilian National Personnel Record Center, St. Louis, Mo.

  O. C. Wenger Personnel Records, Public Health Service

National Archives and Records Administration, Southeast Region, Morrow, Ga.

  Centers for Disease Control Papers, Tuskegee Syphilis Study Administrative Records, 1930–80, Record Group 442

  Tuskegee Syphilis Study Medical Files, Tuskegee Syphilis Study Administrative Records, 1930–80, Record Group 442

  Tuskegee Syphilis Study Photographs

National Library of Medicine, History of Medicine Collection, Bethesda, Md.

Oral History of John R. Heller

U.S. Department of Health, Education, and Welfare, Ad Hoc Advisory Panel on the Tuskegee Syphilis Study Papers

Tuskegee University, Frissell Library, Washingtonian Collection, Tuskegee, Ala.

Eugene H. Dibble Papers

Helen T. Dibble and Lewis W. Jones, "Oral History of Annie Lou Miller," in Statewide Oral History Project, Alabama Center for Higher Education, 1973

Helen T. Dibble and Daniel Williams, audiotape of interview with Eunice Rivers Laurie

Reginald James, "The Mobile Clinic and Syphilis in the Rural Areas of Macon County, Alabama," 1941

John A. Andrew Clinical Society Papers

Ku Klux Klan Clipping File

Eunice Rivers Laurie Papers

Lynching Files

Robert Russa Moton Papers

Frederick Douglas Patterson Papers

School of Nursing Papers

Tuskegee Syphilis Study Clipping File

U.S. Department of Health, Education, and Welfare, Ad Hoc Panel on the Tuskegee Syphilis Study, Bound Books 1 and 2

Myrtle V. Winters, "A Study of the Development and Organization of the Public Health Department of Macon County, Alabama" (master's thesis, Tulane University School of Social Work, 1941)

University of Michigan, Bentley Historical Library, Ann Arbor, Mich.

Reuben Kahn Papers

University of Pittsburgh, Archives Service Center, Pittsburgh, Pa.

John C. Cutler Papers

Thomas Parran Papers

AUTHOR INTERVIEWS AND TELEPHONE INTERVIEWS

Baker, A. Cornelius. April 19, 2007. Washington, D.C. Telephone. April 22, 2007. E-mail message.

Beavers, Irene. January 10, 1994. Tuskegee, Ala.

Bernstein, Walter. February 20, 2007. New York, N.Y. Telephone.

Buxtun, Peter. November 11, 1998. Birmingham, Ala. March 20, 2004. Telephone.

Byron, Don. April 20, 1993. Somerville, Mass.

Detmer, Don. April 13, 2007. Charlottesville, Va. Telephone.

DiIanni, Denise. January 15, 2005. Boston, Mass.

Edgar, Harold. June 12, 1995. New York, N.Y.

Feldshuh, David. June 5, 1992. Ithaca, N.Y. August 16, 2006. Telephone.

Ford, Johnny. January 9, 1995. Tuskegee, Ala.

Foster, Henry. December 13, 2005. Nashville, Tenn.

Gamble, Vanessa Northington. April 13, 2007. Tuskegee, Ala. Telephone.

Geiger, H. Jack. May 3, 2003. New York, N.Y. Telephone.

Glasser, Scott. November 19, 1994. Madison, Wis.

Gray, Fred D. January 10, 1994. Tuskegee, Ala.

Hatch, John. May 13, 2003. Chapel Hill, N.C. Telephone.

Heller, Jean. July 18, 2005, and August 16, 2006. St. Petersburg, Fla. Telephone.

Holguin, Alfonso. August 1, 2005. Galveston, Tex. Telephone.

Hyman, Andrew, and Anna Durant. March 10 and 13, 1995. Washington, D.C. Telephone.

Jenkins, Bill. January 8, 1995. Atlanta, Ga.

Johnson, Francis. July 30, 2008. Tuskegee, Ala.

Jones, James H. November 12, 1998. Birmingham, Ala. July 7, 2004, and July 25, 2005. Telephone.

Julkes, Albert, Jr. November 10, 1998. Tuskegee, Ala.

Katz, Jay. June 2, 1992. New Haven, Conn.

Katz, Ralph. July 7, 2006. New York, N.Y. Telephone.

Leon, Kenny. March 12, 1997. Boston, Mass.

Lindsey, Bryan. October 28, 2007. Atlanta, Ga. Telephone.

Millar, Don. January 12, 2007. Atlanta, Ga. August 8, 2005. Telephone.

Murray, Albert. March 20, 1998. New York, N.Y.

Nelson, Alondra. January 13, 2006. Cambridge, Mass.

Nissen, Steven. February 7, 2006. Cleveland, Ohio.

Noble, Rev. Charles. May 25, 1995. Tuskegee, Ala.

Pack, Amy and Walter. January 15, 1995. Tuskegee, Ala.

Pollard, Charlie Wesley. January 13, 1995. Notasulga, Ala.

Printz, Don. July 12, 2005. Atlanta, Ga. Telephone.

Quinn, Sandra Crouse, and Stephen Thomas. June 8, 2007. Pittsburgh, Pa. Telephone.

Rabb, Louis Mike. July 31, 2008. Tuskegee, Ala.

Rochat, Robert. July 25, 2005. Atlanta, Ga. Telephone.

Schadler, Jay. February 9, 2007. Amesbury, Mass. Telephone.

Schatz, Irwin. April 15, 2003. Honolulu, Hawaii. Telephone.

Schroeter, Arnold. July 11, 2005. Rochester, Minn. Telephone.

Sencer, David. January 12, 2007. Atlanta, Ga. August 1, 2005. Telephone.

Settler, Howard, Jr. August 2, 2005. Tuskegee, Ala. Telephone.

Shaw, Herman. May 15, 1997. Washington, D.C. November 9, 1998. Tallassee, Ala.

Simmons, Fred. May 15, 1997. Washington, D.C.

Sims, Elizabeth. January 17, 2007, and July 29, 2008. Notasulga, Ala.

Snider, Dixie. January 25, 2007. Atlanta, Ga. Telephone.

Story, Robert. January 14, 1995. Tuskegee, Ala.

Strait, George. February 16, 2007. Oakland, Calif. Telephone.

Thompson, A. Lillian. January 13, 1995. Tuskegee, Ala.

Warren, Rueben. June 6, 2007. Atlanta, Ga. Telephone.

Wilson, Cynthia. July 30, 2008. Tuskegee, Ala.

PUBLISHED PRIMARY SOURCES

Alabama, State of. *General Laws of the Legislature of Alabama*. Montgomery: Brown Printing Company, 1927.

Andrews, William L., ed. *Up from Slavery: Booker T. Washington*. New York: W. W. Norton, 1996.

Bauer, Theodore J. "Evaluation of Anti-Syphilitic Therapy with Intensive Follow-Up." *Journal of Venereal Disease Information* 32 (December 1951): 355–70.

Bauer, Theodore J., et al. "Do Persons Lost to Long Term Observation Have the Same Experience as Persons Observed?: Evaluation of Anti-Syphilitic Therapy." *Journal of the American Statistical Association* 49 (March 1954): 36–50.

Beecher, Henry K. "Ethics and Clinical Research." *New England Journal of Medicine* 274 (June 16, 1966): 1354–60.

Blum, Henrik L., and Charles W. Barnett. "Prognosis in Late Latent Syphilis." *Archives of Internal Medicine* 82 (October 1948): 393–409.

Boyd, Mark F., and S. F. Kitchen. "Observations on Induced Falciparum Malaria." *American Journal of Tropical Diseases* 2 (Supplement 1937): 213–35.

Butler, Broadus. "The Tuskegee Syphilis Study." *Journal of the National Medical Association* 65 (July–August 1973): 345–48.

Buxtun, Peter. "Testimony by Peter Buxtun from the U.S. Senate Hearings on Human Experimentation, 1973." In *Tuskegee's Truths: Rethinking the Tuskegee Syphilis Study*, edited by Susan M. Reverby, 150–56. Chapel Hill: University of North Carolina Press, 2000.

Byron, Don. *Tuskegee Experiments*. Elektra Nonesuch 79260–2, 1991.

Caldwell, Joseph G., E. V. Price, A. L. Schroeter, and G. F. Fletcher. "Aortic Regurgitation in the Tuskegee Study of Untreated Syphilis." *Journal of Chronic Diseases* 26 (March 1973): 187–94.

Callis, H. A. "Comparative Therapy in Syphilis." *Journal of the National Medical Association* 21 (January–March 1929). In *Henry Arthur Callis: Life and Legacy*, edited by Charles H. Wesley, 186–204. Chicago: Foundation Publishers, 1977.

———. "The Need for Training of Negro Physicians." *Journal of Negro Education* 4 (January 1935): 32–41.

———. "Primary Syphilis." *Journal of the National Medical Association* 21 (April–June 1929). In *Henry Arthur Callis: Life and Legacy*, edited by Charles H. Wesley, 186–204. Chicago: Foundation Publishers, 1977.

Campbell, Thomas Monroe. *The Movable School Goes to the Negro Farmer*. Tuskegee, Ala.: Tuskegee Institute Press, 1936.

Carley, Paul S., and O. C. Wenger. "The Prevalence of Syphilis in Apparently Healthy Negroes in Mississippi." *Journal of the American Medical Association* 94 (June 4, 1930): 1826–29.

Chester, Benjamin J., John C. Cutler, and Eleanor V. Price. "Serologic Observations Following Penicillin Treatment for Latent Syphilis." *American Journal of Syphilis, Gonorrhea, and Venereal Diseases* 38 (January 1954): 7–17.

Childs, Barton. "Primaquine Sensitivity of Erythrocytes." *Archives of Internal Medicine* 107 (February 1961): 5–53.

Clark, E. Gurney, and Niels Danbolt. "The Oslo Study of the Natural History of Untreated Syphilis." *Journal of Chronic Diseases* 2 (September 1955): 311–44.

Clark, Taliaferro. *The Control of Syphilis in Southern Rural Areas*. Chicago: Julius Rosenwald Fund, 1932.

Cobb, W. Montague. "Special Problems in the Provision of Medical Services for Negroes." *Journal of Negro Education* 18 (Summer 1949): 340–345.

———. "The Tuskegee Syphilis Study." *Journal of the National Medical Association* 65 (July 1973): 345–48.

Collart, Pierre. "Persistence of *Treponema Pallidum* in Late Syphilis in Rabbits and Humans, Not Withstanding Treatment." In *Proceedings of the World Forum on Syphilis and Other Treponematoses.* Washington, D.C.: Public Health Service, 1964.

Curtis, A. C., et al. "Penicillin Treatment of Asymptomatic Central Nervous System Syphilis." *AMA Archives of Dermatology* 74 (October 1956): 355–77.

Cutler, John C. "Venereal Disease: Now and Looking into the Future." *Public Health Nursing* 44 (November 1952): 613–19.

Cutler, John C., and R. C. Arnold. "Venereal Disease Control by Health Departments in the Past: Lessons for the Present." In *Tuskegee's Truths: Rethinking the Tuskegee Syphilis Study,* edited by Susan M. Reverby, 495–506. Chapel Hill: University of North Carolina Press, 2000.

Cutler, John C., R. D. Wright, R. C. Arnold, and S. Levitan. "Local Herxheimer Reaction Following Application of Penicillin Solution to Syphilitic Chancres." *Journal of Venereal Disease Information* 32 (August 1951): 207–8.

Davis, Michael M. "The Ability of Patients to Pay for Treatment of Syphilis." *Journal of Social Hygiene* 18 (October 1932): 380–88.

Deibert, Austin V. "Notes on Cardiovascular Syphilis." *Annual Bulletin of the John A. Andrew Clinic, 1939.* Tuskegee, Ala.: John A. Andrew Clinical Society, 1939: 31–38.

Deibert, Austin V., and M. C. Bruyere. "Untreated Syphilis in the Male Negro: III. Evidence of Cardiovascular Abnormalities and Other Forms of Morbidity." *Journal of Venereal Disease Information* 27 (1946): 301–14.

Denison, George A., and W. H. Y. Smith. "Mass Venereal Disease Control in an Urban Area." *Southern Medical Journal* 39 (March 1946): 195–202.

Dibble, Eugene H. "Statement of Dr. Eugene Dibble." *Report of the President's Commission on the Health Needs of the Nation,* vol. 5, p. 189. Washington, D.C.: Government Printing Office, 1953.

Dibble, Eugene H., Louis Rabb, and Ruth B. Ballard. "John A. Andrew Memorial Hospital." *Journal of the National Medical Association* 53 (March 1961): 103–18.

Dibble, Helen, and Daniel Williams. "An Interview with Nurse Rivers." Transcription by Susan M. Reverby and Carmen Bryant. In *Tuskegee's Truths: Rethinking the Tuskegee Syphilis Study,* edited by Susan M. Reverby, 321–39. Chapel Hill: University of North Carolina Press, 2000.

Diseker, Thomas H., et al. "Long-Term Results in the Treatment of Latent Syphilis." *American Journal of Syphilis, Gonorrhea, and Venereal Diseases* 28 (January 1944): 1–26.

Embree, Edwin R. *Julius Rosenwald Fund Review for the Year.* Chicago: Rosenwald Fund, 1930.

———. *Julius Rosenwald Fund Review for the Two-Year Period 1931–33.* Chicago: Rosenwald Fund, 1933.

———. *Julius Rosenwald Fund: Review of Two Decades, 1917–1936.* Chicago: Rosenwald Fund, 1936.

Feldshuh, David. *Miss Evers' Boys*. New York: Dramatists Play Service Inc., 1995.

Final Report of the Tuskegee Syphilis Study Ad Hoc Advisory Panel. <http://biotech.law.lsu.edu/cphl/history/reports/tuskegee/tus>, accessed February 22, 2009.

Folkes, Homer M. "The Negro as a Health Problem." *Journal of the National Medical Association* 55 (October 8, 1910): 1246.

Fong, T. C. "Therapeutic Quartan Malaria in the Therapy of Neurosyphilis among Negroes." *American Journal of Syphilis, Gonorrhea, and Venereal Diseases* 24 (1940): 133–47.

Friedman, Benjamin. "Syphilitic Aortic Insufficiency." *Alabama Journal of Medical Sciences* 6 (January 1969): 8–17.

Friedman, Benjamin, and Sidney Olansky. "Diagnosis of Syphilitic Cardiovascular Disease." *American Heart Journal* 50 (September 1955): 323–30.

Gjestland, Trygve. *The Oslo Study of Untreated Syphilis*. Oslo, Norway: Akademisk Forlag, 1955.

Goldwater, Leonard J. *Mercury: A History of Quicksilver*. New York: York Press, 1972.

Graves, Marvin L. "The Negro a Menace to the Health of the White Race." *Southern Medical Journal* 9 (May 1916): 407–11.

Guiteras, John. "Experimental Yellow Fever at the Inoculation Station of the Sanitary Department of Havana with a View to Producing Immunization." *American Medicine* 2 (November 23, 1901): 808–17.

Hazen, H. H. *Syphilis in the Negro: A Handbook for the General Practitioner*. Supplement No. 15, Venereal Disease Information. Washington, D.C.: Federal Security Agency, Public Health Service, 1942.

Heller, Jean. "Syphilis Victims in U.S. Study without Therapy for Forty Years." In *Tuskegee's Truths: Rethinking the Tuskegee Syphilis Study*, edited by Susan M. Reverby, 116–18. Chapel Hill: University of North Carolina Press, 2000.

Heller, John R., and P. T. Bruyere. "Untreated Syphilis in the Male Negro: II. Mortality during 12 Years of Observation." In *Tuskegee's Truths: Rethinking the Tuskegee Syphilis Study*, edited by Susan M. Reverby, 119–24. Chapel Hill: University of North Carolina Press, 2000.

Heterington, J. "The Kerato-Cricoid Muscle in the American White and Negro." *American Journal of Physical Anthropology* 19 (1934): 203–12.

Hiltner, Seward. "The Tuskegee Syphilis Study under Review." *Christian Century* 90 (1973): 1174–76.

Hinton, William A. "The Significance of a Positive Blood Test for Syphilis." *New England Journal of Medicine* 217, no. 25 (1937): 978–82.

———. *Syphilis and Its Treatment*. New York: Macmillan, 1936.

Hosty, Thomas S., et al. "Human Anti-Rabies Gamma Globulin." *Bulletin of the World Health Organization* 20 (June 1959): 1111–19.

"Interview with Four Survivors." U.S. Department of Health, Education, and Welfare Study, 1973. In *Tuskegee's Truths: Rethinking the Tuskegee Syphilis Study*, edited by Susan M. Reverby, 132–35. Chapel Hill: University of North Carolina Press, 2000.

Johnson, Charles S. *Shadow of the Plantation*. Chicago: University of Chicago Press, 1934.

———. "The Shadow of the Plantation: Survival." In *Tuskegee's Truths: Rethinking the Tuskegee Syphilis Study*, edited by Susan M. Reverby, 41–58. Chapel Hill: University of North Carolina Press, 2000.

Jordon, James W., and Frank A. Dolce. "Latent Syphilis: Study of 169 Cases Observed Ten Years or More." *Archives of Dermatology and Syphilology* 54 (July 1946): 1–18.

Kahn, Reuben L. "The Inspiration of Research." *Michigan Quarterly Review* 4 (April 1965): 122–30.

Kampmeier, Rudolph H. "Comments on the Present Day Management of Syphilis." *Southern Medical Journal* 46 (March 1953): 226–37.

———. *Essentials of Syphilology*. Philadelphia: J. B. Lippincott, 1943.

———. "The Final Report on the Tuskegee Syphilis Study." *Southern Medical Journal* 67 (November 1974): 56–67.

———. "The Late Manifestations of Syphilis: Skeletal, Visceral, and Cardiovascular." *Medical Clinics of North America* 48 (1964): 667–97.

———. "The Tuskegee Study of Untreated Syphilis." In *Tuskegee's Truths: Rethinking the Tuskegee Syphilis Study*, edited by Susan M. Reverby, 193–201. Chapel Hill: University of North Carolina Press, 2000.

Kenney, John A., Jr. "A Brief History of the Origin of the John A. Andrew Clinics by the Founder." *Journal of the National Medical Association* 26 (January 1934): 65–68.

———. "A Plea for Conservatism in the Use of Anti-Luetic Therapy." *Journal of the National Medical Association* 33 (1941): 272–73.

Laurie, Mrs. Eunice R., Deposition of, September 20, 1974, Tuskegee, Ala. *Pollard v. U.S.*, 384 F. Supp. 304 (U.S. Dist. Ala. 1974).

"Letters to the Editor in Response to Beecher's Essay." In *Ethics in Medicine*, edited by Stanley Joel Reiser, Arthur Dyck, and William J. Curran, 294–96. Cambridge: MIT Press, 1977.

Lewis, Julian Herman. *The Biology of the Negro*. Chicago: University of Chicago Press, 1942.

Lewis, N. D. C., and L. D. Hubbard. "Epileptic Reactions in the Negro Race." *American Journal of Psychiatry* 11 (1932): 647–77.

Limson, M. "Observations on the Bones of the Skull in White and Negro Fetuses and Infants." *Contributions and Embryology* 23 (1932): 136–207.

Logan, Rayford W., ed. *What the Negro Wants*. Chapel Hill: University of North Carolina Press, 1944.

Magnuson, Harold, et al. "Inoculation Syphilis in Human Volunteers." *Medicine* 35 (February 1956): 32–82.

Mahoney, J. F., R. C. Arnold, and A. Harris. "Penicillin Treatment of Early Syphilis: A Preliminary Report." *American Journal of Public Health* 33 (December 1943): 1387–91.

———. "Penicillin Treatment of Early Syphilis: A Preliminary Report." *Venereal Disease Information* 24 (December 1943): 355–57.

Mokotoff, Reuben, William Brams, Louis N. Katz, and Katherine M. Howell. "The Treatment of Bacterial Endocarditis with Penicillin." *American Journal of Medical Sciences* 211 (April 1946): 395–416.

Moore, Joseph Earle. "The Impending Loss of a Partly Won War against Venereal Disease." *American Journal of Syphilis, Gonorrhea, and Venereal Diseases* 38 (May 1954): 237–38.

———. "Management of Syphilis in General Practice." *Journal of Venereal Disease Information* (Supplement 23, 1949): 21–23.

———. *The Modern Treatment of Syphilis.* 2d ed. Springfield, Ill.: Charles C. Thomas, 1947.

———. *Penicillin in Syphilis.* Springfield, Ill.: Charles C. Thomas, 1946.

———. "The Relation of Neuroreoccurrences to Late Syphilis." *Archives of Neurology and Psychiatry* 21 (1929): 117–36.

———. "Venerology in Transition." *British Journal of Venereal Disease* 32 (1956): 217–21.

Moore, Joseph Earle, H. N. Cole, and Paul O'Leary. "Cooperative Clinical Studies in the Treatment of Syphilis." *Venereal Disease Information* 13 (1932): 317–31.

Moore, Joseph Earle, et al. "The Treatment of Early Syphilis with Penicillin: A Preliminary Report of 1,418 Cases." *Journal of the American Medical Association* 126 (September 9, 1944): 67–73.

Moton, Robert Russa. *Finding a Way Out: An Autobiography.* Garden City, N.Y.: Doubleday, Page, 1921.

———. *What the Negro Thinks.* Rev. ed. Garden City, N.Y.: Doubleday Doran, 1932.

Niedelman, Meyer L. "Penicillin in Late Latent Syphilis: Results of Therapy with Procaine Penicillin in Aluminum Monostearate." *AMA Archives of Dermatology* 75 (1955): 503–9.

Olansky, Sidney. "Diagnosis and Treatment of Syphilis." Annual Bulletin of the John A. Andrew Clinic, 12–17. Tuskegee, Ala.: John A. Andrew Clinical Society, April 1952.

———. "Syphilis—Rediscovered." *Disease of the Month* (May 1967): 3–30.

Olansky, Sidney, A. Harris, J. C. Cutler, E. V. Price. "Untreated Syphilis in the Male Negro: Twenty-two Years of Serological Observation in a Selected Syphilis Study Group." *AMA Archives of Dermatology* 73 (May 1956): 519–22.

Olansky, Sidney, L. Simpson, and S. H. Schuman. "Environmental Factors in the Tuskegee Study of Untreated Syphilis." *Public Health Reports* 69 (July 1954): 691–98.

Olansky, Sidney, et al. "Untreated Syphilis in the Male Negro: X. Twenty Years of Clinical Observation of Untreated Syphilitic and Presumably Nonsyphilitic Groups." *Journal of Chronic Diseases* 4 (August 1956): 177–85.

Parran, Thomas. *Shadow on the Land.* New York: Reynal and Hitchcock, 1937.

———. "Syphilis: A Public Health Problem." *Science* 87 (February 18, 1938): 148–49.

———. "Syphilis: The White Man's Burden." In *Tuskegee's Truths: Rethinking the Tuskegee Syphilis Study*, edited by Susan M. Reverby, 59–72. Chapel Hill: University of North Carolina Press, 2000.

Parran, Thomas, and Raymond A. Vonderlehr. *Plain Words about Venereal Disease.* New York: Reynal and Hitchcock, 1941.

Pearl, Raymond. "The Weight of the Negro Brain." *Brain Anthropology* 80 (1934): 431–34.

Pesare, Pasquale J., T. J. Bauer, and G. A. Gleeson. "Untreated Syphilis in the Male Negro: Observation of Abnormalities over Sixteen Years." *American Journal of Syphilis, Gonorrhea, and Venereal Diseases* 34 (May 1950): 201–13.

Peters, J. Jerome, T. J. Bauer, and G. A. Gleeson. "Untreated Syphilis in the Male Negro: Pathologic Findings in Syphilitic and Nonsyphilitic Patients." *Journal of Chronic Diseases* 1 (February 1955): 127–48.

Pollard et al. v. United States of America et al. Civil Action No. 4126-N, Northern Division, Middle District Court of the United States, Montgomery, Ala.

Reynolds, Frank W., and Joseph Earle Moore. "Progress in Internal Medicine—Syphilis." *Archives of Internal Medicine* 80 (1947): 655–90.

Rivers, Eunice, S. H. Schuman, L. Simpson, and S. Olansky. "Twenty Years of Follow-up Experience in a Long-Range Medical Study." In *Tuskegee's Truths: Rethinking the Tuskegee Syphilis Study*, edited by Susan M. Reverby, 125–31. Chapel Hill: University of North Carolina Press, 2000.

Rockwell, Donald H., A. R. Yobs, and M. B. Moore Jr. "The Tuskegee Study of Untreated Syphilis: The 30th Year of Observation." *Archives of Internal Medicine* 114 (December 1961): 792–98.

Rosahn, Paul D. *Autopsy Studies in Syphilis.* Washington, D.C.: Public Health Service, 1949.

———. "Studies in Syphilis VII: The End Results of Untreated Syphilis." *Journal of Venereal Disease Information* 27 (December 1946): 293–301.

Royster, C. L., J. R. Lisa, and J. Carroll. "Anatomic Findings in the Heart in Combined Hypertension and Syphilis." *Archives of Pathology* 32 (1941): 64–75.

St. John, R. K. "Treatment of Cardiovascular Syphilis." *Journal of the American Venereal Disease Association* 3 (December 1976): 148–52.

Schamberg, Jay F., and Carroll S. Wright. *Treatment of Syphilis.* New York: D. Appleton, 1932.

Schuman, Stanley H., et al. "Untreated Syphilis in the Male Negro: Background and Current Status of Patients in the Tuskegee Study." *Journal of Chronic Diseases* 2 (November 1955): 543–58.

"Selections from the Final Report of the Ad Hoc Tuskegee Syphilis Study Panel, Department of Health, Education, and Welfare." In *Tuskegee's Truths: Rethinking the Tuskegee Syphilis Study*, edited by Susan M. Reverby, 157–92. Chapel Hill: University of North Carolina Press, 2000.

Shafer, James K., Lida J. Usilton, and Geraldine A. Gleeson. "Untreated Syphilis in the Male Negro: A Prospective Study of the Effect on Life Expectancy." *Public Health Reports* 69 (July 1954): 691–97.

Shafer, James K., Lida J. Usilton, and Eleanor V. Price. "Long-Term Studies of Results of Penicillin Therapy in Early Syphilis." *Bulletin of the World Health Organization* 10 (1954): 563–78.

Shaw, Herman. "Comments." Annual Meeting of the Southern Historical Association. Birmingham, Ala., November 12, 1998.

———. "Herman Shaw's Remarks." In *Tuskegee's Truths: Rethinking the Tuskegee Syphilis Study*, edited by Susan M. Reverby, 572–73. Chapel Hill: University of North Carolina Press, 2000.

Smith, J. Lawton. *Spirochetes in Late Seronegative Syphilis, Penicillin Notwithstanding.* Springfield, Ill.: Charles C. Thomas, 1965.

———. "Spirochetes in Late Seronegative Syphilis, Penicillin Nothwithstanding." *Optometry and Vision Science* 47 (May 1970): 406.

Smith, W. H. Y., D. G. Gill, and S. R. Damon. "A Preliminary Report of Blood Testing, as Required by Alabama Law, in the First Three Counties Surveyed." *Venereal Disease Information* (November 1944): 332–35.

Snow, William F., Joseph Earle Moore, Wade H. Brown, and Thomas Parran. *Symposium on Research in Syphilis, Reprint No. 11 from Venereal Disease Information 9 (December 20, 1928).* Washington, D.C.: Government Printing Office, 1929.

Solomon, Harry C., and Maida H. Solomon. *Syphilis of the Innocent.* Washington, D.C.: U.S. Interdepartmental Social Hygiene Board, 1922.

Stokes, John M., ed. *Modern Clinical Syphilology.* 2nd ed. Philadelphia: W. B. Saunders, 1934.

Stokes, John M., and Herman Beerman. "The Fundamental Bacteriology, Pathology and Immunology of Syphilis." In *Modern Clinical Syphilology*, 2nd ed., edited by John M. Stokes. Philadelphia: W. B. Saunders, 1934.

"Testimony by Four Survivors from the United States Senate Hearings on Human Experimentation, 1972." In *Tuskegee's Truths: Rethinking the Tuskegee Syphilis Study*, edited by Susan M. Reverby, 136–49. Chapel Hill: University of North Carolina Press, 2000.

Thompson, Lillian A. "Eunice Rivers Laurie Interview, 10 October 1977." In *The Black Women Oral History Project*, edited by Ruth Edmonds Hill, 213–42. New Providence, N.J.: K. G. Saur Verlag, 1992.

Turner, Thomas B. "The Race and Sex Distribution of the Lesions of Syphilis in 10,000 Cases." *Bulletin of the Johns Hopkins Hospital* 46 (1930): 159–184.

Tuskegee News. 100th Anniversary Edition, November 11, 1965.

U.S. Congress. Senate. Committee on Labor and Human Resources. *Henry W. Foster, Jr., of Tennessee, to Be Medical Director in the Regular Corps of the Public Health Service, and to Be Surgeon General of the Public Health Service.* 104th Cong., 1st Sess., May 2 and 3, 1995. Washington, D.C.: Government Printing Office, 1995.

———. Senate. Subcommittee on Health of the Committee on Labor and Public Welfare. *Quality of Health Care—Human Experimentation.* 93rd Cong., 1st Sess. Washington, D.C.: Government Printing Office, 1973.

U.S. Department of Health, Education, and Welfare, Public Health Service. *Syphilis: A Synopsis.* Atlanta: National Communicable Disease Center, Venereal Disease Program, 1968.

"U.S. Health Officer." *Fortune* 23 (May 1941): 84–85, 108–10.

"U.S. Public Health Service." *Fortune* 23 (May 1941): 81–83, 102–8.

U.S. Public Health Service. *Annual Report to the Surgeon General 1933.* Washington, D.C.: Public Health Service, 1933.

———. *The Venereal Disease Handbook for Community Leaders: A Program of Venereal Disease Control.* Washington, D.C.: Government Printing Office, 1924.

Vonderlehr, Raymond A. "A Comparison of Treated and Untreated Syphilis." *John A. Andrew Clinical Society Annual Bulletin*, 1–5. Tuskegee, Ala.: Tuskegee Institute, 1938.

Vonderlehr, Raymond A., T. Clark, O. C. Wenger, and J. R. Heller Jr. "Untreated Syphilis in the Male Negro: A Comparative Study of Treated and Untreated Cases." *Journal of the American Medical Association* 107 (September 12, 1936): 856–60.

Vonderlehr, Raymond A., T. Clark, O. C. Wenger, and J. R. Heller Jr. "Untreated Syphilis in the Male Negro: A Comparative Study of Treated and Untreated Cases." *Venereal Disease Information* 17 (1936): 260–65.

Vonderlehr, Raymond A., and John Heller. *The Control of Venereal Disease*. New York: Reynal and Hitchcock, 1946.

Wenger, O. C. *Caribbean Medical Center: The Organization, Development and Activities of the Caribbean Medical Center at Port of Spain, Trinidad, B.W.I., from February 9, 1943, to March 1, 1945*. Washington, D.C.: Caribbean Commission, 1946.

———. "Untreated Syphilis in the Negro Male." In *Tuskegee's Truths: Rethinking the Tuskegee Syphilis Study*, edited by Susan M. Reverby, 96–99. Chapel Hill: University of North Carolina Press, 2000.

Wenger, O. C., and Ricks, H. C. "The Public Health Aspect of Syphilis in the Negro Race in Certain Southern States." *Southern Medical Journal* (June 1931): 556–61.

Wesley, Charles H. *Arthur Callis: Life and Legacy*. Chicago: Foundation Publishers, 1977.

Yobs, Anne R., S. Olansky, D. H. Rockwell, J. W. Clark Jr. "Do Treponemes Survive Adequate Treatment of Late Syphilis." *Archives of Dermatology* 91 (April 1965): 379–89.

SECONDARY SOURCES

Advisory Committee on Human Radiation Experiments. *Final Report of the Advisory Committee on Human Radiation Experiments*. New York: Oxford University Press, 1996.

Alabama Advisory Committee to the United States Commission on Civil Rights. "Alabama Commission Report." Montgomery: State of Alabama, 1973.

Alcoff, Linda, and Laura Gray. "Survivor Discourse: Transgression or Recuperation?" *Signs* 18 (Winter 1993): 260–90.

Alexander, Adele Logan. "Adella Hunt Logan and the Tuskegee Woman's Club: Building a Foundation for Suffrage." In *Stepping Out of the Shadows: Alabama Women, 1819–1990*, edited by Mary Martha Thomas, 91–113. Tuscaloosa: University of Alabama Press, 1995.

———. *Homelands and Waterways: The American Journey of the Bond Family, 1846–1926*. New York: Pantheon, 1999.

Allen, James, ed. *Without Sanctuary: Lynching Photography in America*. Santa Fe: Twin Palms, 2000.

Altman, Lawrence. *Who Goes First? The Story of Self-Experimentation in Medicine*. Berkeley: University of California Press, 1998.

Anderson, James D. *The Education of Blacks in the South, 1860–1935*. Chapel Hill: University of North Carolina Press, 1988.

Angell, Marcia. "The Ethics of Clinical Research in the Third World." In *Tuskegee's Truths: Rethinking the Tuskegee Syphilis Study*, edited by Susan M. Reverby, 578–83. Chapel Hill: University of North Carolina Press, 2000.

Annas, George J., and Michael A. Grodin, eds. *The Nazi Doctors and the Nuremberg Code*. New York: Oxford University Press, 1992.

Apel, Dora, and Shawn Michelle Smith. *Lynching Photographs*. Berkeley: University of California Press, 2007.

Atkins, Leah Rawls. "From Early Times to the End of the Civil War." In *Alabama: The History of a Deep South State*, edited by William Warren Rogers, 3–203. Tuscaloosa: University of Alabama Press, 1994.

Auchmutey, Jim. "Ghosts of Tuskegee." *Atlanta Journal and Constitution*, September 6, 1992, M01.

Ayers, Edward. *What Caused the Civil War? Reflections on the South and Southern History*. New York: W. W. Norton, 2005.

Baker, Houston A., Jr. *Blues, Ideology, and Afro-American Literature: A Vernacular Theory*. Chicago: University of Chicago Press, 1984.

———. "Meditation on Tuskegee: Black Studies Stories and Their Imbrication." *Journal of Blacks in Higher Education* 9 (Autumn 1995): 51–59.

———. *Turning South Again: Re-Thinking Modernism/Re-Reading Booker T*. Durham, N.C.: Duke University Press, 2001.

Baker, Robert, Arthur L. Caplan, Linda L. Emanuel, and Stephen R. Latham. *The American Medical Ethics Revolution*. Baltimore: Johns Hopkins University Press, 1999.

Baker, Robert, et al. "African American Physicians and Organized Medicine, 1846–1968: Origins of a Racial Divide." *Journal of the American Medical Association* 300 (July 16, 2008): 306–13.

Barthes, Roland. *Camera Lucida*. New York: Hill and Wang, 1982.

Bay, Mia. "The World Was Thinking Wrong about Race." In *W. E. B. Dubois, Race, and the City*, edited by Michael B. Katz, 41–60. Philadelphia: University of Pennsylvania Press, 1998.

Bean, Walter B. "Walter Reed and the History of Medical Experiments." *Bulletin of the History of Medicine* 51 (Spring 1977): 75–82.

Beardsley, Edward. *A History of Neglect*. Knoxville: University of Tennessee Press, 1987.

———. "Making Separate, Equal." *Bulletin of the History of Medicine* 57 (Fall 1983): 382–96.

Beauchamp, Thomas, and James F. Childress. *Principles of Biomedical Ethics*. 6th ed. New York: Oxford University Press, 2008.

Beerman, Herman. "Future Research Needs." In *Proceedings of World Forum on Syphilis and Other Treponematoses*, edited by William J. Brown, 199–208. Washington D.C.: Public Health Service, 1964.

Belmont Oral History Archive. <http://www.hhs.gov/ohrp/belmontArchive.html# histArchive2>, accessed February 22, 2009.

Benedek, Thomas G. "Gonorrhea and the Beginnings of Clinical Research Ethics." *Perspectives in Biology and Medicine* 48 (Winter 2005): 54–73.

———. "The 'Tuskegee Study' of Syphilis: An Analysis of Moral versus Methodologic Aspects." In *Tuskegee's Truths: Rethinking the Tuskegee Syphilis Study*, edited by Susan M. Reverby, 213–35. Chapel Hill: University of North Carolina Press, 2000.

Benedek, Thomas G., and Jonathan Erlen. "The Scientific Environment of the Tuskegee Study of Syphilis, 1920–1960." *Perspectives in Biology and Medicine* 43 (Autumn 1999): 1–30.

Berlin, Ira. "American Slavery in History and Memory and the Search for Social Justice." *Journal of American History* 90 (March 2004): 1251–68.

Bernstein, Walter. *Inside Out: A Memoir of the Blacklist.* New York: De Capo Press, 2000.

Bieze, Michael. *Booker T. Washington and the Art of Self-Representation.* New York: Peter Lang, 2008.

Blakeley, Robert L., and Judith M. Harrington, eds. *Bones in the Basement: Postmortem Racism in Nineteenth-Century Medicine.* Washington, D.C.: Smithsonian Institution Press, 1997.

Blight, David W. *Beyond the Battlefield: Race, Memory, and the American Civil War.* Amherst: University of Massachusetts Press, 2002.

———. *Race and Reunion: The Civil War in American Memory.* Cambridge: Harvard University Press, 2001.

Bond, Horace Mann. *Black American Scholars: A Study of Their Beginnings.* Detroit: Balamp, 1972.

———. *The Education of the Negro in the American Social Order.* New York: Prentice Hall, 1934.

———. *Negro Education in Alabama.* Tuscaloosa: University of Alabama Press, 1994.

Bondeson, William, H. Tristam Englehardt Jr., Stuart F. Spicker, and Joseph M. White Jr. *New Knowledge in the Biomedical Sciences.* Dordrecht, Netherlands: D. Reidel, 1982.

Bowie, Sibyl Kaye. "The Tuskegee Syphilis Study: A Case Study in Crisis Communication in Public Relations." M.A. thesis, University of Georgia, 1986.

Brandon, Dwayne T., Lydia A. Isaac, and Thomas A. LaVeist. "The Legacy of Tuskegee and Trust in Medical Care: Is Tuskegee Responsible for Race Differences in Mistrust of Medical Care." *Journal of the National Medical Association* 97 (July 2005): 951–56.

Brandt, Allan M. "Infernal Medicine." *New Republic* (January 27, 1982): 36–38.

———. *No Magic Bullet.* New York: Oxford University Press, 1987.

———. "Racism and Research: The Case of the Tuskegee Syphilis Study." In *Tuskegee's Truths: Rethinking the Tuskegee Syphilis Study*, edited by Susan M. Reverby, 15–33. Chapel Hill: University of North Carolina Press, 2000.

Brandt, Allan M., and Martha Gardner. "Antagonism and Accommodation: Interpreting the Relationship between Public Health and Medicine in the United States during the 20th Century." *American Journal of Public Health* 90 (May 2000): 707–15.

Braslow, Joel T. "The Influence of Biological Therapy on Physicians' Narratives and Interrogations: The Case of General Paralysis of the Insane and Malaria Fever Therapy." *Bulletin of the History of Medicine* 70 (Winter 1996): 577–608.

Brawley, Otis W. "The Study of Untreated Syphilis in the Negro Male." *International Journal of Radiation Oncology, Biology, Physics* 40 (January 1998): 5–8.

Brown, JoAnne. "Crime, Commerce and Contagionism: The Political Languages of

Public Health and the Popularization of Germ Theory in the United States, 1870–1950." In *Scientific Authority and Twentieth-Century America*, edited by Ronald G. Walters, 53–81. Baltimore: Johns Hopkins University Press, 1997.

Brown, Roger, and James Kulik. "Flashbulb Memories." *Cognition* 5 (March 1977): 73–99.

Brown, Russell W., and James H. M. Henderson. "The Mass Production and Distribution of HeLa Cells at Tuskegee Institute, 1953–55." *Journal of the History of Medicine* 38 (October 1983): 415–31.

Brundage, W. Fitzhugh, ed. *Booker T. Washington and Black Progress.* Gainesville: University of Florida Press, 2003.

———. *The Southern Past: A Clash of Race and Memory.* Cambridge: Harvard University Press, 2005.

———, ed. *Where These Memories Grow.* Chapel Hill: University of North Carolina Press, 2000.

Brunham, Robert C. "Insights into the Epidemiology of Sexually Transmitted Diseases." *Sexually Transmitted Diseases* 32 (December 2005): 722–24.

Burton, Antoinette, ed. *Archive Stories: Fact, Fictions, and the Writing of History.* Durham, N.C.: Duke University Press, 2005.

Butler, Addie. *The Distinctive Black College.* Metuchen, N.J.: Scarecrow Press, 1977.

Cantwell, Alan, Jr. *AIDS and the Doctors of Death: An Inquiry into the Origins of the AIDS Epidemic.* Los Angeles: Aries Rising Press, 1988.

Caplan, Arthur L. "James H. Jones, *Bad Blood.*" *BioSocieties* 2 (June 2007): 276.

———. "When Evil Intrudes." In *Tuskegee's Truths: Rethinking the Tuskegee Syphilis Study*, edited by Susan M. Reverby, 418–23. Chapel Hill: University of North Carolina Press, 2000.

Capshew, James H., et al. "Kinsey's Biographers: A Historiographical Reconnaissance." *Journal of the History of Sexuality* 12 (July 2003): 465–86.

Carby, Hazel. *Reconstructing Womanhood.* New York: Oxford, 1987.

Carmichael, Stokely, and Charles V. Hamilton. *Black Power: The Politics of Liberation in America.* New York: Vintage Books, 1967.

Cave, Vernal G. "Proper Uses and Abuses of the Health Care Delivery System for Minorities with Special Reference to the Tuskegee Syphilis Study." In *Tuskegee's Truths: Rethinking the Tuskegee Syphilis Study*, edited by Susan M. Reverby, 399–403. Chapel Hill: University of North Carolina Press, 2000.

———. "Statement." *Journal of the National Medical Association* 65 (July 1973): 348.

———. "A Tribute to William Augustus Hinton, M.D." *Journal of the American Medical Association* 67 (January 1975): 81–82.

Childress, James F. "Nuremberg's Legacy: Some Ethical Reflections." *Perspectives in Biology and Medicine* 43 (Spring 2000): 347–61.

Childress, James F., Erik M. Meslin, and Harold T. Shapiro. *Belmont Revisited.* Washington, D.C.: Georgetown University Press, 2005.

Clarke, Ellen. "Professional Commitment and Activism in the Lives of Five Southern African American Nurses." Ph.D. diss., Harvard University, 1999.

Claude Moore Health Sciences Library, University of Virginia Health System. "Doing Bad in the Name of Good Conference, 1994." <http://www.healthsystem.virginia

.edu/internet/library/historical/medical_history/bad_blood>, accessed February 22, 2009.

Clayton, Ellen Wright, and Robert J. Levine, eds. *Collected Writings of Jay Katz*. Boston: PRIMR, 2001.

Clendinnen, Inga. *Reading the Holocaust*. New York: Cambridge University Press, 1999.

Clinton, William J. "President William J. Clinton's Remarks." In *Tuskegee's Truths: Rethinking the Tuskegee Syphilis Study*, edited by Susan M. Reverby, 574–77. Chapel Hill: University of North Carolina Press, 2000.

Clover, Carol J. "Law and the Order of Popular Culture." In *Law in the Domains of Culture*, edited by Austin Sarat and Thomas R. Kearns, 97–120. Ann Arbor: University of Michigan Press, 1998.

Colgrove, James, and Ronald Bayer. "Manifold Restraints: Liberty, Public Health, and the Legacy of *Jacobson v. Massachusetts*." *American Journal of Public Health* 95 (April 2005): 571–76.

Cooter, Roger. "Bioethics." *Lancet* 364 (November 13, 2004): 1749.

Coughlin, S. S., G. D. Etheredge, C. Metayer, and S. A. Martin Jr. "Remember Tuskegee: Public Health Student Knowledge of the Ethical Significance of the Tuskegee Syphilis Study." *American Journal of Preventive Medicine* 12 (April 1996): 242–46.

Coulter, Harris L. *AIDS and Syphilis: The Hidden Link*. Berkeley, Calif.: North Atlantic Books, 1987.

Cox, J. D. "Paternalism, Informed Consent, and Tuskegee." *International Journal of Radiation Oncology, Biology, Physics* 20 (January 1998): 1–2.

Cox, James M. "Autobiography and Washington." In *Up from Slavery: Booker T. Washington*, edited by William L. Andrews, 228–39. New York: Norton, 1996.

Crenner, Christopher. "The Tuskegee Syphilis Study and the Concept of Racial Nervous Resistance to Syphilis." Unpublished paper. Copy in author's possession.

Curran, William J. "Law-Medicine Notes: The Tuskegee Syphilis Study." *New England Journal of Medicine* 289 (1973): 730–31.

Curry, Constance, et al. *Deep in Our Hearts: Nine White Women in the Freedom Movement*. Athens: University of Georgia Press, 2000.

Dalton, Harlan L. "AIDS in Blackface." *Daedelus* 118 (Summer 1989): 205–27.

Daniel, Pete. "Black Power in the 1920s: The Case of Tuskegee Veterans Hospital." *Journal of Southern History* 36 (August 1970): 368–88.

Davenport, Walter. "Bad-Blood Wagon." *Collier's National Weekly* (May 27, 1939): 9–10, 27–30.

Davis, Kathy. *The Making of Our Bodies, Ourselves: How Feminism Travels across Borders*. Durham, N.C.: Duke University Press, 2007.

De Kruif, Paul. *The Fight for Life*. New York: Harcourt, Brace, 1938.

Denzin, Norman K. *Reading Race: Hollywood and the Cinema of Racial Violence*. Thousand Oaks, Calif.: Sage, 2002.

Dowling, Harry F. *Fighting Infection: Conquests of the Twentieth Century*. Cambridge: Harvard University Press, 1977.

Dwyer, Ellen. "Psychiatry and Race during World War II." *Journal of the History of Medicine* 61 (April 2006): 117–43.

Edelstein, Ludwig. *The Hippocratic Oath: Text, Translation, and Interpretation.* Baltimore: Johns Hopkins University Press, 1943.

Edgar, Harold. "Outside the Community." In *Tuskegee's Truths: Rethinking the Tuskegee Syphilis Study,* edited by Susan M. Reverby, 489–94. Chapel Hill: University of North Carolina Press, 2000.

Elliott, Carl. "Guinea-Pigging." *New Yorker,* January 7, 2008, pp. 36–41.

Ellison, Ralph. *Invisible Man.* New York: Vintage, 1947.

———. "The Shadow and the Act." In *The Collected Essays of Ralph Ellison,* edited by John F. Callahan. New York: Modern Library, 1995.

Emanuel, Ezekial, et al., eds. *Ethical and Regulatory Aspects of Clinical Research.* Baltimore: Johns Hopkins University Press, 2003.

Embree, Edwin, and Julia Waxman. *The Story of the Julius Rosenwald Fund.* New York: Harper, 1949.

Epstein, Steven. *Inclusion: The Politics of Difference in Medical Research.* Chicago: University of Chicago Press, 2007.

Etter-Lewis, Gwendolyn. *My Soul Is My Own: Oral Narratives of African American Women in the Professions.* New York: Routledge, 1993.

Eyerman, Ron. *Cultural Trauma: Slavery and the Formation of African American Identity.* Port Chester, N.Y.: Cambridge University Press, 2002.

Faden, Ruth R., Tom L. Beauchamp, and Nancy M. P. King. *A History and Theory of Informed Consent.* New York: Oxford University Press, 1986.

Fairchild, Amy. *Science at the Borders.* Baltimore: Johns Hopkins University Press, 2003.

Fairchild, Amy, and Ronald Bayer. "Uses and Abuses of Tuskegee." In *Tuskegee Truths: Rethinking the Tuskegee Syphilis Study,* edited by Susan M. Reverby, 589–604. Chapel Hill: University of North Carolina Press, 2000.

Fairchild, Amy, Ronald Bayer, and James Colgrove. *Searching Eyes: Privacy, the State, and Disease Surveillance in America.* Berkeley: University of California Press, 2007.

Fairclough, Adam. "Civil Rights and the Lincoln Memorial: The Censored Speeches of Robert R. Moton (1922) and John Lewis (1963)." *Journal of Negro History* 82 (Autumn 1997): 408–16.

Fee, Elizabeth. *Disease and Discovery: A History of the Johns Hopkins School of Hygiene and Public Health.* Baltimore: Johns Hopkins University Press, 1987.

———. "Sin versus Science: Venereal Disease in Twentieth-Century Baltimore." In *AIDS: The Burdens of History,* edited by Elizabeth Fee and Daniel M. Fox, 121–46. Berkeley: University of California Press, 1988.

Fletcher, John C. "A Case Study in Historical Relativism: The Tuskegee (Public Health Service) Syphilis Study." In *Tuskegee Truths: Rethinking the Tuskegee Syphilis Study,* edited by Susan M. Reverby, 276–98. Chapel Hill: University of North Carolina Press, 2000.

Forman, James. *Sammy Younge, Jr.: The First Black College Student to Die in the Black Liberation Movement.* New York: Grove Press, 1968.

Foster, Henry W., Jr., with Alice Greenwood. *Make a Difference.* New York: Scribner, 1997.

Fourtner, A. W., C. F. Fourtner, and C. F. Herreid. "Bad Blood: A Case Study of the

Tuskegee Syphilis Project." *Journal of College Science Teaching* 23 (March/April 1994): 277–85.

Frankel, Marc. "Public Policy for Biomedical Research." Ph.D. diss., George Washington University, 1976.

Freidenfelds, Lara. "Recruiting Allies for Reform: Henry Knowles Beecher's 'Ethics and Clinical Research.'" *International Anesthesiology Clinics* 45 (September 2007): 79–103.

Freidenfelds, Lara, and Allan M. Brandt. "Commentary: Research Ethics after World War II: The Insular Culture of Biomedicine." *Kennedy Institute of Ethics Journal* 6 (September 1996): 239–43.

Freimuth, Vicki S., et al. "African Americans' Views on Research and the Tuskegee Syphilis Study." *Social Science and Medicine* 52 (March 2001): 797–808.

Gamble, Vanessa Northington. *Making a Place for Ourselves: The Black Hospital Movement, 1920–1945.* New York: Oxford University Press, 1995.

———. "Trust, Medical Care, and Racial and Ethnic Minorities." In *Multicultural Medicine and Health Disparities*, edited by David Satcher and R. J. Pamies, 437–48. New York: McGraw-Hill, 2005.

———. "The Tuskegee Syphilis Study and Women's Health." *Journal of the American Medical Women's Association* 52, no. 4 (1997): 195–96.

———. "Under the Shadow of Tuskegee: African Americans and Health Care." In *Tuskegee's Truths: Rethinking the Tuskegee Syphilis Study*, edited by Susan M. Reverby, 431–42. Chapel Hill: University of North Carolina Press, 2000.

Gamble, Vanessa Northington, and Deborah Stone. "U.S. Policy on Health Inequities: The Interplay of Politics and Research." *Journal of Health Politics Policy and Law* (February 2006): 93–126.

Garber, Mandy, and Robert Arnold. "Promoting the Participation of Minorities in Research." *American Journal of Bioethics* 6 (May–June 2006): W14–W20.

Gates, Henry Louis, Jr. *Thirteen Ways of Looking at a Black Man.* New York: Random House, 1997.

———. "The Trope of the New Negro and the Reconstruction of the Image of the Black." *Representations* 24 (Autumn 1988): 129–55.

Gerrity, Patricia L. "Public Health Initiatives and the Legacy of Tuskegee: A Case Study." *Family Community Health* 17 (March 1994): 15–22.

Gieryn, Thomas F. "Boundary-Work and the Demarcation of Science from Non-Science." *American Sociological Review* 48 (December 1983): 781–95.

Goodman, James. *Stories of Scottsboro.* New York: Pantheon, 1994.

Goodman, Jordan, Anthony McElligott, and Lara Marks. "Introduction: Making Human Bodies Useful: Historicizing Medical Experiments in the 20th Century." In *Useful Bodies: Humans in the Service of Medical Science in the Twentieth Century*, edited by Jordan Goodman, Anthony McElligott, and Lara Marks, 1–26. Baltimore: Johns Hopkins University Press, 2006.

Graves, Joseph L., Jr. *The Emperor's New Clothes: Biological Theories of Race at the Millennium.* New Brunswick, N.J.: Rutgers University Press, 2001.

Gray, Fred D. *Bus Ride to Justice: Changing the System by the System, the Life Works of Fred Gray.* Montgomery, Ala.: Black Belt Press, 1995.

————. "The Lawsuit." In *Tuskegee's Truths: Rethinking the Tuskegee Syphilis Study*, edited by Susan M. Reverby, 473–88. Chapel Hill: University of North Carolina Press, 2000.

————. *The Tuskegee Syphilis Study: The Real Story and Beyond*. Montgomery, Ala.: Black Belt Press, 1998.

Guinan, M. E. "Black Communities' Belief in 'AIDS as Genocide': A Barrier to Overcome for HIV Prevention." *Annals of Epidemiology* 3 (March 1993): 193–95.

Guzman, Jessie Parkhurst. *Crusade for Civic Democracy: The Story of the Tuskegee Civic Association, 1941–1970*. New York: Vantage, 1984.

Hahn, Richard D. "Obituary for Joseph Earle Moore, 1892–1957." *Maryland State Medical Journal* 7 (February 1958): 128–29.

Halpern, Sydney. "Constructing Moral Boundaries: Public Discourse on Human Experimentation." In *Bioethics in Social Context*, edited by C. Barry Hoffmaster, 69–89. Philadelphia: Temple University Press, 2001.

————. *Lesser Harms: The Morality of Risk in Medical Research*. Chicago: University of Chicago Press, 2004.

Hammonds, Evelynn M. "Black (W)Holes and the Geometry of Black Female Sexuality." *Differences* 6 (1994): 126–45.

————. "The Full-Blooded Negro and the African Past." Paper presented at "The Politics of 'Racial Health': Myths, Maladies, and the History of Policy" Conference, Rutgers University, 2001.

————. "The Logic of Difference: Race, Gender, and 19th Century Gynecological Surgery." Lecture at Wellesley College, Wellesley, Mass., 2002.

————. *The Logic of Difference*. Baltimore: Johns Hopkins University Press, forthcoming.

————. "Your Silence Will Not Protect You: Nurse Eunice Rivers and the Tuskegee Syphilis Study." In *Tuskegee's Truths: Rethinking the Tuskegee Syphilis Study*, edited by Susan M. Reverby, 340–47. Chapel Hill: University of North Carolina Press, 2000.

Hammonds, Evelynn M., and Rebecca M. Herzig, eds. *The Nature of Difference: Sciences of Race in the United States from Jefferson to Genetics*. Cambridge: MIT Press, 2008.

Harkness, Jon M. "Letter to the Editor: The Significance of the Nuremberg Code." *New England Journal of Medicine* 338 (1998): 995–96.

————. "Nuremberg and the Issue of Wartime Experimentation on US Prisoners." *Journal of the American Medical Association* 276 (November 27, 1996): 1672–75.

————. "Research behind Bars." Ph.D. diss., University of Wisconsin, 1996.

Harkness, Jon M., Susan Lederer, and Daniel Wikler. "Laying Ethical Foundations for Clinical Research." *Bulletin of the World Health Organization* 79 (July 2001): 365–66.

Harlan, Louis. *Booker T. Washington: The Making of a Black Leader*. New York: Oxford University Press, 1972.

————. *Booker T. Washington: The Wizard of Tuskegee, 1901–1915*. New York: Oxford University Press, 1983.

————. "The Secret Life of Booker T. Washington." In *Washington in Perspective*,

Essays of Louis R. Harlan, edited by Raymond W. Smock, 110–32. Jackson: University Press of Mississippi, 1988.

Harris, Y., P. B. Gorelick, P. Samuels, and I. Bempong. "Why African Americans May Not Be Participating in Clinical Trials." *Journal of the National Medical Association* 88 (October 1996): 630–34.

Hartman, Saidiya V. *Scenes of Subjection*. New York: Oxford University Press, 1997.

Harvey, A. McGehee. *Science at the Bedside: Clinical Research in American Medicine, 1905–1945*. Baltimore: Johns Hopkins University Press, 1981.

Hayden, Deborah. *Pox: Genius, Madness, and the Mysteries of Syphilis*. New York: Basic Books, 2003.

Hayner, Priscilla B. *Unspeakable Truths: Facing the Challenge of Truth Commissions*. New York: Routledge, 2002.

Health-PAC. *The American Health Empire*. New York: Vintage, 1970.

Hemphill, Essex. "Civil Servant." In *Tuskegee's Truths: Rethinking the Tuskegee Syphilis Study*, edited by Susan M. Reverby, 554. Chapel Hill: University of North Carolina Press, 2000.

Henderson, Mae G. "Speaking in Tongues: Dialogics, Dialectics, and the Black Women Writer's Literary Tradition." In *Changing Our Own Words: Essays on Criticism, Theory, and Writing by Black Women*, edited by Cheryl A. Wall, 16–37. New Brunswick, N.J.: Rutgers University Press, 1989.

Hendricks, Melissa. "Raymond Pearl's 'Mingled Mess.'" *Johns Hopkins Magazine* 58 (April 2006), < http://www.jhu.edu/~jhumag/0406web/pearl.html>, accessed January 27, 2008.

Herzig, Rebecca. *Suffering for Science*. New Brunswick, N.J.: Rutgers University Press, 2005.

Higginbotham, Evelyn Brooks. "African-American Women's History and the Metalanguage of Race." *Signs* 17 (Winter 1992): 251–74.

———. "Beyond the Sound of Silence: Afro-American Women in History." *Gender and History* 1 (Spring 1989): 58–59.

———. *Righteous Discontent: The Women's Movement in the Black Baptist Church, 1880–1920*. Cambridge: Harvard University Press, 1992.

Hine, Darlene Clark. "The Black Professional Class." *Bulletin: American Academy of Arts and Sciences* 60 (Summer 2007): 26–28.

———. *Black Women in White*. Bloomington: Indiana University Press, 1989.

———. "Rape and the Inner Lives of Black Women in the Middle West: Preliminary Thoughts on the Culture of Dissemblance." *Signs* 14 (Summer 1989): 912–21.

———. "Rehearsal for Freedom in Black Country." Nathan Huggins Lectures, Du Bois Institute, Harvard University, March 6–8, 2007.

———, ed. *Black Women's History: Theory and Practice*. Brooklyn, N.Y.: Carlson Publishing, 1990.

Holloway, Karla F. C. "Accidental Communities: Race, Emergency Medicine, and the Problem of PolyHeme®." *American Journal of Bioethics* 6 (May/June 2006): 7–17.

———. *Passed On: African American Mourning Stories*. Durham: Duke University Press, 2002.

Hornblum, Allen. *Acres of Skin*. New York: Routledge, 1999.

Howell, Joel, and Rodney A. Hayward. "Writing Willowbrook, Reading Willowbrook." In *Useful Bodies: Humans in the Service of Medical Science in the Twentieth Century*, edited by Jordan Goodman, Anthony McElligott, and Lara Marks, 190–214. Baltimore: Johns Hopkins University Press, 2003.

Humphreys, Margaret. *Malaria: Poverty, Race, and Public Health in the United States.* Baltimore: Johns Hopkins University Press, 2001.

Hurley, Vic. *The Jungle Patrol: The Story of the Philippine Constabulary.* New York: E. P. Dutton, 1938.

Johansson, S. Ryan. "Food for Thought: Rhetoric and Reality in Modern Mortality History." *Historical Methods* 27 (Summer 1994): 101–25.

Jones, James H. *Alfred Kinsey: A Public Private Life.* New York: W. W. Norton, 1997.

———. *Bad Blood: The Tuskegee Syphilis Experiment.* New York: Free Press, 1981, 1993.

———. "The Tuskegee Legacy: AIDS and the Black Community." *Hastings Center Report* 22 (June 1992): 38–40.

Jonsen, Albert R. "The Belmont Report," <http://www.hhs.gov/ohrp/belmontArchive .html>, accessed February 22, 2009.

———. *The Birth of Bioethics.* New York: Oxford University Press, 1998.

———. "The Birth of the Belmont Report," <http://www.georgetown.edu/nbac/ transcripts/jul98/Belmont.html>, accessed February 22, 2009.

Jonsen, Albert R., and Stephen Toulmin. *The Abuse of Casuistry.* Berkeley: University of California Press, 1990.

Junod, Tom. "Deadly Medicine." In *Tuskegee's Truths: Rethinking the Tuskegee Syphilis Study*, edited by Susan M. Reverby, 509–26. Chapel Hill: University of North Carolina Press, 2000.

Kahn, Jeffrey, Anna Mastroianni, and Jeremy Sugarman. "Introduction: Changing Claims about Justice in Research." In *Beyond Consent*, edited by Jeffrey Kahn, Anna Mastroianni and Jeremy Sugarman, 1–10. New York: Oxford University Press, 1999.

Kahn, Jonathan. "How a Drug Becomes Ethnic." *Yale Journal of Health Policy and Law* 4 (Winter 2004): 1–46.

Kahn, Jonathan, and Pamela Sankar. "BiDil: Race Medicine or Race Marketing." *Health Affairs* (July–December 2005): 455–63.

Katz, Jay. "The Consent Principle of the Nuremberg Code: Its Significance Then and Now." In *The Nazi Doctors and the Nuremberg Code*, edited by George J. Annas and Michael A. Grodin, 227–39. New York: Oxford University Press, 1992.

———. "The Nuremberg Code and the Nuremberg Trial: A Reappraisal." *Journal of the American Medical Association* 276 (November 27, 1996): 1662–66.

———. "The Regulation of Human Experimentation in the United States—A Personal Odyssey." *Institutional Review Board* 9 (January–February 1987): 1–6.

———. *The Silent World of Doctor and Patient.* New York: Free Press, 1984.

Katz, Jay, Alexander Morgan Capron, and Eleanor Swift Glass. *Experimentation with Human Beings.* New York: Russell Sage Foundation, 1972.

Kelley, Robin. *Hammer and Hoe: Alabama Communists during the Great Depression.* Chapel Hill: University of North Carolina Press, 1990.

Kimmelman, Jonathan. "The Therapeutic Misconception at 35: Treatment, Research, and Confusion." *Hastings Center Report* 37 (November–December 2007): 30–42.

King, Patricia A. "The Dangers of Difference." In *Tuskegee's Truths: Rethinking the Tuskegee Syphilis Study*, edited by Susan M. Reverby, 424–30. Chapel Hill: University of North Carolina Press, 2000.

———. "The Dangers of Difference, Revisited." In *The Story of Bioethics*, edited by Jennifer K. Walter and Eran P. Klein, 197–213. Washington, D.C.: Georgetown University Press, 2003.

———. "Race, Justice, and Research." In *Beyond Consent*, edited by Jeffrey Kahn, Anna Mastroianni, and Jeremy Sugarman, 88–110. New York: Oxford University Press, 1999.

———. "Reflections on Race and Bioethics in the United States." *Health Matrix: The Journal of Law-Medicine* 14 (Winter 2004): 149–53.

Kirp, David L. "Blood, Sweat, and Tears: The Tuskegee Experiment and the Era of AIDS." *Tikkun* 10 (March 1995): 50–54.

Kondratas, Ramunas. *Images from the History of the Public Health Service*. Washington, D.C.: U.S. Department of Health and Human Services, Public Health Service, 1994.

Kowalski, Philip J. "No Excuses for Our Dirt: Booker T. Washington and a 'New Negro' Middle Class." In *Post-Bellum, Pre-Harlem*, edited by Barbara McCaskill and Caroline Gebhard, 181–96. New York: New York University Press, 2006.

Kraut, Alan M. *Goldberger's War*. New York: Hill and Wang, 2003.

———. *Silent Travelers: Germs, Genes, and the Immigrant Menace*. New York: Basic Books, 1994.

Kruif, Paul De. *The Fight for Life*. New York: Harcourt, Brace, 1938.

Landecker, Hannah. *Culturing Life: How Cells Became Technologies*. Cambridge: Harvard University Press, 2007.

———. "Immortality, in Vitro: A History of the HeLa Cell Line." In *Biotechnology and Culture: Bodies, Anxieties, Ethics*, edited by Paul Brodwin, 53–72. Bloomington: Indiana University Press, 2000.

Larson, Edward. *Sex, Race, and Science: Eugenics in the Deep South*. Baltimore: Johns Hopkins University Press, 1995.

Lederer, Susan. *Flesh and Blood*. New York: Oxford University Press, 2008.

———. "Hideyo Noguchi's Luetin Experiment and the Antivivisectionists." *Isis* 76 (1985): 31–48.

———. "Hollywood and Human Experimentation: Representing Medical Research in Popular Film." In *Medicine's Moving Pictures*, edited by Leslie J. Reagan, Nancy Tomes, and Paula A. Treichler, 282–306. Rochester, N.Y.: University of Rochester Press, 2007.

———. "'The Right and Wrong of Making Experiments on Human Beings': Udo J. Wile and Syphilis." *Bulletin of the History of Medicine* 58 (1984): 380–97.

———. *Subjected to Science: Human Experimentation in America before the Second World War*. Baltimore: Johns Hopkins University Press, 1995.

———. "The Tuskegee Syphilis Study in the Context of American Medical Research."

In *Tuskegee's Truths: Rethinking the Tuskegee Syphilis Study*, edited by Susan Reverby, 266–75. Chapel Hill: University of North Carolina Press, 2000.

Lederer, Susan, and John Parascandola. "Screening Syphilis: *Dr. Ehrlich's Magic Bullet* Meets the Public Health Service." *Journal of the History of Medicine* 53 (October 1998): 345–70.

Lee, Sandra Soo-Jin. "Racializing Drug Design: Implications of Pharmacogenomics for Health Disparities." *American Journal of Public Health* 95 (December 2005): 2133–38.

Legacy Committee. "Legacy Committee Request." In *Tuskegee's Truths: Rethinking the Tuskegee Syphilis Study*, edited by Susan Reverby, 559–66. Chapel Hill: University of North Carolina Press, 2000.

Lerner, Barron H. "Sins of Omission—Cancer Research without Informed Consent." *New England Journal of Medicine* 351 (August 12, 2004): 628–30.

Leverenz, David. "Booker T. Washington's Strategies of Manliness, for Black and White Audiences." In *Booker T. Washington and Black Progress*, edited by W. Fitzhugh Brundage, 149–76. Gainesville: University Press of Florida, 2003.

Levi, Primo. *The Drowned and the Saved*. New York: Vintage, 1989.

Levinson, Brett. "Obstinate Forgetting in Chile: Radical Injustice and the Possibility of Community." In *Topologies of Trauma: Essays on the Limit of Knowledge and Memory*, edited by Linda Belau and Petar Ramadanovic, 211–32. New York: Other Press, 2002.

Lichtenstein, Browen. "Stigma as a Barrier to Treatment of Sexually Transmitted Infection in the American Deep South: Issues of Race, Gender, and Poverty." *Social Science and Medicine* 57 (2003): 2435–45.

Lie, R. K., E. Emanuel, C. Grady, and D. Wendler. "The Standard of Care Debate: The Declaration of Helsinki versus the International Consensus Opinion." *Journal of Medical Ethics* 30 (April 2004): 190–93.

Litwack, Leon F. *Trouble in Mind: Black Southerners in the Age of Jim Crow*. New York: Alfred Knopf, 1998.

Lombardo, Paul, and Gregory Dorr. "Eugenics, Medical Education, and the Public Health Service: Another Perspective on the Tuskegee Syphilis Experiment." *Bulletin of the History of Medicine* 80 (Summer 2006): 291–316.

London, Alex John. "Justice and the Human Development Approach to International Research." *Hastings Center Report* 35 (January–February 2005): 24–37.

Long, Gretchen. *Doctoring Freedom*. Chapel Hill: University of North Carolina Press, forthcoming.

Love, Spencie. *One Blood: The Death and Resurrection of Charles R. Drew*. Chapel Hill: University of North Carolina Press, 1996.

Maier, Charles S. "Doing History, Doing Justice: The Narrative of the Historian and of the Truth Commission." In *Truth v. Justice: The Morality of Truth Commissions*, edited by Robert I. Rotberg and Dennis Thompson, 261–78. Princeton: Princeton University Press, 1999.

———. "A Surfeit of Memory? Reflections on History, Melancholy, and Denial." *History and Memory* 30 (Fall–Winter 1993): 136–52.

Manjoo, Farhad. *True Enough: Learning to Live in a Post-Fact Society*. New York: John Wiley, 2008.

Marable, Manning. *Black Leadership*. New York: Columbia University Press, 1998.

———. "Tuskegee and the Politics of Illusion in the New South." *Black Scholar* 8 (May 1977): 13–24.

Marks, Harry M. "Epidemiologists Explain Pellagra: Gender, Race, and Political Economy in the Work of Edgar Sydenstricker." *Journal of the History of Medicine and Allied Sciences* 58 (January 2003): 34–55.

———. "Notes from the Underground: The Social Organization of Therapeutic Research." In *Grand Rounds: One Hundred Years of Internal Medicine*, edited by Russell Maulitz and Diana E. Long, 297–338. Philadelphia: University of Pennsylvania Press, 1988.

———. *The Progress of Experiment: Science and Therapeutic Reform in the United States, 1900–1990*. New York: Cambridge University Press, 1997.

Martin, Waldo. "In Search of Booker T. Washington." In *Booker T. Washington and Black Progress*, edited by Fitzhugh Brundage, 38–57. Gainesville: University Press of Florida, 2003.

Maschke, Karen J. "Human Research Protections: Time for Regulatory Reform?" *Hastings Center Report* 38 (March–April 2008): 19–22.

Mastroianni, Anna, and Jeffrey Kahn. "Swinging on the Pendulum." *Hastings Center Report* 31 (May–June 2001): 21–28.

McAdams, Don. *The Stories We Live By*. New York: W. W. Morrow, 1993.

McBride, David. *From TB to AIDS: Epidemics among Urban Blacks since 1900*. Albany: SUNY Press, 1991.

McCully, Audrey Wenger. "The United States Public Health Service Venereal Disease Clinic and Government Free Bath House (1919–1936)." *The Record: Annual Publication of the Garland County Arkansas Historical Society* (1981): 95–105.

McDonald, Charles J. "The Contribution of the Tuskegee Study to Medical Knowledge." In *Tuskegee's Truths: Rethinking the Tuskegee Syphilis Study*, edited by Susan Reverby, 202–12. Chapel Hill: University of North Carolina Press, 2000.

McDonald, Leroy. *Tuskegee Subject No. 626*. Dallas, Tex.: Leroy McDonald, 1991.

Mercer, Kobena. *Welcome to the Jungle: New Positions in Black Cultural Studies*. New York: Routledge, 1994.

Miles, Toni P., and David McBride. "World War I Origins of the Syphilis Epidemic among 20th Century Black Americans: A Bio-Historical Analysis." *Social Science & Medicine* 45 (January 1997): 61–69.

Mitscherlich, A., and F. Mielke. *The Death Doctors*, translated by James Cleugh. London: Elek Books, 1962.

More, Ellen Singer, and Maureen A. Milligan, eds. *The Empathic Practitioner: Empathy, Gender, and Medicine*. New Brunswick, N.J.: Rutgers University Press, 1994.

Moreno, Jonathan. "Protectionism in Research Involving Human Subjects." *Technical and Policy Issues in Research Involving Human Subjects*. National Bioethics Advisory Commission 2 (August 2001): 13–121.

Moreno, Jonathan, and Susan Lederer. "Revising the History of Cold War Research Ethics." *Kennedy Institute of Ethics Journal* 6 (September 1996): 223–37.

Mugleston, William F. "Booker T. Washington." In *African American National Biography*, edited by Henry Louis Gates Jr. and Evelyn Brooks Higginbotham, 8:124–25. New York: Oxford University Press, 2008.

Mullan, Fitzhugh. *Plagues and Politics: The Story of the United States Public Health Service*. New York: Basic Books, 1989.

Murray, Albert, and John F. Callahan, eds. *The Selected Letters of Ralph Ellison and Albert Murray*. New York: Modern Library, 2000.

Mustafa, Hudita. "Portraits of Modernity: Fashioning Selves in Dakarois Popular Photography." In *Images and Empires: Visuality in Colonial and Postcolonial Africa*, edited by Paul Stuart Landau, 188–201. Berkeley: University of California Press, 2002.

Naipaul, V. S. *A Turn in the South*. New York: Alfred A. Knopf, 1989.

Neiman, Susan. *Evil in Modern Thought*. Princeton, N.J.: Princeton University Press, 2002.

Nelson, Sioban. "Ethical Expertise and the Problem of the Good Nurse." In *The Complexities of Care: Nursing Reconsidered*, edited by Suzanne Gordon, 69–87. Ithaca, N.Y.: Cornell University Press, 2006.

Norrell, Robert J. *Reaping the Whirlwind: The Civil Rights Movement in Tuskegee*. New York: Vintage, 1986.

———. "Understanding the Wizard: Another Look at the Age of Booker T. Washington." In *Booker T. Washington and Black Progress*, edited by W. Fitzhugh Brundage, 107–30. Gainesville: University Press of Florida, 2003.

O'Meally, Robert, and Genevieve Fabre, eds. *History and Memory in African-American Culture*. New York: Oxford University Press, 1994.

Osler, William W. "Internal Medicine as a Vocation." In *Aequanimitas, with Other Addresses to Medical Students, Nurses, and Practitioners of Medicine*, 131–46. Philadelphia: Blakiston Company, 1904.

Palmer, Larry I. "Paying for Suffering: The Problem of Human Experimentation." *Maryland Law Review* 56 (1997): 604–23.

Parascandola, John. "John Mahoney and the Introduction of Penicillin to Treat Syphilis." *Pharmacy in History* 43 (January 2001): 3–13.

———. *Sex, Sin, and Science: A History of Syphilis in America*. New York: Praeger, 2008.

———. "Syphilis at the Cinema: Medicine and Morals in VD Films of the U.S. Public Health Service in World War II." In *Medicine's Moving Pictures*, edited by Nancy Tomes, Leslie J. Reagan, and Paula A. Treichler, 71–92. Rochester, N.Y.: University of Rochester Press, 2007.

———. "VD at the Movies: PHS Films of the 1930s and 1940s." *Public Health Reports* 111 (March–April 1996): 173–75.

Parker, Lisa S., and Hilary K. Alvarez. "The Legacy of the Tuskegee Syphilis Study." In *Ethics and Public Health: Model Curriculum*, edited by Bruce Jennings, Jeffrey Kahn, Anna Mastroianni, and Lisa S. Parker, 37–73. Washington, D.C.: Association of Schools of Public Health, 2003.

Pernick, Martin S. *A Calculus of Suffering*. New York: Columbia University Press, 1985.

———. "Eugenics and Public Health in American History." *American Journal of Public Health* 87 (November 1997): 1767–72.

———. "The Patient's Role in Medical Decision-Making: A Social History of Informed Consent in Medical Therapy." In *Making Health Care Decisions: The Ethical and Legal Implication of Informed Consent in the Patient-Practitioner Relationship*, 1–35. Washington, D.C.: Government Printing Office, 1982.

Pickle, Kathryn, Sandra Crouse Quinn, and J. D. Brown. "HIV/AIDS Coverage in Black Newspapers, 1991–1996: Implications for Health, Communication, and Health Education." *Journal of Health Communications* 7 (October–December 2002): 427–44.

Poirier, Suzanne. *Chicago's War on Syphilis, 1937-1940: The Times, the Trib, and the Clap Doctor*. Champaign-Urbana: University of Illinois Press, 1995.

Portelli, Alessandro. *The Death of Luigi Trastulli and Other Stories*. Albany: SUNY Press, 1990.

Proctor, Robert. "Nazi Doctors, Racial Medicine, and Human Experimentation." In *The Nazi Doctors and the Nuremberg Code*, edited by George J. Annas and Michael A. Grodin, 17–32. New York: Oxford University Press, 1992.

———. *Racial Hygiene*. Cambridge: Harvard University Press, 1988.

Quetel, Claude. *History of Syphilis*. Baltimore: Johns Hopkins University Press, 1990.

Radolf, Justin D., and Sheila A. Lukehart, eds. *Pathogenic Treponema*. New York: Caister Academic Press, 2006.

Reverby, Susan M. "Herman Shaw." In *African American National Biography*, edited by Henry Louis Gates Jr. and Evelyn Brooks Higginbotham, 7:165–67. New York: Oxford University Press, 2007.

———. "History of an Apology: From Tuskegee to the White House." *Research Nurse* 3 (July/August 1997): 1–9.

———. "Inclusion and Exclusion: The Politics of History, Difference, and Medical Research." *Journal of the History of Medicine* 63 (January 2008): 103–13.

———. "Infecting with Syphilis: The U.S. Public Health Service and the Post-War Experiments in Guatemala." Forthcoming.

———. "'Misrepresentation of the Tuskegee Study'—Distortion of Analysis and Facts." *Journal of the National Medical Association* 97 (August 2005): 1180–81.

———. "More Than Fact and Fiction: Cultural Memory and the Tuskegee Syphilis Study." *Hastings Center Report* 31 (September–October 2001): 22–28.

———. *Ordered to Care: The Dilemma of American Nursing*. New York: Cambridge University Press, 1987.

———. "Rethinking the Tuskegee Syphilis Study: Nurse Rivers, Silence, and the Meaning of Treatment." In *Tuskegee's Truths: Rethinking the Tuskegee Syphilis Study*, edited by Susan M. Reverby, 365–85. Chapel Hill: University of North Carolina Press, 2000.

———. "'Special Treatment': BiDil, Tuskegee, and the Logic of Race." *Journal of Law, Medicine, and Ethics* 36 (Fall 2008): 478–84.

———. "Syphilis of the Innocent." *Women's Review of Books* 25 (November–December 2008): 11.

———. "Tuskegee: Could It Happen Again?" *Postgraduate Medicine Journal* 77 (September 2001): 553–54.

———, ed. *Tuskegee's Truths: Rethinking the Tuskegee Syphilis Study*. Chapel Hill: University of North Carolina Press, 2000.

Reverby, Susan M., and Elizabeth Sims. "Charlie Wesley Pollard." In *African American National Biography*, edited by Henry Louis Gates Jr. and Evelyn Brooks Higginbotham, 6:387–88. New York: Oxford University Press, 2007.

Richardson, Ruth. *Death, Dissection, and the Destitute*. 2nd ed. Chicago: University of Chicago Press, 2000.

Rocchio, Vincent F. *Reel Racism: Confronting Hollywood's Construction of Afro-American Culture*. Boulder, Colo.: Westview, 2000.

Rogers, Naomi. "Race and the Politics of Polio: Warm Springs, Tuskegee, and the March of Dimes." *American Journal of Public Health* 97 (May 2007): 784–95.

Rogers, William Warren, and Robert David Ward. "From 1865 through 1920." In *Alabama: History of a Deep South State*, edited by William Warren Rogers, Wayne Flynt, Leah R. Atkins, and Robert D. Ward, 225–392. Tuscaloosa: University of Alabama Press, 1994.

Rosenberg, Charles E. "Meanings, Policies, and Medicine: On the Bioethical Enterprise and History." *Daedalus* 128 (Fall 1999): 27–46.

———. *No Other Gods*. Baltimore: Johns Hopkins University Press, 1997.

Rosengarten, Theodore. *All God's Dangers*. Chicago: University of Chicago Press, 2000.

Rosenkrantz, Barbara. "Non-Random Events." In *Tuskegee's Truths: Rethinking the Tuskegee Syphilis Study*, edited by Susan M. Reverby, 236–50. Chapel Hill: University of North Carolina Press, 2000.

Rothman, David. "Research Ethics at Tuskegee and Willowbrook [Letter]." *American Journal of Medicine* 77 (June 1984): A49.

———. "The Shame of Medical Research." *New York Review of Books* 47 (November 30, 2000): 60–64.

———. *Strangers at the Bedside*. New York: Basic Books, 1991.

———. "Were Tuskegee and Willowbrook 'Studies in Nature'?" *Hastings Center Report* 12 (February 1982): 5–7.

Roy, Benjamin. "The Julius Rosenwald Fund Syphilis Seroprevalence Studies." *Journal of the National Medical Association* 88 (May 1996): 315–22.

———. "The Tuskegee Syphilis Experiment: Biotechnology and the Administrative State." In *Tuskegee's Truths: Rethinking the Tuskegee Syphilis Study*, edited by Susan M. Reverby, 299–320. Chapel Hill: University of North Carolina Press, 2000.

———. "The Tuskegee Syphilis Experiment: Medical Ethics, Constitutionalism, and Property in the Body." *Harvard Journal of Minority Health* 1 (Fall–Winter 1995): 11–15.

Sadiq [Bey, Sadiq]. "Tuskegee Experiment." In *Tuskegee's Truths: Rethinking the Tuskegee Syphilis Study*, edited by Susan M. Reverby, 552–53. Chapel Hill: University of North Carolina Press, 2000.

Savage, Kirk. *Standing Soldiers, Kneeling Slaves*. Princeton, N.J.: Princeton University Press, 1997.

Savitt, Todd. *Race and Medicine*. Kent, Ohio: Kent State University Press, 2007.

Schacter, Daniel. *Searching for Memory: The Brain, the Mind, and the Past*. New York: Basic Books, 1996.

Schafer, Elizabeth D. "Eugene Heriot Dibble, Jr." In *African American National Biography*, edited by Henry Louis Gates Jr. and Evelyn Brooks Higginbotham, 2:666–67. New York: Oxford University Press, 2007.

Schmidt, Ulf. *Justice at Nuremberg*. London: Palgrave Macmillan, 2004.

Schoen, Johnna. *Choice and Coercion*. Chapel Hill: University of North Carolina Press, 2005.

Schuklenk, U. "The Standard of Care Debate: Against the Myth of an 'International Consensus Opinion.'" *Journal of Medical Ethics* 30 (April 2004): 194–97.

Schwartz, Marie Jenkins. *Birthing a Slave: Motherhood and Medicine in the Antebellum South*. Cambridge: Harvard University Press, 2006.

Scott, Joan. "The Evidence of Experience." In *Feminists Theorize the Political*, edited by Judith Butler and Joan W. Scott, 22–40. New York: Routledge, 1992.

Scythes, John B., Colman M. Jones, and Robert H. Notenboom. "A New Gold Standard for Syphilis." Poster presentation for the European Academy of Dermatology and Venerology—II, Spring Conference, May 2004, Budapest, Hungary, <http://colman.net/eadv/index.html>, accessed February 22, 2009.

Sedwick, Judith. *Women of Courage*. Cambridge: Radcliffe College, 1984.

Seegal, David. "In Memoriam: Joseph Earle Moore, 1892–1957." *Journal of Chronic Diseases* 7 (February 1958): 93–94.

Segrest, Dale. *Conscience and Command*. Atlanta: Scholars Press, 1994.

Segrest, Mab. *Memoir of a Race Traitor*. Boston: South End Press, 1994.

Shelton, Deborah L. "Legacy of Tuskegee." *American Medical News* (June 3, 1996): 24–30.

Shick, Tom W. "Race, Class, and Medicine: 'Bad Blood' in Twentieth-Century America." *Journal of Ethnic Studies* 10 (Summer 1982): 97–105.

Shweder, Richard. "The Idea of Moral Progress: Bush versus Posner versus Berlin." *Philosophy of Education Yearbook* (Urbana, Ill.: Philosophy of Education Society, 2003): 29–56.

———. "Tuskegee Re-Examined." *Spiked* online. January 8, 2004. <http://www.spiked-online.com/Articles/0000000CA34A.htm>, accessed February 22, 2009.

Siddique, Irtaza Husain. "Life Expectancy of Untreated Syphilis Cases: A Prospective Study." M.A. thesis, University of Alabama in Birmingham, 1978.

Sidel, Victor, and Ruth Sidel. *Reforming Medicine: The Lessons of the Last Quarter Century*. New York: Pantheon, 1984.

Silver, George A. "The Infamous Tuskegee Study." In *Tuskegee's Truths: Rethinking the Tuskegee Syphilis Study*, edited by Susan M. Reverby, 507. Chapel Hill: University of North Carolina Press, 2000.

Smith, Susan L. "Neither Victim nor Villain: Nurse Eunice Rivers, the Tuskegee Syphilis Experiment, and Public Health Work." In *Tuskegee's Truths: Rethinking*

the Tuskegee Syphilis Study, edited by Susan M. Reverby, 348–64. Chapel Hill:
University of North Carolina Press, 2000.

———. 'Sick and Tired of Being Sick and Tired': Black Women's Health Activism in
America, 1890–1950. Philadelphia: University of Pennsylvania Press, 1995.

Smitherman, Geneva. Talkin and Testifyin: The Language of Black America. Boston:
Houghton Mifflin, 1977.

Solomon [Watson], Martha. "Commentary: The Rhetoric of Dehumanization: An
Analysis of Medical Reports of the Tuskegee Syphilis Project." In Critical Questions:
Invention, Creativity, and the Criticism of Discourse and Media, edited by William L.
Nothstine, Carole Blair, and Gary A. Copeland. New York: St. Martin's, 1994.

———. "The Rhetoric of Dehumanization: An Analysis of Medical Reports of the
Tuskegee Syphilis Project." In Tuskegee's Truths: Rethinking the Tuskegee Syphilis
Study, edited by Susan M. Reverby, 251–65. Chapel Hill: University of North
Carolina Press, 2000.

Stanfield, John H. "Venereal Disease Control Demonstrations among Rural Blacks in
the American South." Western Journal of Black Studies 5 (Winter 1981): 246–53.

Steinbock, Bonnie, John D. Arras, and Alex John London, eds. Ethical Issues in
Modern Medicine. 6th ed. New York: McGraw-Hill, 2003.

Steingroot, Ira. "Lauding Byron." Tikkun 9 (March–April 1994): 76–79.

Studdert, David M., and Troyen A. Brennan. "Clinical Trials in Developing
Countries: Scientific and Ethical Issues." Medical Journal of Australia 169 (1998):
545–48.

Sutton, Karen. "Sam Doner." In African American National Biography, edited by
Henry Louis Gates Jr. and Evelyn Brooks Higginbotham, 3:27. New York: Oxford
University Press, 2007.

Talone, P. "Establishing Trust after Tuskegee." International Journal of Radiation
Oncology, Biology, Physics 40 (January 1998): 3–4.

Taper, Bernard. Gomillion v. Lightfoot: The Tuskegee Gerrymander Case. New York:
McGraw-Hill, 1962.

Tapper, Melbourne. "An 'Anthropathology' of the 'American Negro': Anthropology,
Genetics, and the New Racial Science, 1940–1952." Social History of Medicine 10
(August 1997): 263–89.

Termini, Benedict, and Stanley I. Music. "The Natural History of Syphilis: A Review."
Southern Medical Journal 65 (February 1972): 21–45.

Thomas, Henry M., Jr. "Memorial: Joseph Earle Moore." Transactions of the American
Clinical and Climatological Association 71 (1960): xlix.

Thomas, Stephen B., and Sandra Crouse Quinn. "The Tuskegee Syphilis Study, 1932
to 1972: Implications for HIV Education and AIDS Risk Education Programs in
the Black Community." In Tuskegee's Truths: Rethinking the Tuskegee Syphilis Study,
edited by Susan M. Reverby, 404–17. Chapel Hill: University of North Carolina
Press, 2000.

Thomas, Stephen B., and James W. Curran. "Tuskegee: From Science to Conspiracy to
Metaphor [Editorial]." American Journal of the Medical Sciences 317 (January 1999):
1–4.

Thornton, Shirley A. "African Americans Moving into the 21st Century: Accepting the

Responsibility for Our Own Destiny." *Journal of Negro Education* 64 (Spring 1995): 104–10.

Tomes, Nancy. *The Gospel of Germs*. New York: Cambridge University Press, 1998.

Turner, Patricia. *I Heard It through the Grapevine*. Berkeley: University of California Press, 1993.

U.S. Department of Health and Human Services. *Prevention and Beyond*. Washington, D.C.: Department of Health and Human Services, 1988.

———. *Report of the Secretary's Task Force on Black and Minority Health*. Washington, D.C.: Department of Health and Human Services, August 1985.

Varmus, Harold, and David Satcher. "Ethical Complexities of Conducting Research in Developing Countries." In *Tuskegee's Truths: Rethinking the Tuskegee Syphilis Study*, edited by Susan M. Reverby, 584–88. Chapel Hill: University of North Carolina Press, 2000.

Veressayev, Vikenty. *The Memoirs of a Physician*. New York: Alfred Knopf, 1916.

Vessey, J. A., and S. Gennaro. "The Ghost of Tuskegee." *Nursing Research* 43, no. 2 (1994): 67.

Wailoo, Keith. *Drawing Blood: Technology and Disease Identity in Twentieth-Century America*. Baltimore: Johns Hopkins University Press, 1997.

———. *Dying in the City of Blues: Sickle Cell Anemia and the Politics of Race and Health*. Chapel Hill: University of North Carolina Press, 2001.

Wall, Lewis L. "The Medical Ethics of J. Marion Sims." *Journal of Medical Ethics* 32 (June 2006): 346–50.

Walls, Edwina. "Hot Springs Waters and the Treatment of Venereal Diseases: The U.S. Public Health Service Clinic and Camp Garraday." *Journal of the Arkansas Medical Society* 91 (February 1995): 430–37.

Ward, Thomas J., Jr. *Black Physicians in the Jim Crow South*. Fayetteville: University of Arkansas Press, 2003.

Washington, Harriet. *Medical Apartheid*. New York: Doubleday, 2007.

Wasunna, Angela. "Researchers Abroad." *Hastings Center Report* 35 (January–February 2005): 3.

Weindling, Paul. *Nazi Medicine and the Nuremberg Trials*. London: Palgrave Macmillan, 2006.

———. "The Origins of Informed Consent: The International Scientific Commission on Medical War Crimes and the Nuremberg Code." *Bulletin of the History of Medicine* 75 (Spring 2001): 37–71.

Weisbord, Robert. *Genocide? Birth Control and Black America*. Westport, Conn.: Greenwood Press, 1975.

Weiss, Ellen. "Robert R. Taylor of Tuskegee: An Early Black American Architect." *Arris: Journal of the Southeast Chapter of the Society of Architectural Historians* 2 (1991): 3–19.

Wendler, David, Ezekial Emanuel, and Robert K. Lie. "The Standard of Care Debate." *American Journal of Public Health* 94 (June 2004): 923–28.

White, Robert M. "Grand Dragon or Windmill: Why I Opposed the Presidential Apology for the Tuskegee Study." *Journal of the National Medical Association* 89 (November 1997): 719–20.

———. "Misinformation and Misbeliefs in the Tuskegee Study of Untreated Syphilis Fuel Mistrust in the Health Care System." *Journal of the National Medical Association* 95 (November 2005): 1566–73.

———. "Misrepresentations of the Tuskegee Study of Untreated Syphilis." *Journal of the National Medical Association* 97 (April 2005): 564–81.

———. "Sociocultural Issues in Clinical Research: Unraveling the Tuskegee Syphilis Study." Letter to the Editor. *Arthritis Care and Research* 47 (August 2002): 457.

———. "Unraveling the Tuskegee Study of Untreated Syphilis." *Archives of Internal Medicine* 160 (March 13, 2000): 585–98.

Whitrow, Magda. "Wagner-Jauregg and Fever Therapy." *Medical History* 34 (July 1990): 294–310.

Whorley, Twyanna. "The Tuskegee Syphilis Study: Access and Control over Controversial Records." In *Political Pressure and the Archival Record*, edited by Margaret Procter, Michael G. Cook, and Caroline Williams, 109–18. Chicago: Society of American Archivists, 2005.

———. "The Tuskegee Syphilis Study: Access and Control over Controversial Records." Ph.D. diss., University of Pittsburgh, 2006.

Wickman, Patricia R. *Osceola's Legacy*. Tuscaloosa: University of Alabama Press, 1991.

Wilkerson, Karen Buhler. *False Dawn: The Rise and Decline of Public Health Nursing, 1900–1930*. New York: Garland, 1990.

Williams, Linda. *Playing the Race Card: Melodramas of Black and White from Uncle Tom to O. J. Simpson*. Princeton, N.J.: Princeton University Press, 2001.

Williams, Patricia. "American Kabuki." In *Birth of a Nation'hood*, edited by Toni Morrison and Claudia Brodsky Lacour, 273–92. New York: Pantheon, 1997.

Williams, Ralph Chester. *The United States Public Health Service, 1798–1950*. Washington, D.C.: Commissioned Officers Association of the United States Public Health Service, 1951.

Wilson, Ruth Dannehower. *Jim Crow Joins Up*. New York: William J. Clark, 1944.

Wolf, Susan. "Erasing Difference: Race, Ethnicity, and Gender in Bioethics." In *Embodying Bioethics: Recent Feminist Advances*, edited by Anne Donchin and Laura M. Purdy, 65–81. Lanham, Md.: Rowman and Littlefield, 1999.

Wolinsky, Howard. "Steps Still Being Taken to Undo Damage of 'America's Nuremberg.'" *Annals of Internal Medicine* 127 (August 15, 1997): 143–44.

Wright, Richard. *White Man, Listen!* New York: Doubleday, 1957.

Yoon, Carol Kaesuk. "Families Emerge as Silent Victims of Tuskegee Syphilis Experiments." In *Tuskegee's Truths: Rethinking the Tuskegee Syphilis Study*, edited by Susan M. Reverby, 457–62. Chapel Hill: University of North Carolina Press, 2000.

Zuberi, Tukufu. *Thicker Than Blood: How Racial Statistics Lie*. Minneapolis: University of Minnesota Press, 2001.

AUDIOTAPES, DVDS, VIDEOS, AND TELEVISION PROGRAMS

Alabama Stories: Shiloh Community, a Church, a School, a Cemetery. DVD. Alabama Public Television. Directed by Rhonda Colvin. Birmingham: Alabama Public Television, 2008.

Bad Blood. VHS. London: a Diverse Production for Channel 4, in association with the Arts and Entertainment Network, 1992.

A Conversation on Moral Intuition at the National Bioethics Center. DVD. Tuskegee: Tuskegee University, 1999.

Critical Thinking in Nursing: Lessons from Tuskegee. VHS. New York: National League for Nursing, 1993.

"The Deadly Deception." *Nova.* DVD. PBS. Directed by Denise DiIanni. Boston: WGBH Educational Foundation Films for the Humanities and Sciences, 1993.

Feldshuh, David, and Walter Bernstein. *Miss Evers' Boys.* DVD. Directed by Joseph Sargent. New York: HBO. February 22, 1997.

Living Black and White: Tuskegee Alabama. VHS. Tuscaloosa: University of Alabama Center for Public Television, 1996.

Race Prejudice and Health Care: The Lessons of the Tuskegee Syphilis Experiment. Audiotapes. Minneapolis: Illusion Theater, 1993.

Saturday Night Live. NBC. Hosted by Hugh Laurie. Season 32, Episode 4. October 28, 2006.

Susceptible to Kindness: "Miss Evers' Boys" and the Tuskegee Syphilis Study. VHS. Ithaca: Cornell University Media Services, 1993.

"The Tuskegee Study." *Primetime Live.* ABC. February 6, 1992.

Voices of the Tuskegee Syphilis Study. DVD. Directed by Deborah Gray. Atlanta: Centers for Disease Control, 2005.

"White House Apology for the Tuskegee Syphilis Study." *CNN Live,* May 16, 1997.

Index

African American men in Study: ages of, 113, 258–60; amount of time between first lesion and first exam, 117, 260; autopsy agreements, 1, 48, 52, 53, 56, 66, 118, 171, 242, 296–97 (n. 39); as blue-collar workers, 113, 114; burial fund for, 1, 53, 79, 150, 171, 210, 242, 306 (n. 62), 308 (n. 100); cash incentives for, 73, 172, 206, 244; certificates for, 73, 172; children examined and treated during Study, 130; chosen as poor and black, 105, 292–93 (n. 97); and compensation, 91, 92, 101–2, 103, 104, 291 (n. 74), 292 (n. 89); concentration camp victims comparison, 6, 87, 192–93; and confidentiality, 112–13; contagion, possibility of, for families of, 2, 105, 117, 124, 129, 232, 264 (n. 5), 299–300 (n. 94), 305–6 (n. 58); control group, 48–50, 79, 113; control group, syphilitic infection in, 59, 61, 279 (n. 31); control group switched to syphilitic group, 61, 113, 117, 119, 124, 126, 296 (n. 32), 305–6 (n. 58), 321–22 (n. 53); cooperation denied, 69, 74, 115–16; deaths from other diseases, 68, 118–19, 126, 261, 296 (nn. 36, 38), 297 (n. 50); deaths from syphilis, 2, 62–63, 64, 67, 68, 71–72, 80, 82, 90, 91, 116, 117–20, 133, 232, 261, 288 (nn. 25–26), 296 (nn. 36–38), 297 (n. 50); deaths useful to Study, 47,

52, 139, 275 (n. 122), 276 (n. 144), 283 (n. 4); deceived, 1, 48, 51, 55, 63, 70, 72, 75–76, 79, 82, 84, 87, 105, 116, 132, 150, 198, 207, 233, 287–88 (n. 23); deceived about spinal taps, 45–46, 59, 144, 275 (n. 110); and diet, 68, 282 (n. 75); disease histories, 39, 42, 45, 305–6 (n. 58); in documentaries, 149, 206–8; family members and closure, 10, 265 (n. 32); as farmers, 111, 113, 114–15; and federal apology, 224–25, 247; and fictionalizing, 210–11, 213–15, 224–25; follow-ups on controls and subjects, 56, 62, 67, 74, 84, 280 (n. 36); given hot meals for participating, 73, 79, 307 (n. 77); individuals, 8, 9, 111–12, 113, 134, 226, 233, 251–55, 256, 294 (nn. 4, 6, 7), 295 (n. 12), 301 (n. 117); and informed consent, 38, 48, 99, 100; knowledge of having syphilis, 71, 79, 88–89, 91, 95, 96, 97, 98, 105, 121–22, 125, 128, 171–72, 287 (n. 13); as latent syphilitics, untreated, 1, 46, 48, 71, 78, 86, 98, 117, 124, 129, 242, 282 (n. 88), 299 (n. 93); and lawsuit, 103–8, 292 (n. 89); and lawsuit and settlement, 107–8, 198, 246, 293–94 (n. 112), 326 (n. 24); media and, after Study exposure, 88, 104–5, 132, 133; medical records of, 6, 8, 112, 232, 294 (nn. 4, 7), 294–95 (n. 9); memorial/museum to, 238, 248; and mental asylum possibilities, 44; migration from rural South, 56, 62, 113, 283 (n. 4); misdiagnosis of, 143, 305–6 (n. 58); neurological symptoms in, 116; nontreatment as cause of death, 2, 62–63, 64, 67, 80, 82, 90, 116, 119–20, 133, 288 (nn. 25–26); recruitment of, 41–44, 46, 56, 58–59, 111, 113, 238, 257, 278 (n. 19), 296 (n. 24); schooling of, 114, 295 (n. 17); service, participation seen as, 67, 69, 78–79, 84, 144, 148, 207, 208, 212; and settlement, 108, 132–33, 198, 292 (n. 89), 293–94 (n. 112); sexual partners other than wives, no tracking of, 41, 131; and spinal taps, 45–46, 59, 119–20, 173, 242, 275 (n. 110), 276 (n. 144); spokesman for after Study exposure, 111–12, 294 (n. 3); as subjects, not syphilitic, 117; as subjects and controls, 1, 8, 38, 51, 52, 55, 104, 113, 242, 258–60, 295 (n. 12); as subjects and controls, mortality rates of, 71–72, 96, 116–17, 118, 176–77, 293 (n. 109); as subjects *vs.* patients, 50, 51, 56; and syphilis and cardiovascular disease, 48, 49, 53–54, 60–61, 68, 74, 107, 118–19, 125, 126, 127, 128, 148, 177, 297 (n. 56), 298 (n. 70); treatment, expected to ask for, 46, 49, 55, 78, 95, 97, 318 (n. 85); treatment, receiving, 51–52, 58–59, 62, 75, 84, 86, 87, 95, 105, 106, 120, 121–22, 145, 179–82, 183, 299 (n. 89), 321–22 (n. 53); treatment after Study exposure, 92, 100–101, 103, 131, 246, 291 (n. 76); treatment at beginning of Study, 1, 39, 41–44, 59, 71, 90, 116, 120, 242; treatment denied, 2, 57, 96, 97, 101, 102, 105, 122–23, 175, 179–80, 242, 298 (nn. 62, 66), 317–18 (n. 84), 318 (n. 85); treatment for early-stage infectious syphilis, 39, 41, 42–43, 44, 94, 97, 120, 143, 175; treatment for other diseases, 81, 82, 84, 173; treatment from local doctors, 97, 120–21, 126; "treatments," 1, 46, 47, 51, 55, 57, 70, 73, 173–74, 242; treatment

with heavy metals, 94, 98, 120, 171; treatment with penicillin, 68, 71–72, 74, 80, 106–7, 120, 145, 173, 316 (n. 49); treatment with penicillin for other ailments, 124–28, 299 (nn. 79, 82), 300 (n. 96); treatment with penicillin from local doctors, 77, 84, 102, 125, 127–28, 164, 297 (n. 56), 299 (n. 82), 300 (n. 96); treatment with penicillin "not offered," 87, 99; treatment with penicillin outside Macon County, 122–23, 124–27, 299 (n. 80); treatment with penicillin not prescribed for latent syphilis, 124, 150, 232; untreated, 58–59, 84, 107, 125, 127, as victims, 87, 106, 134, 191, 277 (n. 2); volunteers, thought of as, 53–54, 70, 78, 92, 146, 191, 197; wives and children, and lawsuit by, 130–31, 300 (n. 103); wives and children treated after Study exposed, 131, 247, 291–92 (n. 79), 300–301 (n. 104), 301 (nn. 106, 108); wives examined, 129–30, 298 (n. 70), 300 (n. 95); wives treated, 94, 125, 129–31; and World War II draft, 61, 122, 243, 279 (nn. 28, 30)

African Americans, 16, 22, 31, 86; and AIDS research and legacy of Tuskegee, 198–200, 322–23 (n. 71); and health care, 5, 17–19, 80, 152, 160, 162, 166, 178, 217, 219–20, 285 (n. 29); and medical research after Tuskegee, 198–200, 227, 234–35, 265 (n. 14); as physicians, 17, 156–57, 160, 165–66, 216–20, 310 (n. 31), 313 (n. 78); and pregnancy, abortion, and sterilization, 217, 327 (n. 4), 328 (n. 6); syphilis expectations among, 3, 43, 44, 45, 54, 264 (n. 9); syphilis in populations of, 24, 27, 140–41, 269 (n. 93); and syphilis treatment and research, 65, 140–41, 162; testifying, 7; "Tuskegee" as symbol for oppression of, 204, 324 (n. 2); "unplotted" lives of, 30; and venereal disease as threat to whites, 26–28, 269 (n. 90); World

War I, syphilis and black soldiers in, 18, 25, 39, 269 (n. 83). *See also* Racialism; Racism

African Americans in Macon County: and automobile ownership, 30, 111, 270 (n. 8), 294 (n. 2); and "bad blood" terminology, 88–89; black population in 1930, 29; canvassing for men with latent syphilis for Study, 1, 41–43; child mortality among, 31, 271 (n. 20); community hospital for, 17, 19; currently, 237–39, 248; death of, 31, 32, 271 (n. 20), 275 (n. 122); and doctors, 32–33; education of, 15–18; and health care, 18–19, 29, 31–33, 154–56, 158–59, 165, 166; history of, 13–18; and malaria, 32, 63, 88, 161–63, 279 (n. 23); and malnutrition, 31, 33, 36; and migration, 14, 56, 62, 67, 113; and miscarriages and stillbirths, 31, 34, 270 (n. 14); and rural poverty, 29–30, 31–32, 114–15; professional control of veterans' hospital by, 18–19; and sanitation, 29–30, 36; and syphilis, neurological symptoms of, 44, 45, 54; and syphilis education, 121–22; and syphilis rate, 33, 35, 43, 175, 241; syphilis treatment and Rosenwald Fund Demonstration Project, 31–37, 241, 270 (n. 2), 273 (n. 63), 300–301 (n. 104); syphilis treatment for early-stage infection, 39, 41, 42–43, 44, 57, 96, 97, 120, 121, 175, 179, 242, 278 (n. 9); veterans, 18–19; women, 43, 44, 57, 131, 242, 278 (n. 9), 300–301 (n. 104), 327 (n. 4)

AIDS, 194, 217, 221, 224, 247, 269 (n. 91), 280 (n. 44), 329 (n. 20); and African Americans and legacy of Tuskegee, 198–200, 322–23 (n. 71); anti-HIV drug trial in Uganda, 227, 228–30, 304 (n. 38)

Alabama: African Americans in, history of, 13–15; Black Belt, 14, 17, 111, 192, 237, 266 (n. 5); civil rights movement in, 75, 103, 105–6, 115, 132, 165, 244, 245, 284 (n. 11); expresses regret for Study, 134; health care in, 17, 41, 116, 154–56, 170; Jim Crow and white supremacy in, 17, 30–31, 41, 115, 116, 153–54, 213, 241, 270 (n. 12), 305 (n. 53); lawsuit against, 103, 104, 107, 246; as prison, 192–93, 281 (n. 59); racism in, 30–31, 41, 105–6, 115, 213–14, 293 (n. 102), 305 (n. 53); Study, cooperation in, 39, 81, 273 (n. 72), 305 (n. 53); and syphilis blood test before marriage, 129; and syphilis research on blacks other than Study men, 147; and syphilis treatment in 1930s, 39, 43, 47, 96, 107, 142; and Tuskegee Institute, 15, 158–59; venereal disease, state laws on, 63, 95, 105, 122, 272 (n. 41), 279 (n. 31); venereal disease control in 1940s, 122–24

Alabama Historical Register, 239

Alabama Shakespeare Company, 207

Alabama Trust for Historic Preservation, 248

Allen, James B., 91, 104, 107

Alliance Theater, Atlanta, 213

American Heart Association, 48, 55

American Medical Association, 17, 26, 53, 54, 156, 159, 310 (n. 31)

Aneurysms, 74, 118, 119, 261; aortic aneurysm, 107

Angell, Marcia, 228, 229, 230

Aortic regurgitation, 59, 246

Aortic valvular disease, 125, 127

Aortitis, 42, 48, 60, 117, 119, 145, 261, 282 (n. 81), 293 (n. 110), 298 (n. 70), 299 (n. 89)

Arsenical drugs, 23, 27, 60, 90, 98, 125, 137, 162, 164, 273 (n. 63), 297 (n. 56), 303 (n. 27), 308 (n. 101); arsphenamine, 4, 24, 95, 140, 272 (n. 49), 303 (nn. 48–49); neoarsphenamine, 34, 35–36, 42–43, 46, 51, 54, 57, 122, 127, 141, 272 (n. 49)

Arteriosclerosis, 48, 68, 118, 119, 276 (n. 128), 297 (n. 56), 299 (n. 85)

Aspirin, 1, 46, 47, 49, 51, 55, 57, 70, 73, 173, 242, 283 (n. 2)

Brandt, Allan M., 195, 196–97, 206, 247, 321 (n. 52), 328 (n. 9)

Brown, William J., 78–80, 82, 83, 90–91, 95–96, 128, 250, 283 (n. 4)

Bruce, Dick, 118, 296 (n. 38)

Burial insurance, 1, 53, 79, 171, 210, 242, 277 (n. 153), 306 (n. 62)

Burney, Leroy E., 73, 250

Butler, Broadus, 92, 93, 100, 249, 290 (n. 53), 291 (n. 73)

Buxtun, Peter, 208, 222, 284 (nn. 17, 20), 286–87 (n. 10); and breaking news on Study, 84, 246, 249; hearing appearances, 100, 102; initial concern about Study, 76–79, 82, 83, 195, 245

Byron, Don, 204–5, 206, 215, 325 (nn. 7, 11, 12)

Caldwell, Joseph G., 81, 83–84, 95, 96, 126–27, 181, 246, 249

Callis, H. A., 161

Caplan, Arthur, 197–98

Capron, Alexander Morgan, 190

Cardiovascular disease: aortic regurgitation, 59, 246; aortic valvular disease, 125, 127; and latent syphilis, penicillin and, 64–65, 126, 147, 148, 293 (n. 110), 299 (n. 78); as symptom of syphilis, 26, 49, 58, 75, 107, 116, 118, 128, 138, 177, 257, 307–8 (n. 91); and syphilis, differences assumed between blacks and whites, 3, 43, 269 (n. 85); and syphilis, differences between blacks and whites researched, 136; vs. syphilitic symptoms, 42, 48, 53–54, 55, 68, 117, 118–19, 145, 269 (n. 93), 276 (nn. 127–28), 296 (nn. 36, 38), 297 (n. 43); treatments for syphilitics reveal, 60–61, 65. See also Aneurysms; Aortitis; Arteriosclerosis; Hypertension

Carley, Paul S., 27

Carlson, Tucker, 200, 323 (n. 77)

Carver, George Washington, 97–98, 132, 158, 225, 290 (n. 63)

Carver Research Foundation, 158, 310 (n. 40)

Cave, Vernal, 289 (n. 36), 292 (n. 83), 293 (n. 104), 299 (n. 80); and HEW Ad Hoc Panel, 92, 93, 102, 106, 107, 249, 281 (n. 56), 288–89 (n. 34), 289 (n. 39); Rivers, interview with, 93, 290 (n. 62)

CDC (Communicable Disease Center; Centers for Disease Control after 1970), 77, 84, 85, 105, 113, 118, 181, 236, 239; and anti-HIV drug trial in Uganda, 227, 228, 229; and breaking news on Study, 87, 88, 94; and congressional hearings, 100, 102; and criticisms of Study, 76, 78–79, 82–83, 208, 245; and federal apology for Study, 221, 223–24, 226; latent syphilis, and controversy over, 90–91, 150; lawsuit against, 103–8, 219, 246; and minority health, 199, 221–22; nontreatment of subjects defended, 93–94, 95–96; and public relations relative to Study, 81, 82, 217, 245; records of, 92, 107, 196, 197; reevaluation of Study in 1965, 74–75, 245; reevaluation of Study in 1969, 79–82, 147, 164, 208, 218–19, 237, 245, 285 (nn. 29–30); treatments for men after Study exposure, 100–101, 103, 131, 133, 246, 291–92 (n. 79), 301 (n. 108); treatments for men in Study in last years, 96, 107, 128, 173; Venereal Disease Division, 78–79, 87, 150; wives and children treated, 130–31, 300–301 (n. 104); wives and children treated after Study exposed, 301 (n. 106)

Centers for Disease Control. See CDC

Central Alabama Veterans Health Care System, 238, 264 (n. 4). See also Tuskegee Veterans' Administration Hospital

Chancres, 3, 40, 176, 242, 316 (n. 44)

Chicago: syphilis treatment programs in, 143, 305 (n. 57)

Civil rights movement, 74, 245; in Alabama, 75, 105–6, 115, 132, 165, 244, 245,

Hypertension, 43, 48, 68, 117, 118, 119, 177, 276 (n. 128), 296 (n. 36)

Illiteracy, 29, 39, 45, 149
Influenza, 31, 127, 261
Intrauterine devices (IUDs), 158, 163–64
Iodide pills. *See* Mercury; Protiodide of mercury
Iron tonic, 1, 55, 73, 173, 242, 283 (n. 2)
Iskrant, Albert P., 63
Ivy, Andrew, 66

Jakin, Ga., 41, 168, 169
James, Reginald G., 250, 291 (n. 68), 298 (n. 61); and "bad blood wagons," 96, 98, 121, 179, 278 (nn. 9–10); and hearings, 96–97, 98–99, 121, 179, 290 ·(n. 62), 298 (n. 62), 317–18 (n. 84)
Japanese medical experiments in China, 78
Jenkins, Bill, 82–83, 131, 208, 246, 249, 285 (nn. 36, 37, 39)
Jessup wagon. *See* Movable School program
Jewish Chronic Disease Hospital, 190, 191
John A. Andrew Clinical Society, 17, 60, 155, 156–57, 158, 166, 266–67 (n. 31), 311 (n. 44)
John A. Andrew Memorial Hospital, 29, 90, 101, 120, 128; autopsies done at, 48; closing of, 156, 184, 238, 310 (n. 29); Dibble's tenure at, 39, 41, 51, 153, 155–59, 166; Foster and, 216, 217, 327 (n. 4); programs and expansion at, 155–56; research at, 163–64; Rivers at, 41, 170; Study, cooperation with, 41, 48, 90, 158, 159–60, 163, 166; syphilis penicillin treatment given at, 164; syphilis treatment given at, 39, 51, 61, 97, 125. *See also* Tuskegee Institute
Johns Hopkins University, 37, 39, 40, 43, 49, 50, 59, 68, 120, 302 (n. 3); syphilis clinic, 24, 58, 65, 136, 303 (n. 23)
Johnson, Charles S., 29, 31, 33, 88, 89, 145, 270 (n. 11), 270–71 (n. 17), 287 (n. 14)

Johnson, Frank M., Jr., 105–6, 107, 293 (n. 106)
Johnson, Price, 149, 206
Jones, James H., 48, 183, 206, 208, 209, 222, 282–83 (n. 90), 321 (n. 48), 322 (n. 57), 328 (n. 9); and *Bad Blood*, 195–96, 197–98, 200, 201, 217, 219, 247, 287 (n. 18), 324 (n. 2); and interviews for book, 66, 148, 181, 193, 205, 287 (n. 14); and lawsuit, 105, 107, 196, 321 (n. 50)
Julkes, Albert, Jr., 132, 133, 134, 226
Junod, Tom, 132, 149

Kahn, Reuben L., 163, 312 (n. 67)
Kaiser, Clyde, 80
Kampmeier, Rudolph H., 65, 281 (n. 55), 305 (n. 50)
Katz, Jay, 66, 190, 191, 291 (n. 71), 292 (n. 93), 319 (n. 20), 328 (n. 9); and HEW Ad Hoc Panel, 92, 93, 99–100, 102, 197, 249, 288–89 (n. 34), 289 (nn. 39, 41); and Rivers, 290 (n. 45), 291 (n. 73), 316 (n. 59)
Katz, Ralph V., 221, 329 (n. 25)
Keidel tubes, 42, 274 (n. 88)
Kennebrew, Elizabeth M., 84, 103, 172, 245, 250
Kennedy, Edward M., 92, 100–103, 104, 191, 212, 246, 289 (n. 41), 292 (n. 93)
Kenney, John A., Sr., 17, 153, 156, 266–67 (n. 31)
Kidney disorders, 68
King, Martin Luther, Jr., 79, 89, 103, 245
King, Patricia, 5, 194, 320 (n. 41)
Ku Klux Klan, 18, 154

Lancaster, Rosa, 32
Laurie, Eunice Rivers. *See* Rivers, Eunice Verdell
Laurie, Hugh, 236
Laurie, Julius, 174
Lederer, Edith, 84, 249
Lederer, Susan, 21, 52, 143, 191
Lee, Phil, 221
Lee, Spike, 200, 323 (n. 77), 327 (n. 42)

Neoarsphenamine. *See* Arsenical drugs: Neoarsphenamine

Neurological complications, 26, 65, 116, 296 (n. 31); blacks and whites, differences supposed between, 3, 44, 45, 54, 63, 136, 264 (n. 9), 269 (n. 85), 307–8 (n. 91)

Neurosyphilis, 118, 137, 164, 257; malaria as "cure" for, 4, 63, 161–63, 279 (n. 23), 307–8 (n. 91); penicillin in treatment of, 65, 147; spinal taps to test for, 44–45, 54, 69, 279 (n. 23). *See also* Syphilis; Syphilis treatments

New Deal, 114

New England Journal of Medicine, 190, 228, 229, 245

New York Undercover: "Bad Blood," 222, 329 (n. 27)

Nissen, Steven, 234

NitroMed company, 234

Notasulga, Ala., 13, 42, 88, 115, 213, 237, 239, 248

Nova: "The Deadly Deception," 148, 149–50, 205–7, 247, 285 (nn. 37, 39), 306–7 (n. 71), 325 (nn. 13, 18), 326 (n. 19)

Nuremberg Code, 66, 189, 193, 243

Nuremberg Trials, 66, 77, 189, 220, 281 (n. 59)

Obama, Barack, 215, 322–23 (n. 71)

Olansky, Sidney, 76, 306 (n. 70), 308 (n. 97); in documentaries, 148–50, 206, 207, 220, 306–7 (n. 71); nontreatment, reevaluation of, 80–81; and penicillin, 106, 206; as PHS physician in charge of Study in 1950s, 69, 70–72, 74–75, 106, 144, 145–48, 244, 249; son of, 150; syphilis, and other research on, 146–47, 307 (n. 83), 324 (n. 83)

Osceola, 237

Osler, William, 1, 143, 264 (n. 1)

Oslo Study, 176, 232, 241, 303 (n. 23); comparison with Study, 58, 69, 125, 146, 172, 178; as nontreatment study,

25–26, 64, 67, 99, 125, 137, 138, 172; reexamination of, 26, 69, 137, 146, 244, 302 (n. 2); as study on whites, 37, 146, 172

Oveta Culp Hobby Award, 73, 167, 182–83, 184, 244, 313 (n. 1), 328 (n. 10)

Palmer, Larry I., 106, 108, 293 (n. 103)

Paresis, 44–45

Parks, Rosa, 103, 132, 244

Parran, Thomas, Jr., 40, 115, 136, 250, 269 (nn. 74, 79); and syphilis education, 25, 88; and syphilis treatments, 4, 23–24, 56, 57, 61–62, 141–42

Patterson, Frederick D., 156, 159

Payton, Benjamin, 223

Pearl, Raymond, 22

Pellagra, 21, 36, 88, 267–68 (n. 51)

Penicillin: dangers of, 94, 144, 147, 150, 175; and Herxheimer reaction, 81, 144, 147, 150, 175; for latent syphilis, 65, 68, 72, 74, 120, 127–28, 138–39, 146–48, 164, 173, 176, 181–82, 232, 299 (n. 83), 307 (n. 81); for latent syphilis, controversy over, 81, 87, 90–91, 92–93, 102, 106, 124, 148, 149, 150, 206, 299 (n. 78), 307 (n. 80), 325 (n. 16); for latent syphilis, current reexamination of, 231, 331 (n. 17); for latent syphilis and cardiovascular disease, 64–65, 293 (n. 110), 297 (n. 56), 299 (n. 78); for latent syphilis before organ damage, 4, 126, 151, 293 (n. 110); for latent syphilis combined with malaria treatment, 162–63; for neurosyphilis, 65; for other ailments, 124–28, 299 (n. 82), 300 (n. 96); syphilis, for early-stage, 65, 124, 144, 243; syphilis, post–World War II treatment for, 2, 63, 64–65, 67, 71–72, 77, 80, 99, 106–7, 122–23, 125, 281 (n. 69); syphilis treatments before, 23–24, 120, 124, 137–38, 140, 142. *See also* African American men in Study

Perry, William B., 57, 96, 250

Scottsboro Boys, 30, 241, 270 (n. 12)

Scrofula. *See* Tuberculosis

Segregation, 16, 18, 30, 62, 153–56, 213–14, 243; and health care in Alabama, 17–19, 41, 95, 116, 154–56, 165, 194

Sencer, David J., 131, 150, 237, 250, 291–92 (n. 79), 326 (n. 23); in documentaries, 207, 208; and reevaluation of Study in 1969, 80, 81–82, 219, 285 (n. 29)

Settler, Howard, 133, 218

Shadow on the Land (Parran), 25

Sharecroppers, 30, 39, 102, 112, 154, 206

Sharecroppers' Union, 30, 115, 154, 242

Shaw, Herman, 101–2, 126, 134, 215, 270 (n. 8), 298 (n. 70); denied treatment, 122–24, 132, 133; in documentaries, 149, 207–8; early life and background, 111, 114–15; and federal apology, 224–25, 226; and Rivers, 167, 213; as spokesman for Study men, 111–12, 294 (n. 3)

Shiloh Community Restoration Foundation, 237, 248

Shiloh Missionary Baptist Church, 13, 42, 115, 213, 237, 238–39, 248

Shweder, Richard, 230, 233

Sickle cell traits, 62

Simmons, Fred, 113, 125

Sims, Liz, 237, 239

Sing Sing prison syphilis study, 146–47, 201, 299 (n. 83), 307 (n. 83), 324 (n. 83)

Smallpox, 36, 141, 150, 159

Smith, J. Lawton, 80, 81, 249, 277 (n. 156)

Smith, Murray, 48, 52, 61, 93, 121, 122, 159, 170, 249; Study, assists with, 39, 44, 45, 46, 111; and treatments for Study participants, 125, 127–28, 299 (n. 89), 300 (n. 96)

Snider, Dixie, 223

Sparkman/Allen bill, 104, 107

Spinal taps, 39, 49, 119–20, 173, 242, 274 (n. 100), 276 (n. 144); deceiving men of Study about, 45–46, 59, 144, 275 (n. 110); neurosyphilis, and testing for, 44–45, 54, 69, 279 (n. 23)

Spirochetes, 3, 4, 23, 54, 151; and blood

tests, 36, 39; deliberate injections of, 146–47, 201; and Herxheimer reaction, 81, 144, 147; penicillin for killing, 64, 81, 139, 146–47, 243, 307 (n. 81)

Stillbirths, 31, 34, 270 (n. 14)

Stokes, John H., 26, 34, 98, 116, 137, 272 (n. 58)

Stokes, Louis, 223, 224

Stollerman, Eugene, 79–80, 81, 208, 249

Story, Robert, 126, 128, 299 (n. 79)

Strait, George A., Jr., 148, 206, 207, 208, 325 (n. 18)

Syphilis: African American rate in Macon County, 33, 35, 43, 175, 241; Alabama law, blood tests for before marriage and, 129; as "bad blood," 22, 23; in black soldiers during World War I, 18, 25, 39, 269 (n. 83); blacks and whites, differences between researched, 136, 139; blindness caused by, 3, 133, 314 (n. 6); and cause of death, 64, 67, 68, 80, 82, 90, 117–20, 261, 296 (nn. 36–38); congenital, 23, 35, 40, 71, 131, 264 (n. 8); documentaries, intricacies of lost in, 207; education about, 25, 61, 88, 121–22; and eugenics, 22, 142, 268 (n. 67); and gender differences, 3, 136, 139; human history of, 2–3; and infants, 3, 23, 24, 264 (n. 8), 268 (n. 71); and infection of "innocent" spouse, 23, 268 (n. 71); infectious early-stage, 1, 3, 23–26, 28, 41, 57, 65, 264 (nn. 5, 8); infectiousness of, 2, 201, 287 (nn. 19–20); latent, 3, 60, 64, 98, 151; latent forms of believed not to be fatal, 137, 147, 231; latent noninfectious, 1, 3, 35–36, 46, 55, 91; medical fascination with, 136, 139, 141; medical questions about, 23, 24; as menace from blacks, 26–28; modes of infection, 3, 264 (n. 8); mortality after twelve years, 62–63, 243; mortality rates, 67, 71–72, 75, 116–17, 118, 176–77, 293 (n. 109); natural history of, 3, 8, 24, 37, 63, 303 (n. 26); necessity for long-term study of, 147–48; "not too bad" as disease, 149, 177; and pregnancy, 3, 24, 57, 264 (n. 8); rates of, 25, 27, 28, 33, 35, 43; second-stage, 3, 25–26; silence about, 23, 25, 58, 88; stigma about, 3, 133, 158, 209, 214; survival of, 2, 3, 26, 137; third-stage noninfectious, 3, 150, 299 (n. 93). *See also* Aneurysms; Aortitis; Blood tests; Cardiovascular disease; Medical research studies; Neurological complications; Neurosyphilis; Racialism; Syphilis treatments; U.S. Public Health Service; U.S. Public Health Service Study at Tuskegee

"Syphilis in the South: New Ideas, New Partners" conference, 221

Syphilis treatments, 3–4, 23, 278 (n. 14); Alabama public health officials and, 39, 43, 47, 96, 107, 122–24, 273 (n. 72), 305 (n. 53); blood purifiers, 23, 268 (n. 68); Chicago programs, 143, 305 (n. 57); and disease histories, 39, 40–41, 42, 45; education for local doctors, 34, 271 (n. 33); expense of, 24–25, 39, 42, 44; heavy metals injections, 2, 34, 95, 120, 125, 297 (nn. 41, 54), 299 (n. 78); heavy metals used in, side effects of, 34, 35, 36, 94, 98, 137, 171, 290 (n. 52); "inadequate" treatment, adequate therapy, 58–59, 60, 62, 63, 64, 69–70, 120, 136, 137; for infectious stage, 23–25, 28, 34, 39, 41, 42–43, 44, 47, 57, 71, 81, 94, 96, 97, 141–42, 143, 175; at Johns Hopkins clinic, 24, 58, 65, 136, 303 (n. 23); for latent syphilis, 34, 65, 81, 98, 107, 139, 142, 151, 293 (n. 110), 303 (n. 27), 308 (n. 101); for latent syphilis before penicillin, 23–24, 120, 124, 137–38, 173, 316 (n. 44); long-term before penicillin, 54, 65, 137–38, 140, 142, 305 (n. 50); malaria as "cure," 4, 63, 161–63, 279 (n. 23), 307–8 (n. 91); medical questions about, 23–25; minimal treatment for latent syphilis, 142, 273 (n. 63), 305 (nn. 48–49); nontreatment as, 2, 26, 27, 38, 63, 65, 75, 80, 136, 146–47, 307 (n. 88); nontreatment for latent syphilis, 35–36, 37, 38, 40, 46, 55, 78, 82, 98–99, 106, 137, 257; nontreatment for latent syphilis, current reexamination of, 231, 331 (n. 17); nontreatment for latent syphilis, findings on, 54, 63, 64, 67, 68, 96, 147, 280 (n. 44); overtreatment, concern with, 60, 137, 151, 303 (n. 27), 308 (n. 101); San Francisco venereal disease program, 76–77; World War II draft and, 61, 122, 243. *See also* Arsenical drugs; Bismuth; Cardiovascular disease; Mercury; Penicillin; Rapid treatment centers; Rosenwald Fund Demonstration Project

"Syphilis Victims in U.S. Study Went Untreated for 40 Years" headline, 85

Syphilology, 23, 25, 26, 65

Talladega County, Ala., 30, 242

Tallapoosa County, Ala., 30, 111, 242

Tallasee, Ala., 13, 111, 124

Taylor, Helen, 153, 315 (n. 33). *See also* Dibble, Eugene H., Jr.

Testifying, 7, 8

Testimony, 7

Thomas, Stephen, 199, 235

Tissue samples, 49, 56, 57–58, 68, 69, 74, 80, 112, 116, 119, 280 (n. 42)

Treponema pallidum bacterium, 2, 147. *See also* Syphilis

Tuberculosis, 31, 128, 261, 269 (n. 93), 271 (n. 19)

Turner, Thomas B., 136

Tuskegee, Ala., 1, 14, 111, 112, 113, 115, 132, 166, 212; civil rights movement affects, 165, 245; museums planned for, 6, 238, 248; and Native Americans, 13, 237, 265 (n. 3); segregation in, 16, 154; transportation in, 30

Tuskegee Airmen, 62, 92, 132, 200, 204, 215, 237, 243, 291 (n. 73)

Tuskegee Airmen, The (film), 215, 323 (n. 79)

21, 267–68 (n. 51); and laboratory work, 20, 267 (n. 45); lawsuit against, 103–8, 293 (n. 106), 293–94 (n. 112); Macon County, and syphilis treatment and "bad blood wagon" in, 57, 96, 121, 179, 242, 278 (n. 9); Macon County, and syphilis treatment and Rosenwald Fund Demonstration Project in, 31–37, 241, 270 (n. 2), 300–301 (n. 104); Macon County, and syphilis treatment for early-stage infectious syphilis in, 39, 41, 42–43, 44, 84, 97, 120, 175; Macon County, early interest in, 28, 29, 37–38; and medical research, 19, 20–22, 267–68 (n. 51); and mental asylum studies, 20, 267–68 (n. 51); and nontreatment of syphilis as breaking law, 63, 279 (n. 31); and physicians in field, 66–67, 139, 304 (n. 30); and prisoner studies, 20, 146–47, 299 (n. 83); and professional connections, 21, 268 (nn. 57–58); and public health work, 19–22, 269 (n. 74); and racism of southern medical system, 47; records from early in Study, 92, 104, 105, 195, 289 (n. 43), 292 (n. 93); and reevaluation of Study in 1950s, 73, 243, 244, 283 (n. 1); Study, and public relations relative to, 81, 82, 217, 245; Study, and service of participants and, 67, 69, 78–79, 84, 144, 148, 207, 208; syphilis, concern about, 7, 19, 23, 24–25, 28, 37, 56, 60; syphilis, concern about at infectious stage, 61, 65, 76–77, 130, 141–42, 280 (n. 53); syphilis, desire to understand, 55, 58, 69, 135–36, 302 (n. 2); syphilis, fight against, 24, 37, 139, 141, 144, 148, 272 (n. 58); syphilis education, 25, 34, 61, 88, 121–22, 157, 271 (n. 33), 298 (n. 61); and Tuskegee Institute, 13, 18–19, 24, 56, 158, 159, 208; and venereal disease control, 164, 172, 207; white physicians of, 1, 8, 9, 66–67, 135–51, 192; and withholding of treatment for syphilis, 2, 54, 61, 70, 87,

95, 116, 232. *See also* African American men in Study; Blood tests; CDC; Medical research studies; Rapid treatment centers; Rosenwald Fund Demonstration Project; U.S. Public Health Service Study at Tuskegee; Venereal Disease Clinic; Venereal Disease Division of PHS; Venereal Disease Research Laboratory

U.S. Public Health Service (PHS) Commissioned Corps, 19, 20–21, 135, 267 (nn. 46, 50), 327 (n. 2)

U.S. Public Health Service (PHS) Study at Tuskegee: African American men as participants in, 40–41; and AIDS research and African Americans, 198–200; anti-HIV drug trial in Uganda comparison, 228–30, 248; and "bad blood wagons," 57, 121–22, 174–75; beginnings of, 21, 37–46, 138, 242; and beginnings of long-term Study, 46–55, 242; black physicians' complicity with, 4, 8, 83, 97–98, 107, 158–66, 196, 214, 217–20; breaking news on, 6, 8, 84–85, 86–91, 190, 246, 286 (n. 7), 287 (n. 12); and civil rights movement, 75, 78, 79, 83, 86, 89–90, 103, 178; cooperation with local health institutions, 39, 45, 46, 48, 50, 51, 52–53, 56, 57, 81, 83, 158, 159–60, 163, 166, 170, 242, 308 (n. 2); and deaths caused by nontreatment of men, 2, 62–63, 64, 67, 82, 90, 91, 133, 288 (nn. 25–26); and deceiving of participants, 1, 53–54, 79, 87, 198, 279 (n. 31), 287–88 (n. 23); and deceiving of participants about spinal taps, 45–46, 59, 144, 275 (n. 110); and defending of Study after breaking news on, 87, 286 (nn. 6–7), 291 (n. 67); and defending of Study twenty years later, 148–50; and deliberate infections story, 2, 38, 89–90, 192, 200–203, 213, 273 (n. 65), 287 (nn. 19–20), 321 (n. 46), 323 (nn. 78–79); documentaries about, 134, 148–49, 205–9, 220, 247, 306–7 (n. 71),

325 (nn. 13, 14, 16), 326 (n. 20); ethical concerns about in mid-1950s, 70–72, 244, 282 (n. 85), 282–83 (n. 90); ethical concerns about in mid-1960s, 73–79, 82–84, 245, 246, 284 (nn. 12, 15, 16, 20); ethics of, 47, 48, 56, 60–61, 202, 324 (n. 89); and eugenics, 268 (nn. 65, 67), 305 (n. 53); family members' illnesses blamed on, 131; fictionalizing of, 202–3, 207–8, 209–15, 247, 323 (n. 79), 327 (n. 42); follow-ups on controls and subjects, difficulties with, 69, 74, 82, 121, 298 (n. 58); follow-ups on controls and subjects, failure to report on difficulties with, 62, 280 (n. 36); and funding, 40, 42, 44, 49, 50, 56–57, 62, 274 (n. 98); as "golden moment" never to be repeated, 81; as good public health practice, 143–44, 202; halting of, 8, 91, 92, 246; and health care for African Americans, 158–59; hiatus in 1934, 56, 277 (n. 3); and incentives for participants, 73, 78, 146, 172, 307 (n. 77); and informed consent, 41, 48, 143, 144, 150, 163, 193, 194–95, 198, 274 (n. 84), 306 (n. 62); invisibility of, 70, 191, 219; and Kennedy hearings, 100–103, 104, 191, 246; knowledge of by health professionals elsewhere, 127; and lawsuit, 103–8, 292 (n. 89); and lawsuit and settlement, 198, 246, 293–94 (n. 112); lawsuits emerge, 88, 101, 286 (n. 9); legality of, 63, 143–44, 279 (n. 31); and local doctors, 47, 50, 52–53, 90; and morality, 138, 148–49, 182–83, 191, 303 (n. 23); naming of, 8–9, 41; Nazi death camps comparison, 6, 87, 286 (n. 4); Nazi medical experiments comparison, 65–66, 77–78, 189, 192–93, 281 (n. 59); nontreatment of subjects defended, 75, 98–99, 106, 107, 176, 317 (n. 65); nontreatment thought not to be harming participants, 48, 78, 106, 136, 146, 150, 231, 308 (n. 100);

as nontreatment study, 40–41, 46, 56, 62, 80–81, 88, 99, 142–43, 207, 231, 282 (n. 88), 305 (n. 54); "official" stories of, 195–98, 321 (n. 46), 322 (n. 59); Oslo Study comparison, 58, 69, 125, 146, 172, 178; and penicillin, 87, 92–93, 99, 102, 126–27, 149, 150, 151, 176, 206, 317 (n. 65); photographs of, 184, 201, 287–88 (n. 23); PHS doctors not in field for, 47–48; PHS responsibility moved to CDC, 74; physicians of not punished, 9–10, 209, 226, 265 (n. 32), 326 (n. 24); population rather than individuals studied, 232–33; protocol, lack of, for, 38, 58; publicity about from *Bad Blood*, 197, 322 (n. 55); public relations relative to, 81–82, 83; racial assumptions in, 7, 28, 37, 43, 54, 60, 63, 91, 97, 99, 119, 150, 151, 232; racism and, 1, 2, 4–5, 8, 91, 95, 133–34, 149, 178, 193, 194, 195; racism seen as Study exposed, 79, 80, 82, 83, 94, 98–99, 102–3, 105, 106, 150–51, 196–97, 198, 202–3, 208–9, 225–26, 285 (n. 29); records from early in Study, 92, 104, 105, 195, 292 (n. 93); recruitment of African American men for, 1, 41–43, 58–59, 113; reevaluation in 1950s, 73, 243, 244, 283 (n. 1); reevaluation in 1965, 74–75, 245; reevaluation in 1969, 79–82, 95–96, 147, 164, 208, 217, 218–19, 237, 245, 285 (nn. 29–30); reports of, 6, 68, 77, 85, 113, 138, 145, 177, 243, 244, 277 (n. 160), 281 (n. 69), 303 (n. 22); reports, first, 53–54, 58, 242; reports, second, 62–63, 243; reports, third, 63, 243; reports, fourth, 67, 243; reports, fifth, 175, 243, 316 (n. 59); reports, final (thirteenth), 83–84, 126–27, 246, 286 (n. 48); Rivers employed in, 8, 41, 47, 50, 170–71, 242; Rosenwald Fund Demonstration Project as forerunner of, 29–37, 270–71 (n. 17); Rosenwald Fund Demonstration Project patients *vs.* subjects for, 40,